Restaurant
CONFIDENTIAL

Restaurant
CONFIDENTIAL

The Shocking Truth About What You're Really Eating When You're Eating Out

Michael F. Jacobson, Ph.D., Jayne G. Hurley, RD,
and the Center for Science in the Public Interest

WORKMAN PUBLISHING • NEW YORK

Library of Congress Cataloging-in-Publication Data

Jacobson, Michael F.
Restaurant Confidential / by Michael F. Jacobson and Jayne Hurley.
p. cm.
Includes index.
ISBN 0-7611-0035-0
1. Restaurants—United States. 2. Food—Composition. I. Hurley, Jayne. II. Title
TX945. J33 2002
613.2—dc21 2002019767

Workman Publishing Company, Inc.
708 Broadway
New York, NY 10003-9555
www.workman.com

Manufactured in the United States of America

First Printing: May 2002
10 9 8 7 6 5 4 3 2 1

Contents

To my parents, Larry and Belle Jacobson

*To my mom, Mildred Greer, for her love,
her support . . . and her wonderful baked beans*

Acknowledgments

Producing *Restaurant Confidential* was really a group effort. The nutrition analyses of various types of restaurant foods were organized by Jayne Hurley, senior nutritionist at the Center for Science in the Public Interest (CSPI). Since 1993, Jayne has been CSPI's impresario of restaurant nutrition. To design the studies, she oftentimes relied upon advice from Gary Beecher, Joanne Holden, Margaret Hoke, and other researchers at the Beltsville (Maryland) Human Nutrition Research Center of the U.S. Department of Agriculture. We thank them for their help. Identifying the kinds of foods to analyze and determining which restaurants to visit was a major task that Jacqueline Adriano, Daved Alexander, Nona Alter, Maxine Anderson, Adam Arenson, Victoria Dolby, Kathryn Fitzgerald, Tamar Genger, Jacob Kaplan, Karen Orville, Anne Pokorny, Wendie Rosofsky, Beth Sumrell, Patricia Treanor, and Michelle Werkstell undertook with skill and persistence. CSPI members helped purchase many of the meals in cities around the country. We thank Juliann Goldman for coordinating much of that work and Ingrid VanTuinen and Heather Jones DeMino for compiling the results and doing a tremendous amount of research for and proofreading of this book. In addition, Bonnie Liebman (chapter 2), Stephen B. Schmidt, Geneva Collins, and Mimi Harrison helped write and edit sections of this book. Also, we are grateful to the dozens of people at restaurants large and small for providing (however reluctantly!) a great deal of useful information. Lastly, we thank Peter Workman, Jennifer Griffin, Margot Herrera, Cindy Schoen, and others at Workman Publishing for their care and patience in producing this book.

Michael F. Jacobson, Ph.D.
Executive Director
Center for Science in the Public Interest

Preface

Dinnertime in America exists in the collective memory of the nation as a scene that could have been painted by Norman Rockwell: Mom, Dad, and the children gathered around the table after a day of work and study, eating nutritious and sustaining food lovingly prepared at home. Whether or not that food was actually quite as nutritious as the image suggests, that warming scene is today mostly a myth.

Family life has changed, and there just isn't as much time available for the careful preparation of food at home. Americans now spend about 41 percent of their food dollars on meals prepared outside the home, and the American Restaurant Association estimates that we spend more than $225 billion annually at restaurants. There are more than 800,000 food outlets in this country, ranging from street-corner vendors, cafeterias, and take-out establishments to family-style and upscale restaurants. There are 177,000 fast-food outlets and 196,000 table-service restaurants. The result is that the food-service industry now influences national eating habits to a degree that nutrition experts consider to be dangerous. Thirty-four percent of our calories are consumed outside the home; this figure rises to 45 percent for men in the 18- to 39-year-old age bracket. Much of our eating is, indeed, casual and capricious . . . a doughnut grabbed on the run, a cappuccino drunk on the way to work . . . but much more of it is a necessary part of our lives, a slice of time inserted into a frantic schedule.

One obvious problem with eating out is that most restaurants serve large portions loaded with calories, fat, saturated fat, and salt. A healthy plate of broiled fish is likely to be accompanied by a baked potato drenched in butter and sour cream. A stir-fried chicken and peanut dish from a Chinese restaurant may have as much fat as four fast-food burgers. Breakfast-to-go has begun to look a lot like dessert. Movie theaters offer vats of popcorn drenched in highly saturated coconut oil. Soft drinks are loaded with sugar. And all of this is being served at a time when obesity and diabetes have become dual threats to the national health.

But it need not be this way. Michael F. Jacobson and Jayne G. Hurley are executive director and senior nutritionist, respectively, of the Center for Science in the Public Interest, a nonprofit organization that focuses on improving the safety and nutritional quality of our food supply. In this book they have turned their attention to the risks inherent in restaurant eating today—and to strategies for avoiding those risks. The authors are careful to point out that not all restaurant foods present the diner with excessive amounts of undesirable ingredients. But all too many do, and one of the functions of this book is to distinguish between the excessive and the sensible.

Thus, the reader is presented with lists of such items as the ten best and worst restaurant meals, the worst snacks, the foods highest in calories, and the foods lowest in saturated fat and calories. And the authors have looked hard at some of the most popular foods—including Chinese, Mexican, Italian, and Greek cuisine, steak, seafood, pizza, and sandwiches—and told us in unflinching detail what we would be wise to order and what we should avoid.

But these advisories are only part of the message that Jacobson and Hurley deliver. They also urge restaurant owners to offer "lite" or "healthy" servings, to allow reasonable substitutions (such as a baked potato for french fries), to use liquid vegetable oils for frying, and to offer fat-free milk and whole-wheat breads. And they make a case for requiring restaurants to provide nutritional information about their meals.

The key to the problem, however, lies not only in what restaurants offer but also in what customers demand. So long as there is a demand for self-indulgent serving sizes and ingredients, restaurants, particularly fast-food chains, will continue to cater to those indulgences. On the other hand, it has been shown that informed and health-conscious consumers can influence the products that are offered for their consumption. What Jacobson and Hurley have given us in this book is a much-needed guide to bring about such changes, as well as an approach to sensible, enjoyable dining outside the home.

Dr. David Kessler
Dean of the Yale University School of Medicine
and former Commissioner of the
U.S. Food and Drug Administration

Chapter 1

Introduction: Eating Out as a Way of Life

N ot so very long ago, going to a restaurant was considered an occasion, an exciting experience saved for celebrations. Maybe the family "gave" Mom the day off on Mother's Day, or everyone gathered together to dine out after a graduation. What went on behind the scenes in restaurant kitchens was invisible and kind of intriguing, and the whole experience came with a dash of glamour and anticipation.

For most people these days, eating out is neither exotic nor much of an event. In fact, eating out regularly seems to have become part of nearly everyone's daily routine. Overextended, time-crunched Americans increasingly rely on restaurants and take-out shops, and some kids practically grow up in fast-food outlets or on take-out food.

The proof is in the percentages: In 1955 Americans spent 19 percent of their food dollar on food that was prepared outside the home—today that figure has risen to about 41 percent, and it's still climbing. Hundreds of thousands of eateries dot the landscape, sprouting up everywhere from malls and airports to schools and gas stations. The U.S. Department of Agriculture (USDA) estimates that we're spending more than $222 billion annually at restaurants and cafeterias, including $118 billion at fast-food restaurants.

In many restaurants, food is no longer simple, straightforward fare. Menus are filled with dishes that are masterpieces of overwrought excess. Slick marketing campaigns encourage us to crave increasingly bigger and richer dishes. Portions of meat have gotten larger, layers of melted cheese have gotten fatter, salt and sugar are abundant, and even salads have been corrupted by silly additions like nuggets of fried chicken. We may count on health departments to ensure sanitation in restaurants, but who is looking after our interests when it comes to the nutritional consequences of what those restaurants serve? Neither health inspectors nor anyone else out there seeks to protect us from the growing extremes of calories, fat, and salt.

Good, reliable information about what we're being offered—and eating—in restaurants is virtually nonexistent. You'll rarely find nutrition information on menus, and restaurant critics don't address the health impact of the dishes they recommend. Even some popular books about restaurant nutrition are wildly inaccurate. But as we depend more and more upon restaurants for our meals, the nutritional quality of what we eat is increasingly important.

USDA surveys find that food eaten outside the home is nutritionally worse than home-cooked food in practically every way. For example, restaurant meals are, on average, 20 percent fattier than home cooking, and they're about 15 percent higher in saturated fat, which promotes heart disease. They're also higher in sodium and cholesterol and much lower in calcium, dietary fiber, and iron. In its understated way, the USDA notes, "Away-from-home foods generally contain more of the nutrients overconsumed and less of the nutrients underconsumed by Americans. As a result, the increased popularity of dining out may make it more difficult for Americans to improve the overall nutritional quality of their diets, particularly in terms of reducing intakes of fat and saturated fat." As we'll discuss in greater detail in the next chapter, eating out, if one is not careful, may increase the risk of heart disease, high blood pressure, obesity, and other health problems.

In 1993, the Center for Science in the Public Interest (CSPI), a nonprofit, consumer-advocacy organization where the authors of this book work, launched an investigation into restaurant nutrition. We began with a study of Chinese-restaurant meals, having no idea what we'd find. We were shocked when the lab analysis revealed sky-high amounts of calories, fat, and sodium in many popular dishes. A single entrée, kung pao chicken with rice, contained 1,600 calories, 76 grams of fat, and 2,600 milligrams of sodium. That's more than enough fat and sodium for an entire day, and it doesn't take into account the usual accompaniments, such as soup, an egg roll, and extra soy sauce. We were also astounded to discover how large the portion sizes were, only to learn in subsequent studies that such huge servings are the norm—regardless of the type of cuisine—in the midpriced restaurants we visited.

The media found our results as hot as a wok during the evening rush. The *Washington Post* trumpeted "Moo Shu Madness." "Restaurateurs Sizzle over Kung Pao Study," reported the *Los Angeles Times*.

Media controversy flared after we announced the results of each new study of a restaurant cuisine—Italian, Mexican, seafood, and many others. Our news conferences became standing room–only events. Local TV newscasters staked out targeted restaurants to solicit patrons' reactions. The *Oprah* show, CBS's *48 Hours*, *Dateline NBC*, ABC's *20/20*, and many other news and talk shows featured our studies. Headline writers had a field day. (Some of our favorites: "The Taco Belly!" in the *New York Post* after our Mexican study; "Avoiding the Fatter Breakfast Platter Is Sometimes a Matter of Batter" in the *Washington Post* about our breakfast investigation; "Study: The Buns Can Add Tons" in *New York Newsday* following our tests of sweets.) The studies also provided plenty of rich material for Jay Leno, David Letterman, and editorial cartoonists, all of whom helped spread the message.

Public-relations flacks for the restaurant industry swiftly mounted a counterattack, because the notion that restaurant dining could be unhealthful wasn't exactly the sort of publicity the industry liked. When sales at Chinese restaurants plummeted right after our report, restaurateurs blamed CSPI. The National Restaurant Association labeled us nutrition terrorists. Sometimes the media joined in, calling us the Food Police and peppering their stories with wisecracks and puns. But even some of the journalists who lampooned us eventually took our message to heart. Hefty Rush Limbaugh, for instance, began exercising and eating a lower-fat, no-sugar, and no-alcohol diet, and found that his weight dropped back down toward the healthy zone.

Restaurants by the Numbers

- There are 844,000 eateries in the United States, ranging from street-corner hot-dog vendors to cafeterias to fancy restaurants.
- There are 177,000 fast-food restaurants.
- There are 196,000 table-service restaurants.
- 29 percent of our meals are purchased outside the home.
- 22 percent of our snacks are purchased outside the home.
- 41 percent of our food dollars were spent outside the home in 2000 (compared to 19 percent in 1955).
- $222 billion is spent annually at restaurants; another $117 billion is spent at company and school cafeterias, stadiums, and other venues.
- 34 percent of our calories are consumed outside the home (restaurants, vending machines, snack bars, etc.), compared to 18 percent in 1977–78.
- 45 percent of calories eaten by 18- to 39-year-old men are consumed outside the home.

Sources: U.S. Department of Agriculture and the National Restaurant Association

Despite what some critics charged, CSPI's mission was never to ban high-calorie restaurant meals or take the fun out of eating out. (Hey, we eat out, and fairly frequently, but we order judiciously!) And, no, it was not our intention to make everyone eat nothing but broccoli and bean sprouts. Our goal has always been to provide reliable information so that health-conscious consumers can make informed choices when they eat out and to encourage restaurants to provide more healthful options. And that's the intent of this book.

Of course, no matter how much information they've been given, some people will continue eating what we've dubbed a "coronary bypass special" (those double cheeseburgers at fast-food outlets) or the "heart attack on a plate" (fettuccine Alfredo). That's their right. In some cases it may not even be a problem—if such meals are rare events. Our arteries can, indeed, withstand an occasional indulgence.

CSPI's restaurant studies have proved vital for the many people who want the facts about restaurant nutrition. After all, neither the government nor the restaurant industry itself is providing the data. (The only exceptions are a few major restaurant chains, mostly fast-food ones, that voluntarily publish nutrition information. As we explain in the next chapter, restaurants are required to disclose nutrition information only when they make nutritional claims for a dish.)

As our studies continued to shock the public (and us) over the next few years, the National Restaurant Association kept pooh-poohing the findings. In 1996, Jeffrey Prince, then director of communications for the organization, urged a convention of public-relations executives to launch "a concerted effort to make the case against CSPI."

Such protests from the restaurant industry were all too familiar to us. A decade earlier, CSPI had fought a similar battle with the fast-food giants. McDonald's and the other major players boasted that their patrons didn't care about the nutritional quality of their meals or the ingredients from which they were made. After we began focusing the national spotlight on the abysmal dining options that McDonald's, Burger King, and others offered, several state attorneys general ordered McDonald's, Wendy's, Burger King, and several other major companies to halt deceptive ads and to provide customers with ingredient and nutrition information.

Once the public began learning more about the foods those multibillion-dollar corporations were serving, the companies started making changes. McDonald's and most other major hamburger chains stopped cooking their french fries in beef tallow, a practice that put more beef fat in an order of fries than in a hamburger. (Ironically, instead of switching from beef tallow to vegetable oil, as we had urged, companies switched to hydrogenated vegetable shortening, which was soon discovered to be about as bad as beef fat. You'll find more on that shortening in the next chapter.) Grilled chicken sandwiches, salads, baked potatoes, fruit and yogurt parfaits, and a few other healthful alternatives to fried or grilled beef patties have since appeared at many chains. (See chapter 16, On the Run, for the latest on what chains are offering.)

Nutrition information on core menu items is now available from the largest chains—plastered on restaurant walls, printed in brochures, and posted on company Web sites. Unfortunately, the lion's share of the typical fast-food menu remains as harmful as it ever was, although at least consumers can find out what they're getting. That option is simply not available at most midpriced and upscale restaurants, where, shockingly, it turns out that many meals are far worse for your health than the fattiest fast foods.

The Often Surprising Results of Our Studies

Some restaurant-industry officials and journalists have derided CSPI's restaurant studies as merely stating the obvious. They said, of course people know that an Original Grand Slam break-

A Message to Restaurateurs

···

Restaurants could do a lot to help people eat a more healthful diet. Please consider the following:

☞ Offer a "healthy" or "lite" section on your menu.

☞ Allow patrons to make reasonable substitutions, such as a baked potato instead of french fries.

☞ Make available low-fat versions of foods like ham, sausages, hot dogs, cheeses, mayonnaise, ice cream, and hamburgers. Offer 1 percent, low-fat, or fat-free milk, vegetable burgers, and whole wheat bread and rolls. Provide fruit and vegetable side dishes that go beyond fries and coleslaw.

☞ Use vegetable oil instead of solid shortenings for frying.

☞ List calorie content next to each item on fast-food menu boards.

☞ Provide nutrition information for standard dishes.

☞ Note on the menu when there is a possible presence of allergens like nuts.

☞ Lower the prices of salads and fruit, making up for any loss by small increases in the prices of less healthful items.

☞ Provide half portions at a lower price.

fast at Denny's (two eggs, two hotcakes, two sausage links, and two strips of bacon) or a fried seafood platter is high in fat. And, they argued, no one eats sweets for nutrition, so what harm is one Cinnabon going to do? The answer, as we discovered, is plenty! Countless people, including journalists, *were* shocked to learn from our sweets study that what most people consider a snack to tide them over until mealtime—an Au Bon Pain Sweet Cheese Danish, for example—actually packs as many calories as a McDonald's Quarter Pounder with Cheese. And we're confident that few people suspected that some of the sweets, including Au Bon Pain's Pecan Roll and The Cheesecake Factory's Original Cheesecake, harbored at least *an entire day's* worth of saturated fat.

Indeed, our studies have provided one eye-popping surprise after another. Who would have guessed that spaghetti with meat sauce would be one of the *better* entrée options at an Italian restaurant? Who could imagine that we'd be giving the thumbs-up to a roast beef sandwich with mustard from a deli or that a typical sandwich-shop tuna salad sandwich with mayo on the bread has more fat and calories, and nearly as much saturated fat, as an overstuffed corned beef sandwich with mustard? And who wouldn't be taken aback by our discovery that some salad entrées, like a chef's salad, can deliver half a day's calories, largely because of the amazing amount of dressing restaurants add to them?

In fact, those facts *aren't* obvious, even to trained nutritionists. A survey conducted by New York University and CSPI nutritionists at the 1996 annual meeting of the American Dietetic Association found that dietitians greatly underestimated the calorie and fat content of restaurant meals. The researchers showed 203 dietitians five meals (lasagna, grilled chicken Caesar salad, a tuna salad sandwich, a hamburger with onion rings, and a porterhouse steak dinner) and asked them to estimate the calorie and fat content. The dietitians, who should be better able than anyone to accurately gauge the nutrient content of foods, underestimated the calorie contents by an average of 37 percent and the fat content by a whopping 49 percent. For example, they thought that the tuna salad sandwich provided 375 calories, but it actually provided 720 calories. They said it contained 18 grams of fat, whereas it actually contained 43 grams. They believed the hamburger and onion rings to contain 865 calories and 44 grams of fat; but they actually contained about twice those amounts. "The survey proves that even nutrition professionals can't estimate accurately the calorie and fat content of restaurant meals," said Marion Nestle, Ph.D., chair of New York University's Department of Nutrition and Food Studies. "If nutritionists can't tell what's in restaurant meals, consumers certainly can't."

One of the most shocking things we discovered about many restaurant meals is their gargantuan size. The entrées at places like The Cheesecake Factory, for example, are big enough to feed a family—a *slice* of carrot cake weighs almost a pound and has 1,560 calories. Adam Drewnowski, Ph.D., then director of the Human Nutrition Program at the University of Michigan, said, "People have a mental image of a 200-calorie muffin, but what they're in fact served is a huge 900-calorie muffin."

Even Jeffrey Prince, the former restaurant association official, has observed: "If any of you have been to Europe lately, and have come back to the U.S., you are absolutely flabbergasted at the discrepancy in the size of what we serve. Probably at home, but certainly in restaurants. And when you analyze these foods, 'Hey, there's a lot of calories in them!' because there's six times [or] three times as much food on the plate as there used to be. The biggest-selling item in the restaurant supply industry today is the 12-inch plate because the 10- or 11-inch plate won't hold the food anymore."

The American Dietetic Association may mean well when it states that "there are no good or bad foods" and that the "keys to a good diet are balance, variety, and moderation," but it misses an important point. If you're eating out 4.2 times a week—which the National Restaurant Association says is average—balance and moderation are pretty hard tricks to pull off in a land where 1,000-calorie meals are the norm. Let's be realistic. People who are downing fried seafood platters for dinner are not eating spinach salads at other meals. They're more likely to be eating cheeseburgers, "super-sized" orders of fries, pizza, kung pao chicken, or lasagna, and washing them down with quart-size sodas.

The Master
"Make It Better" Strategy

A 10-Point Plan for Eating Out More Healthfully

1. **Check the menu before you walk in.** There ought to be a law requiring restaurants to post menus in their windows! If you discover that everything is deep fried only after you sit down, you'll have a hard time leaving.

2. **If the menu is vague, ask a server to explain it.** You may think the chicken salad will be topped with grilled chicken, but instead you are served a bowl of romaine lettuce and other salad fixings, topped with fried, breaded nuggets. Always ask first to avoid surprises.

3. **Look for the "healthy" or "light" section on menus.** These items are likely to be better choices than other dishes.

4. **Don't be shy about requesting changes.** Feel free to ask for sauce on the side, to have an item grilled rather than fried, to order the beef with broccoli heavy on the broccoli and light on the beef, or to request that fatty toppings like cheese and dressing be left off. Most restaurants will honor your request.

5. **Ask about substitutions.** Restaurants may let you replace your coleslaw and fries with a side salad and baked potato, get your omelette made with egg whites or an egg substitute, or provide light dressing in place of a full-fat one on your entrée salad. They may say no, or they may charge extra, but you won't know unless you ask.

6. **Watch for hidden fats.** Two major sources of fat in the American diet are salad dressings and red meat. Although full-fat dressings are not harmful to the heart, they can bump up the calories in an entrée salad from 650 to 950. Unfortunately, many restaurants don't have light dressing substitutes

for their specialty salads. Steak cuts can vary astronomically in the amount of fat they contain, ranging from a relatively lean filet mignon or sirloin to the very fatty porterhouse and prime rib.

7. **Use doggie bags to create tomorrow's lunch.** Take home half of what you're served and you save not only calories and fat, but also the cost of tomorrow's meal. Alternatively, you and a friend could share an entrée or dessert.

8. **Beware the buffets.** All-you-can-eat salad and breakfast bars can be terrific if you choose wisely, but you may overeat in order to feel that you're getting your money's worth. Ordering à la carte is often a better choice, or take a piece of fruit or a yogurt from the buffet for a snack later in the day.

9. **Eat out less often.** Instead of eating lunch out every day, brown-bag it once or twice a week, or cruise the salad bar (or fruit and yogurt aisles) at the supermarket. If you are going for an outing, pack a cooler with sandwiches, yogurt, and fruit. Your wallet as well as your waistline will thank you.

10. **Be an advocate.** Restaurants change in response to consumer demand. If you keep pestering your favorite lunch and dinner spots to offer light Caesar dressing, whole wheat sandwich rolls, or a tossed salad that goes beyond iceberg lettuce, maybe they will make some changes. Fill out those response cards, request those nutrition brochures, and be candid when the manager or server asks if everything is okay. If you speak up, some of those wishes are bound to be fulfilled because restaurants want you to return. On a broader scale, you can urge your city council to require that chain restaurants provide a modicum of nutrition information. Menus could easily indicate whether liquid oil or solid shortening is used for deep-fat frying, and fast-food restaurants could list calories on the menu board.

How We Conduct Our Studies

In almost every chapter we identify which restaurant chains were chosen for the analysis of a particular cuisine or category of food. The chapters on mall food and fast food don't list that information because most of the nutrition information presented is from the restaurants' own lab analyses. Here is a more detailed explanation of how we conducted our studies.

CSPI nutritionists designed its studies with advice from scientists at the USDA's Human Nutrition Information Service and USDA's Beltsville (Maryland) Human Nutrition Research Center. Those are the experts who supervise the collection and testing of thousands of food samples for the government's Nutrient Data Base. They helped us determine the number of cities and restaurants to visit, the number of food samples to collect, and the appropriate procedures for handling the samples and preparing the composites. Here's what we did.

Step 1: Identifying the dishes. We used industry trade data (such as *Restaurants and Institutions*'s biennial menu census) to determine the 15 or so most popular dishes in a given cuisine type, as reported by the restaurants themselves (for example, lasagna, spaghetti with meatballs, and so on for the Italian study). To make sure we'd have some promising dishes to recommend, we selected at least two relatively nutritious dishes for analysis, whether or not they were among the most popular items. The Chinese and Greek studies were conducted somewhat differently. Since Chinese and Greek cuisines are almost exclusively the domain of mom-and-pop restaurants, rather than chains, no industry-wide data were available. To determine the most popular dishes, we conducted informal surveys of restaurants around the country. For sweets and pizza, the companies told us what their best-selling items were.

Step 2: Choosing the restaurants. CSPI again used industry trade data (such as *Restaurants and Institutions*'s Top 400 list) to determine the largest chains for the targeted cuisine type (for example, Outback and Lone Star for steak houses; Denny's and Shoney's for family-style restaurants). We then selected chain restaurants in at least three major cities (one city each on the East Coast, West Coast, and in the Midwest). When appropriate, we also chose some of the busiest independent restaurants in the same cities.

Step 3: Buying the food. For each survey, CSPI staffers (or a commercial pickup service) purchased approximately 135 dishes or meals. Typically, in each of three cities, we selected the same 15 dishes from each of at least three restaurants. The meals were boxed with cold packs in insulated containers and express shipped to an independent laboratory or to CSPI.

Step 4: Determining basic ingredient amounts for the composite samples. Technicians dissected each meal and weighed the major ingredients (for example, how many ounces each of chicken, bacon, and cheese went into the bacon-and-cheese grilled chicken sandwich analyzed in the dinner-house study). That let us estimate the variability of dishes going into the composite sample and allowed us to eliminate any dishes that varied greatly from the norm.

Step 5: Creating and analyzing the composite samples. Composites of each dish were made from the six to twelve samples (equal portions of nine steak houses' cheese fries were mixed together, for example) and shipped to a second independent laboratory. That laboratory analyzed the samples for calories, fat, saturated fat (and, in most cases, *trans* fat), cholesterol, and sodium, and sent the results to CSPI. (For sweets and desserts, sugar content also was analyzed.)

It's important to note that our composites do not tell you exactly what you're being served when you order a particular dish at a specific restaurant. A composite provides a snapshot overview of the "average" dish being served. When we found wide variations in the composition of a dish—such as the amount of peanuts served in the kung pao chicken or the quantity of breading on the fried clams—we have noted that fact in the description of our findings.

Although some restaurant industry officials have charged that our studies are irrelevant because they provided composite nutritional values, the fact is that nutrient levels are almost always based on composites because that is the only economical way to present data. We use composites because the alternative—analyzing each sample of a given dish separately—is prohibitively expensive and still wouldn't tell you what the restaurant in your neighborhood serves.

Although no single nutritional analysis is accurate for every restaurant meal, we believe that our numbers are the most accurate that you'll find anywhere. Actually, it would delight us if restaurateurs (starting with chain restaurants) provided their patrons with accurate information, at least for calories and saturated fat, about the dishes they offer. Indeed, we have urged state and local governments to require chains to do so.

So much for the behind-the-scene look at CSPI's studies. It's time now to look at the health consequences of the foods we eat and then turn to the restaurants—from Denny's to your local Mexican place—and find out just how good (or bad) your favorite meals are. The purpose of this book is to guide you to the healthier selections. In each chapter, we tell you about some fabulous, great-tasting meals—and we offer our advice for overhauling troublesome dishes in summary tips provided in a section we call the "Strategy."

Bon appétit—but caveat emptor!

Chapter 2

Nutrition: Eating Out—
Healthfully

Restaurant food has a lot to offer: taste, convenience,
entertainment, the experience of sampling unfamiliar
cuisines, a chance to socialize without doing the dishes.
But if we eat out frequently without being careful, we
may pay for those benefits twice: first with our wallets and later
with our health. An occasional dining-out splurge isn't a problem.
But a steady diet of typical restaurant meals—together with similar meals at home—increases the risk of many major illnesses.

For decades, health authorities have warned that an unhealthy diet promotes heart disease, cancer, stroke, diabetes,
osteoporosis, and obesity. The National Academy of Sciences,
the U.S. surgeon general, the National Cancer Institute, the
American Cancer Society, the American Heart Association, and
others agree on how to improve the typical American diet. You
can boil down their advice to two simple messages:

• **Eat more** fruits, vegetables, beans, whole grain breads and
cereals, and other plant foods that supply not just vitamins and
minerals, but also the fiber, antioxidants, and other phytochemicals that are missing from animal foods and heavily processed
junk foods. Also, eat more fish, poultry, and low-fat dairy products.

• **Eat less** of foods that are high in saturated or *trans* fat, cholesterol, sodium, refined sugars, or calories. This includes whole

and 2 percent reduced-fat milk, cheese, ice cream, butter, hamburgers, hot dogs, and baked goods made with butter. It also means cutting back on fried foods, pastries, stick margarine, and other foods made with hydrogenated vegetable oil. You also should consume fewer egg yolks, soft drinks and other sweets, and high-sodium processed foods.

That's nutrition in a nutshell. Smart eating isn't that complicated. Here's a rundown of the scientific evidence that makes the advice to eat healthfully so compelling.

Calories, Calories, Calories

Health experts keep lengthening the list of reasons not to be overweight: diabetes, heart disease, stroke, gout, gallbladder disease, arthritis, and cancers of the breast, colon, and uterus. What's more, being overweight often leads to psychological problems, difficulty getting a job, and other social problems. Yet Americans are becoming fatter and fatter. In 1960 one out of every eight American adults was obese. Today, more than one out of every four adults is obese. Over that same period, the percentage of adults who are either obese or overweight jumped from about two out of five to three out of five, and much of that increase occurred since 1990.

"Can we explain the increase because we have less willpower than we did ten years ago?" asks Yale University's Kelly Brownell, one of the nation's leading obesity experts. "Has the gene pool changed in ten years?" Clearly, that's not the explanation. "Evolution takes millions of years," he points out.

Most Americans want to be lean. We join gyms, we read diet books, and we buy diet foods and supplements, but nothing seems to work. Fattening food—in enormous quantities—beckons us at every restaurant, not to mention every shopping mall, gas station, amusement park, airport, vending machine, and convenience store. If it's a place with people, it's a place with junk food.

Meanwhile, technology is systematically eliminating every reason for us to move our muscles. From automobiles to escalators to remote-control television sets, it seems that our only body parts that get exercise are our fingers . . . and our jaws.

Daily Limits for Adults

Health experts recommend that most people over the age of two eat a diet that gets no more than 30 percent of its calories from fat. Even more important than limiting total fat is limiting saturated fat. *Less than* 10 percent of calories should be your target. That's why this chart shows 9 percent of calories from saturated fat. But getting lower levels may be even better. That's why food labels (and this book) use 20 grams of saturated fat as a population target. It works out to roughly 9 percent of calories for women and for men over 50 and to only 6 percent for men aged 19 to 50— a reasonable target, since men are at greater risk for heart attacks at an early age.

Age	19–50 females	50+ females	19–50 males	50+ males
Calories	2,200	1,900	2,900	2,300
Fat (grams)	73	63	97	77
Saturated fat (grams)	22	19	29	23

Calorie data: Recommended Dietary Allowances, National Academy of Sciences, 10th edition (1989).

Baby on Board:
Dining Out with Children

No matter what kind of restaurant, special menus for children always seem to offer the same fatty or sugary junk: grilled cheese sandwiches, soft drinks, chips, hot dogs, burgers, fries, fish or chicken fingers, and maybe a small cheese pizza. Of course, the obvious inclination is to order something—*anything*—fast to satisfy your hungry, impatient child.

But if you know what you're doing, you can turn eating out into an opportunity to expand your children's eating horizons and prepare them for a lifetime of healthier eating.

Here are some suggestions for making the best of an often-difficult situation.

☛ Ask for something to eat immediately if your child is cranky. Any wise waiter will gladly bring a cup of soup, fruit, salad, or a roll.

☛ Skip the children's menu and select something from the adults'. Some restaurants may serve half-orders at a lower price. Or, if your child is not very hungry, he or she can share some of your meal.

☛ While your children are very young, help them develop a taste for ... water! Water (fizzy or tap) can be dressed up with slices of orange, lemon, or lime. Combined with cranberry, orange, or unsweetened pineapple juice, it becomes a wholesome soft drink. The current epidemic of obesity in children is attributed in part to the endless flow of sweetened drinks—especially the oceans of sodas—that kids consume. If you start early, your children may develop a taste for less-sweet alternatives—and save themselves thousands of empty calories over a lifetime.

☛ If there's a salad bar, use it—but keep an eye out for pitfalls like shredded cheese, bacon bits, Jell-O cubes, and gobs of creamy dressings. Most salad bars offer raw carrots, celery sticks, peppers, cucumbers, garbanzo beans, and many other cool and crunchy things your children can dip into some low-fat dressing.

☛ When children are still young, take them to ethnic restaurants that offer selections well beyond the standard American fare. If they're not adventurous eaters, start with simple foods that feature mild flavors. Often, it's easier (and cheaper) to order a side dish instead of a main meal.

For example:

• **Mexican:** Order a side of beans (not refried, if possible) that the child can either wrap in a flour tortilla or eat with rice. A few strips of chicken or vegetables from an order of fajitas might also go over well.

• **Indian:** Try flat bread, like whole wheat chapati and a side dish of dal (lentils). Mix it with rice if it's too spicy. (To get your children used to spicy foods, start them with a favorite ingredient like potatoes, mildly spiced. As they get used to stronger flavors, they can move on to tandoori chicken, curried vegetables, and many other delicacies.)

• **Middle Eastern:** Try some hummus and pita bread. The grilled chicken and rice from an order of souvlaki are also good bets.

• **Chinese:** Create your own side dish by extracting a sampling of favorite foods like broccoli, carrots, baby corn, snow pea pods, or chicken from the main dishes you order. Add rice or lo mein (noodles).

Of course, nothing succeeds as well as a good example from you. If you eat healthy foods in restaurants and at home, your child will follow your lead.

"Animals—and people—evolved in an environment where food was scarce and calorie expenditures were high," explains Brownell. "Under those conditions, being programmed to eat high-calorie food is adaptive. Those ancient genes wouldn't be a problem if the environment weren't so damaging." And restaurants are a huge part of that environment. "Serving sizes in restaurants have exploded," says Marion Nestle, chair of the Department of Nutrition and Food Studies at New York University. "Food is cheap relative to other costs like rent and labor," she explains. "So it's easy to throw in a bit more food to provide more 'value' to diners."

"A bit more" is an understatement. It is not at all unusual for a typical restaurant meal to pack 1,000 calories, not counting appetizers or dessert, each of which could run another 1,000. Yet, most women need only about 2,000 calories per day, whereas men need about 2,500. (See Restaurant Hall of Shame, page 23; Ten of the Worst Restaurant Meals, page 39; and Foods Highest in Calories, page 56.)

Here are some figures from our research that put those daily calories in perspective. A typical 3½-cup serving of spaghetti and meatballs has 1,160 calories. Kung pao chicken—4½ cups if you count the rice—provides 1,620 calories. A fried seafood platter—including french fries, coleslaw, biscuits, and tartar sauce—goes over the top with more than 2,100 calories. Even a standard deli sandwich provides about 550 calories (for chicken salad or ham) to about 730 (tuna salad or a turkey club).

Among the more popular appetizers are cheese nachos (about 800 calories), fried mozzarella sticks (about 800 calories), stuffed potato skins (about 1,100 calories, *without* sour cream), and a fried whole onion (about 1,700 calories *without* the dipping sauce). Desserts, of course, are high in calories, too. A slice of The Cheesecake Factory Original Cheesecake has about 700 calories, whereas a fudge brownie sundae weighs in at around 1,100 calories.

Soft drinks are a particular problem. A 12-ounce can has about 150 calories. But at many restaurants and convenience stores, a 12-

ounce drink is the "kiddie" version. Some restaurants offer single servings that are as large as two quarts—the size of a half-gallon milk carton—and others offer free refills. Moreover, research suggests that the calories in liquid foods contribute more to obesity than calories in solid foods (see chapter 14, In the Drink: Beverages).

All those calories help explain why frequent restaurant-goers are more likely to be overweight. "We asked people how many times they ate at different restaurants, like Chinese and Mexican restaurants, or places that serve pizza, hamburgers, fried chicken, or fried fish," says Megan McCrory of the Jean Mayer U.S. Department of Agriculture Human Nutrition Research Center on Aging at Tufts University in Boston. "The more often they ate out, the fatter they were."

But a careful diner can beat the odds. If you order from the "healthy" or "light" menus offered at some restaurants, you can slash the calories. Dishes like The Olive Garden's Garden Fare Capellini Pomodoro or Shrimp Primavera, T.G.I. Friday's Garden-burger, or Applebee's Lemon Chicken Pasta fall in the 500- to 700-calorie range. And there is a bonus: Most light or healthful dishes aren't just lower in calories, they're also richer in vegetables. Dishes loaded with lots of vegetables can make it easier to limit calories, because vegetables have low calorie density—in other words, their bulk makes you feel full.

And watch those beverages. Always ask for water. You can also order seltzer water either plain or mixed with orange juice, or have fat-free milk. If you do order a soft drink, get a small size (even if the larger sizes are temptingly close in price) with ice or a diet soda.

Restaurant Hall of Fame

These foods keep the saturated fat at reasonable levels and, in most cases, supply some fruit or vegetables. (Unfortunately, even the best restaurant foods contain too much sodium.)

	Calories	Total Fat (g)	Saturated Fat (g)
1. Subway's "7 Subs with 6 Grams of Fat or Less"*	260	5	1
2. Blimpie's Veggie Max Sub	400	7	1
3. McDonald's Fruit 'n Yogurt Parfait with granola	380	5	2
4. Turkey sandwich with lettuce, tomato, and mustard	370	6	*2*
5. Grilled or broiled chicken or seafood (average, without side dishes)	270	8	*2*
6. Szechuan shrimp or chicken with rice*	930	19	2
7. Chicken, lamb, or pork souvlaki with rice*	290	10	*3*
8. Chinese stir-fried spinach, broccoli, or mixed vegetables with rice *	750	19	3
9. Pasta with red clam or marinara sauce*	870	20	4
10. Fajitas (chicken, shrimp, or vegetable) with tortillas*	840	24	5

*Numbers are an average of the items listed.

Note: Saturated fat numbers in *italics* include artery-clogging *trans* fat.

Restaurant Hall of Shame

Each of these foods has more than 1,000 calories and one to *four* days' worth of saturated fat.

	Calories	Total Fat (g)	Saturated Fat (g)
1. Cheese fries with ranch dressing	3,010	217	*91*
2. Movie theater popcorn with "butter" topping (large)	1,640	126	*73*
3. Prime rib, untrimmed (16 oz.)	1,280	94	*52*
4. Fettuccine Alfredo	1,500	97	48
5. Stuffed potato skins with sour cream	1,260	95	*48*
6. Fudge brownie sundae	1,130	57	*30*
7. Beef and cheese nachos with sour cream and guacamole	1,360	89	*28*
8. Denny's Meat Lover's Skillet (ham, bacon, and sausage over fried potatoes with cheddar and two eggs)	1,150	93	26
9. The Cheesecake Factory Carrot Cake (1 slice)	1,560	84	23
10. Pizzeria Uno Chicago Classic (½ pizza)	1,500	74	*30*

Note: Saturated fat numbers in *italics* include artery-clogging *trans* fat.

Protecting Your Heart

One out of three Americans will die of heart disease. It kills more men—*and* women—than any other illness, including cancer.

Despite these grim statistics, there is actually some good news about heart disease. Americans, both male and female, are dying of heart attacks at less than *half* the rate we did in 1965. Coronary-bypass operations, clot-busting drugs, and hospital cardiac-care units have saved the lives of countless people whose arteries had already become clogged. Prompt medical attention and effective new medications also are helping to lower the mortality rate. Best of all, researchers have figured out how to *prevent* heart disease in the first place. Not smoking cigarettes, keeping blood pressure under control, and getting enough exercise are one part of the equation. Diet is another.

Protect Your Heart with Fruits, Vegetables, Beans, and Whole Grains

The American Heart Association advises people to "choose a diet with plenty of vegetables, fruits, and whole-grain products" to reduce the risk of heart disease. What's more, the association urges people to "choose a diet moderate in sugar" to make room for those healthier foods. Junk foods—even fat-free or low-fat ones like soft drinks, SnackWell's cookies, and fat-free frozen yogurt—can crowd out those beneficial fruits, vegetables, and whole grains.

Many Chinese, Thai, and other Asian restaurants serve a wide variety of vegetables, but the typical American restaurant rarely goes beyond the vegetable of the day. The only time you're likely to find whole grains and fruits is at breakfast, when some restaurants offer fresh fruit or orange juice and a cereal like shredded wheat, bran flakes, or oatmeal.

"The four vegetables that Americans eat most are potatoes (mostly as french fries), tomatoes (mostly as sauce or ketchup), onions, and iceberg lettuce," says Marion Nestle of New York University. "That's not my idea of fruits and vegetables—that's garnish on burgers."

Plant foods like broccoli, oranges, berries, dark leafy greens, carrots, melons, and other good choices protect the heart in three ways. First, unless buried in butter, they're low in heart-damaging fat. Second, the dietary fiber and some of the chemicals in plants—called phytochemicals—may protect the heart. Finally, when we fill up on plant foods, we're likely to eat less of other things.

Good Stuff Comes in Plant Packages

• **Insoluble fiber.** Insoluble fiber, which cannot be digested by the body's digestive enzymes, is found in many fruits, vegetables, and whole grain breads and cereals. Wheat bran is an especially good source. In a study of more than 43,000 American male health professionals, those who reported eating an average of 29 grams of fiber (most of it insoluble) a day had about a 40 percent lower risk of heart attack than those who averaged 12 grams a day, which is more typical for Americans. Fiber from all grains was "most strongly associated with a reduced risk [of heart disease]," noted the researchers. A study of 22,000 Finnish men came up with similar findings: Eating more bran cereal, whole wheat bread, and other grains that are loaded with insoluble fiber was linked to a lower risk of heart attacks.

• **Soluble fiber.** "To reduce your risk of heart disease, you may want to eat more beans, peas, oats, and barley," says David Jenkins, a fiber expert at the University of Toronto. (The beans he refers to are not green beans, but include kidney, black, garbanzo, and pinto beans, lentils, split peas, and black-eyed peas.) The "sticky" water-soluble fiber in those foods cannot be digested by the body. This enables it to help lower blood cholesterol by binding to cholesterol and carrying it out of the body.

You can also get soluble fiber from vegetables like peas, corn, baked potatoes *with* the skin, prunes, oranges, artichokes, pears, and many other fruits and vegetables, as well as oats. Eating one or two of those foods occasionally or even daily won't make much of a dent in blood cholesterol, but a diet that's loaded with fruits, vegetables, and whole grains can make a big difference.

• **Antioxidants.** Some studies suggest that cholesterol in blood damages arteries only when it combines with oxygen. One reason antioxidants may be beneficial is that they may block that reaction. "Many fruits and vegetables are rich in antioxidants," notes Tim Byers, professor of preventive medicine at the University of Colorado Health Science Center in Denver. Those antioxidants

---

The Fat Culprits

Some of the biggest sources of nasty saturated or *trans* fats are:

☞ cheese, pizza, cheeseburgers, macaroni and cheese, nachos and cheese, cheese fries

☞ beef and pork, including hamburgers, sausages, hot dogs, bologna

☞ whole and 2 percent reduced-fat milk, cream, butter

☞ baked goods, such as doughnuts, cinnamon rolls, cakes, pies, cookies, croissants, icing

☞ regular and premium ice cream, chocolate candy, chocolate coating

☞ fried restaurant foods, including french fries, onion rings, fried chicken, and fried fish, which are usually fried in solid shortening

☞ movie-theater popcorn that is popped in coconut oil

include vitamin C, flavonoids, and carotenoids like lycopene and beta-carotene. Whereas vegetables and fruit are the best sources of antioxidants, whole grain breads and cereals also contain more than their refined counterparts.

• **Folate.** Folate (sometimes called folic acid) is best known for its ability to reduce the risk of spina bifida and similar birth defects, but it also may reduce the risk of heart disease. Folate, a B vitamin, lowers blood levels of a harmful amino acid called homocysteine. Fruits and vegetables—particularly orange juice, spinach, asparagus, and beans (other than green beans)—are among the richest sources of folate. You can also get a day's worth of folate from vitamin supplements and smaller amounts from breads, cereals, pasta, and other foods that are fortified with the vitamin.

Saturated and *Trans* Fat

Cutting back on saturated fat and *trans* fat should be a top priority if you want to cut your risk of heart disease.

Saturated fat raises blood cholesterol, especially the "bad" LDL cholesterol. (**LDL** stands for **low-density lipoproteins.**) The evidence that diets rich in saturated fat can cause heart disease is overwhelming. For instance:

• Blood-cholesterol levels rise when people are fed saturated fats. People with high levels of blood cholesterol are at high risk of heart attack.
• When monkeys (whose physiology is similar to that of people) are fed diets high in saturated fat, their arteries end up resembling those of people with heart disease.
• When patients are given drugs that lower blood cholesterol or are put on diets with low levels of saturated fat and cholesterol, their risk of heart disease drops dramatically.

Whereas saturated fat occurs naturally in meat and dairy products, most of the *trans* fat we eat is created when manufacturers use "partially hydrogenated" liquid oils. Hydrogenation is the process that makes liquid oils more solid, more stable, and less greasy tasting. Hydrogenated oils are used to make stick margarines and shortenings like Crisco and are found in thousands of processed foods.

Trans fat raises LDL ("bad") blood cholesterol about as much as saturated fat does, and it also might lower HDL ("good")

Fat Attack Dishes

☛ A **grilled cheese sandwich** from a typical sandwich shop has about 500 calories and 17 grams of saturated or *trans* fat (or three-quarters of a day's worth).

☛ An order of **stuffed potato skins**—a popular appetizer at dinner-house chains like Bennigan's and Planet Hollywood—has about 1,100 calories and 40 grams of saturated or *trans* fat, which is two days' worth.

☛ A serving of **fried mozzarella sticks**, another popular appetizer, has 800-some calories and 28 grams of saturated fat or *trans* fat.

☛ A large order of **french fries at Burger King** packs 500 calories and 13 grams of saturated or *trans* fat. (A king-size order has 600 calories and 16 grams of saturated or *trans* fat.)

☛ The **cheese fries** served with ranch dressing at many steak houses is another example of excessive restaurant fare. Its 91 grams of saturated or *trans* fat are bad enough. Add 3,000 calories, and you'll wonder why health departments don't require restaurants to have a defibrillator on hand.

Fat Attack Meals
●●

And those foods are all *individual* items. Figures for some typical *meals*, which would seem like modest choices, also are shocking. For example:

☞ A **mushroom cheeseburger** plus an order of **french fries**—a popular item on most dinner-house menus—supplies 1,500 calories and 40 grams of saturated fat or *trans* fat. That one meal would fill your quota of artery-clogging fat for two days.

☞ A trimmed 12-ounce **sirloin steak** (one of the leanest items on steak-house menus) plus a **Caesar salad** (a popular side dish offered at most steak houses) and a **baked potato with butter** provide 1,100 calories and 24 grams of saturated or *trans* fat. Other steak dinners are even worse.

☞ A **fried seafood platter** (which includes french fries, coleslaw, biscuits, and tartar sauce), a popular meal at places like Red Lobster, has about 2,200 calories and 39 grams of saturated or *trans* fat.

blood cholesterol. (**HDL** stands for **h**igh-**d**ensity **l**ipoprotein.) People with high levels of LDL have a higher risk of heart disease; people with high levels of HDL have a lower risk of heart disease. Thanks to *trans* fat, some baked goods and most fried versions of potatoes, fish, and chicken pose the same threat to your heart as beef, ice cream, and other foods rich in saturated fat.

The less saturated and *trans* fat you consume, the better. On average, Americans consume about 26 grams of saturated fat, plus 5 grams of *trans* fat, per day. Your goal ought to be no more than 20 grams per day of saturated and *trans* fat—less if you already have heart disease or high cholesterol levels. (Throughout this book, the "saturated fat" column in our charts includes *trans* fat when the number appears in italics. If the number is not in italics, we had no information on *trans* fat in the food.) Some of the foods lowest in saturated fat are listed in the charts on pages 22 and 31.

When you're in the supermarket, informative food labels can help you limit your saturated fat (though labels don't yet disclose *trans* fat). The problem with restaurant eating is that the menus don't offer nutrition information, so unsuspecting diners don't realize that many dishes have close to a whole day's worth of saturated and *trans* fat (see Restaurant Hall of Shame, page 23, and Foods Highest in Saturated Fat, page 33).

Not all fats are bad. The polyunsaturated and monounsaturated fats found largely in oils, salad dressing, and mayonnaise can help lower LDL ("bad") cholesterol, although they are calorie-dense foods that most Americans can afford only in modest quantities. More impressive are the omega-3 fats found largely in fish oils. They may help prevent heart attacks and strokes by preventing blood clots and abnormal heart rhythms. See chapter 10, Catch of the Day: Seafood Restaurants, page 189.

Foods Lowest in Saturated Fat and Calories

··

To keep your saturated fat at (or below) the 20-gram limit, look for salads (except taco salad), broiled or grilled chicken or fish, and Chinese dishes that aren't deep fried or meat laden. Several Taco Bell items made the list because they are too small to contain much meat or cheese.

Item	Calories	Saturated Fat (g)
Panda Express Mixed Vegetables with steamed rice	300	0
Subway's "7 subs with 6 grams of fat or less" (6-inch)*	260	1
Broiled, blackened, or grilled seafood*	270	1
Schlotzsky's Light & Flavorful Dijon Chicken Sandwich (small)	330	1
Schlotzsky's Light & Flavorful Pesto Chicken Sandwich (small)	350	1
Blimpie Vegi Max Sub (6-inch)	400	1
Au Bon Pain Thai Chicken Sandwich	420	1
Hot or cold cereal with reduced-fat 2% milk	210	2
Wendy's Grilled Chicken Sandwich	300	2
Blimpie Turkey Sub (6-inch)	330	2
Schlotzsky's Light & Flavorful Chicken Breast Sandwich (small)	360	2
Turkey sandwich with mustard	370	2
McDonald's Fruit 'n Yogurt Parfait with granola	380	2
Panda Express Chicken with Mushrooms with steamed rice	390	2
Blimpie Grilled Chicken Sub (6-inch)	400	2

Foods Lowest in Saturated Fat and Calories

·······························

(Continued)

Item	Calories	Saturated Fat (g)
Panda Express Chicken with String Beans with steamed rice	400	2
Au Bon Pain Honey Smoked Turkey Wrap	540	2
McDonald's McSalad Shakers with fat-free dressing*	140	3
Taco Bell Chicken Soft Taco	190	3
Barbecue or grilled chicken breast*	280	3
Taco Bell Chicken or Steak Gordita Nacho Cheese	290	3
KFC Tender Roast Sandwich	350	3
Blimpie Roast Beef Sub (6-inch)	390	3
Panda Express Beef & Broccoli with steamed rice	400	3
McDonald's Chicken McGrill Sandwich	450	3
Au Bon Pain Oriental Chicken Salad with lite dressing	500	3
Crispy or soft chicken taco*	220	4
Taco Bell Steak Soft Taco	280	4
Taco Bell Bean Burrito	370	4
Taco Bell Chicken or Steak Fiesta Burrito	380	4
Au Bon Pain Pesto Chicken Salad with lite dressing	460	4
Roast beef sandwich with mustard	460	4

*Numbers are an average of the items listed.
Note: Saturated fat numbers in *italics* include artery-clogging *trans* fat.

Foods Highest in Saturated Fat

••••••••••••••••••••••••••••••••••

Aim for no more than 20 grams of saturated fat in a day. Less is better. Any single food with more than 4 grams of saturated fat should sound an alarm. Meat and full-fat dairy products explain the high levels of saturated fat in these foods

Item	Saturated Fat (g)
Cheese fries with ranch dressing	*91*
Fried whole onion with dipping sauce	*57*
Prime rib, untrimmed	*52*
Fettuccine Alfredo	48
Stuffed potato skins with sour cream	*48*
Porterhouse steak, untrimmed	*40*
The Cheesecake Factory Original Cheesecake	*31*
Fried mozzarella sticks	*28*
Burger King Double Whopper with Cheese	*27*
Cheese nachos	25
Taco Bell Mucho Grande Nachos	25
Cheese quesadillas with sour cream, pico de gallo, and guacamole	24
Au Bon Pain Sweet Cheese Danish	*23*
Onion rings	*23*
Burger King Double Whopper	*22*
BBQ baby back ribs	*21*
Lasagna	21
Au Bon Pain Pecan Roll	*20*
Taco salad with sour cream and guacamole	20
Burger King Double Cheeseburger	*19*

Note: Saturated fat numbers in *italics* include artery-clogging *trans* fat.

Cholesterol

"If you're healthy, go right ahead and enjoy your eggs. Your cholesterol will probably stay about the same." That's what one advertising campaign by the American Egg Board claimed. Yet the industry's own studies show that eggs *do* raise blood cholesterol levels. "Saturated fat affects blood cholesterol levels more than dietary cholesterol does," claim the ads. That's true. But it does not mean that cholesterol in food is unimportant.

Eating two eggs—the serving size shown in the ads—every day would raise blood cholesterol by close to nine points, according to studies analyzed in a study funded by the egg industry. (A higher-quality study by Oxford University found an eleven-point rise.) In either case, researchers found roughly a 5-percent rise in cholesterol.

"Every 1-percent rise in blood cholesterol translates into a 2-percent rise in the risk of heart disease," says Jeremiah Stamler, a world-renowned expert on heart disease who is now professor emeritus at the Northwestern University School of Medicine in Chicago. "So adding two egg yolks to your daily diet means nearly an 11 percent rise in heart-disease risk. That's an important increase." Eating fewer eggs would pose a proportionally smaller problem. The culprit: cholesterol in the egg yolk. The egg whites (and egg-white omelettes) are harmless. One yolk has 215 milligrams of cholesterol—more than two-thirds the 300-milligram daily maximum recommended for everyone aged two or older by the American Heart Association, the National Heart, Lung and Blood Institute (NHLBI), and others. For people with high LDL ("bad") cholesterol, the heart association and NHLBI recommend no more than 200 milligrams of cholesterol a day.

Eggs aren't the only high-cholesterol food served in restaurants. One serving of lasagna, chicken chow mein, beef and cheese nachos (with sour cream and guacamole), or The Cheesecake Factory's Original Cheesecake has about as much cholesterol as one egg yolk. A porterhouse steak, kung pao

Foods Highest in Cholesterol
··

Limit yourself to 300 milligrams of cholesterol a day.

Item	Cholesterol (mg)
Egg salad sandwich without mayo	520
Moo shu pork with rice	465
Denny's Original Grand Slam (eggs, two pancakes, two strips of bacon, and two sausage links)	460
Scrambled eggs	440
Fettuccine Alfredo	420
House fried rice	345
General Tso's chicken with rice	340
Seafood casserole	320
Fried calamari	925
Denny's Breakfast Dagwood (ham, eggs, sausage, bacon, and three cheeses inside boule bread)	800
Denny's French Slam (French toast with margarine and syrup, two eggs, two strips of bacon, and two sausage links)	775
Denny's T-bone Steak & Eggs	655
Ham and cheese omelette	650
Denny's Moons Over My Hammy (ham and egg sandwich with cheese on sourdough bread)	580
Dunkin' Donuts Bacon and Cheddar Omwich on Biscuit	300
Orange (crispy) Beef with rice	295
McDonald's Steak, Eggs, & Cheese Bagel	290

chicken, chef salad, and moo shu pork have even more cholesterol, ranging from 260 to 465 milligrams.

What's more, studies in animals and in human populations
indicate that the cholesterol in foods may promote heart disease
by means *other* than raising blood cholesterol. When monkeys
and other animals are fed amounts of cholesterol that are too
small to cause high blood cholesterol, the animals still develop
harmful lesions in their arteries.

Finding Lower-Fat Meals

Some restaurant meals are reasonably low in saturated and
trans fat, and plenty of restaurant fare is nearly *trans*-free. The
trouble is finding it. Unless the chef invites you into the kitchen
to inspect the cooking oils, your best bet is to order meals and
snacks that are packed with fruits or vegetables *and* low in *all*
fats (see Restaurant Hall of Fame, page 22, and Best Snacks,
page 58). For example:

- At most delis, a **turkey sandwich with mustard** has only six
  grams of *any* fat—and only two of them are either *trans* or
  saturated.
- When dining at seafood (or other) restaurants, instead of fried
  fish and french fries, order **grilled fish** and a baked potato
  with a tablespoon of sour cream.
- At a steak house or dinner-house chain like Applebee's, try the
  barbecue or **grilled chicken breast** instead of steak. At
  McDonald's, order a Chicken McGrill sandwich instead of a
  burger.
- Try lower-fat Chinese dishes like **Szechuan shrimp** or **stir-
  fried vegetables** instead of deep-fried pork or beef dishes
  that have few vegetables. To save calories at a Chinese restaurant, you can ask the server to tell the kitchen to "Please fry it
  with very little oil." Fortunately, Chinese restaurants ordinar-
  ily use liquid oil, so you would not get much *trans* fat.

- At Mexican restaurants, order **chicken, shrimp,** or **vegetable fajitas** or **chicken tacos** or **burritos.** Avoid (or eat sparingly) the chips (ask for warm tortillas instead), cheese, and sour cream.
- Take off at least some of the breading and skin from **fried chicken,** since that's where most of the fat resides.
- At an Italian restaurant, **spaghetti with marinara sauce** and **linguine with red or white clam sauce** are better bets than dishes like lasagna, which has meat or cheese, or both.

Ten of the Best Restaurant Meals

••

You can find other healthful meals at restaurants if you know what to look for: more fruits and veggies, fewer fried foods, and less meat, cheese, and cream.

	Calories	Total Fat (g)	Saturated Fat (g)
Au Bon Pain Bagel with preserves and yogurt with berries	660	4	1
Wendy's Grilled Chicken Sandwich and salad with fat-free dressing	430	7	2
Subway "7 under 6" Sub and baked potato chips*	390	7	1
The Olive Garden Chicken Giardino and Minestrone Soup	560	9	3
Denny's Slim Slam (Egg Beaters, ham, and two hotcakes with fruit topping)	600	12	3
Turkey sandwich with mustard and garden salad with light dressing	460	13	3
Chinese stir-fried spinach, broccoli, or mixed veggies and steamed rice*	750	19	3
McDonald's Grilled Chicken Caesar McSalad Shaker with Fat Free Herb Vinaigrette and Fruit 'n Yogurt Parfait	520	8	4
Grilled chicken or seafood, baked potato with sour cream (1 Tb.), and vegetable*	640	14	5
Pasta with marinara or clam sauce and salad with light dressing*	940	24	5

*Numbers are an average of the items listed.

Note: Saturated fat numbers in *italics* include artery-clogging *trans* fat.

Ten of the Worst Restaurant Meals

•••••••••••••••••••••••••••••••••••••••

The best of the losers has more than 1,000 calories and 1½ days' worth of saturated fat.

	Calories	Total Fat (g)	Saturated Fat (g)
Prime rib, Caesar salad, and loaded baked potato	2,210	151	78
Fettuccine Alfredo, salad with dressing, and half an order of garlic bread	2,210	146	57
Burger King Double Whopper with Cheese, king fries, and king Coca-Cola Classic	2,050	95	43
Fried seafood combo with fries, coleslaw, and two biscuits	2,170	130	39
BBQ baby back ribs, french fries, and coleslaw	1,530	99	36
Starbucks White Chocolate Mocha (venti–20 oz.) and Cinnamon Scone	1,130	51	31
Lasagna, salad with dressing, and half an order of garlic bread	1,670	102	30
Denny's Meat Lovers Skillet and two slices of toast with margarine	1,420	105	28
KFC Extra Crispy Chicken (drumstick and two thighs), Potato Wedges, and Biscuit*	1,420	89	28
Beef Burrito, refried beans, rice, sour cream, and guacamole	1,640	79	28

*Includes trans fat from the biscuit only.

Note: Saturated fat numbers in *italics* include artery-clogging *trans* fat.

Avoiding High Blood Pressure

Don't have high blood pressure? There's more than a fifty-fifty chance that someday you will. By their sixties, one out of two Americans has blood pressure that's high enough to treat with drugs. Millions more have blood pressure that's high enough to increase their risk of a heart attack or stroke.

Over the past several decades, the death rate due to stroke has dropped by a whopping 60 percent. Drugs, less cigarette smoking, diet, exercise, and other factors contributed to that enormous improvement in health. But stroke remains the third leading cause of death, after heart disease and cancer. And high blood pressure is the biggest risk factor. "We're talking about a problem which, if you live long enough, only a minority of Americans escape," says Jeffrey Cutler, an epidemiologist at the National Heart, Lung and Blood Institute. "All families will be touched by it. If it's not me, it's my spouse."

High blood pressure, or hypertension, can kill people in several ways. The most common are:

• **Heart Disease.** High blood pressure speeds artery clogging. This makes it one of the Big Three risk factors for heart disease (along with high blood cholesterol and smoking).

• **Stroke.** High blood pressure increases the risk of stroke in two ways. "It accelerates artery clogging in the brain, and it causes blood vessels to burst," says Jeremiah Stamler of Northwestern University Medical School.

"Among the risk factors for stroke and heart disease, one of the most preventable is high blood pressure," says Paul Whelton, hypertension expert and senior vice president for Health Sciences at Tulane University in New Orleans. In addition, "treatment is effective in lowering the risk."

Most people never think about their blood pressure until the doctor says it's high. *"High"* blood pressure" means that the systolic (higher number) is at least 140, *or* the diastolic (lower number) is at least 90. Once you have hypertension, it needs to be managed by a physician for the rest of your life. And while drugs that lower blood pressure are lifesavers, they come with a cost— financial and otherwise. In men, sexual impotence is the most common side effect.

Even so-called *normal* blood pressure (120 to 129 systolic or 80 to 84 diastolic) or *high-normal* blood pressure (130 to 139 systolic or 85 to 89 diastolic) raises the risk of heart attack and stroke. Despite the name, people with normal or high-normal blood pressure need to lower it, or at least keep it from rising as they get older. And people with *optimal* blood pressure (less than 120 systolic *and* less than 80 diastolic) need to keep it that way. Here are some ways to lower the risk of high blood pressure:

1. Cut the salt. "In the U.S., the average person's systolic blood pressure rises by 15 points between the ages of 25 and 55," says heart disease expert Jeremiah Stamler. "If Americans' average salt intake were lower by about one teaspoon a day [we currently average one and a half teaspoons per day], the rise would be 6, not 15, points. That could mean a 16 percent drop in coronary heart disease deaths and 23 percent fewer stroke deaths at age 55."

Stamler is recommending a steep reduction, but even smaller reductions would be beneficial. However, cutting salt isn't easy. At least 75 percent of the sodium we consume comes not from the saltshaker, but from the salt in processed foods like canned soups, frozen dinners, frozen pizza, processed meat, cheese, and, of course, restaurant foods.

You should aim to consume no more than 2,400 milligrams of sodium, which is the equivalent of a little more than one teaspoon of salt, in a day. Less is better, of course, but it is nearly impossible to walk out of a restaurant without having consumed 1,000 to 3,000 milligrams of sodium (see Foods Highest in

Sodium, opposite). A single order of spaghetti with meatballs or lasagna typically tops 2,000 milligrams. A platter of chicken fajitas with rice, beans, sour cream, and guacamole often hits 3,660 milligrams of sodium.

Some of the lower-sodium dishes are listed in our Restaurant Hall of Fame (page 22), and Best Snacks (page 58), but even those are not low in sodium. You can get away with roughly 750 milligrams by ordering broiled fish (like flounder) accompanied by a baked potato (with a tablespoon of sour cream), a tossed salad (with one tablespoon of light dressing), and a dinner roll. Substituting a small portion of sirloin steak or filet mignon for the fish should yield comparable numbers.

2. Lose weight. If you're overweight, lose weight, even if it's only about 10 pounds. In a major study, people who lost an average of eight pounds by dieting and modest exercise cut their risk of high blood pressure in half.

3. Exercise. Walk briskly, jog, swim, cycle, or do other aerobic exercise for at least 30 minutes on most days. Exercise may lower blood pressure even if you don't lose weight.

4. Limit alcohol. Men should drink no more than two servings of beer, wine, or liquor a day. Women should limit themselves to one a day.

Foods Highest in Sodium

Most restaurant foods are high in sodium—making it difficult to limit your intake of sodium to 2,400 milligrams (or less). These foods are either Chinese dishes or dishes made with ham, corned beef, or other processed meats.

Item	Sodium (mg)
Cheese fries with ranch dressing	4,890
Schlotzsky's Large Original sandwich	4,400
Denny's Lumberjack Slam (two eggs, three hotcakes with margarine and syrup, ham, two strips of bacon, and two sausage links)	4,170
Fried whole onion with dipping sauce	3,840
House lo mein	3,460
Reuben sandwich	3,270
Beef with broccoli with rice	3,150
General Tso's chicken with rice	3,150
Orange (crispy) beef with rice	3,140
Overstuffed corned beef sandwich with mustard	3,130
Dunkin' Donuts Salt Bagel	3,030
Shrimp with garlic sauce with rice	2,950
Denny's Moons Over My Hammy (ham and egg sandwich with Swiss and American cheese on sourdough bread)	2,810
House fried rice	2,680
Kung pao chicken with rice	2,610
Moo shu pork with rice	2,590
Denny's Meat Lover's Skillet (ham, bacon, and sausage over fried potatoes with cheddar and two eggs)	2,510
Buffalo wings with blue cheese dressing and celery sticks	2,460
Spaghetti with sausage	2,440
Beef and cheese nachos with sour cream and guacamole	2,430

Until 1997, these four strategies were the only proven ways to prevent high blood pressure. Then a new study called Dietary Approaches to Stop Hypertension (DASH) showed that a diet rich in certain foods and lower in others could lower blood pressure significantly. In people who already had hypertension, blood pressure dropped as much as it would have on medication. The DASH diet was:

• **Low in fat, saturated fat, cholesterol, and refined sugars.** That meant a maximum of 6 ounces of skinless poultry, seafood, or very lean meat a day. To the dietitians who worked on DASH, that's two 3-ounce portions, but in restaurants—and probably most homes—a typical serving of meat, fish, or poultry is 6 ounces or *more*. Any dairy products in the DASH diet were low in fat, and sweets were kept to a minimum.

• **Rich in fruits, vegetables, and low-fat dairy products.** "Rich" meant eight to ten servings of fruits and vegetables (a serving is usually half a cup or one piece of fruit) and two or three servings of *low-fat* milk, yogurt, or cheese a day.

The DASH diet probably lowered blood pressure for a number of reasons. Low-fat dairy products helped, but it's not clear whether their calcium, potassium, or protein was responsible. Fruits and vegetables also helped, but it's not certain whether their phytochemicals, magnesium, fiber, or lower fat content made the difference. One thing is clear, though: You can keep your blood pressure from rising by eating a DASH-like diet.

And that's not all. A DASH diet has everything you need to cut your risk of other life-threatening illnesses: fruits and vegetables to cut your risk of cancer, calcium to lower your risk of osteoporosis, less saturated fat and cholesterol to cut your risk of heart disease, and a control on calories to help prevent obesity and diabetes. "It's not a diet for one disease," says DASH investigator Lawrence J. Appel of The Johns Hopkins University in Baltimore. "It's a diet for *all* diseases."

The DASH Diet

Participants in the DASH study found the diet easy to follow. Granted, when it came to the food, all they had to do was eat, since the researchers did all the planning, shopping, and cooking. Still, the foods weren't unusual—you could buy everything at a local supermarket.

Here's *how many* servings of *which* kinds of foods were in the DASH study's 2,000-calorie-a-day "Combination Diet." You can ensure that it is low in sodium by choosing lower-salt versions of breads, cereals, nuts, salad dressings, vegetable juices, and other foods.

DASH DIET—SERVING SIZES

Food and Servings	Examples of 1 Serving
Grains and grain products* 7 to 8 a day	1 slice bread ½ cup dry cereal ⅓ cup cooked rice, pasta, or cereal
Vegetables 4 to 5 a day	1 cup raw leafy vegetables ¼ cup raw nonleafy vegetables ⅓ cup cooked vegetables ½ cup vegetable juice
Fruits 4 to 5 a day	¾ cup fruit juice 1 medium fruit ½ cup fresh, frozen, or canned fruit ¼ cup dried fruit
Low-fat or nonfat dairy foods 2 to 3 a day	1 cup fat-free or 1% low-fat milk 1 cup low-fat yogurt 1½ oz. nonfat cheese
Meats, poultry, and fish 2 or less a day	3 oz. broiled or roasted lean meat, skinless poultry, or seafood
Nuts, seeds, and beans 4 to 5 a week	½ cup cooked beans ⅓ cup nuts 2 Tb. sunflower seeds
Fats, oils, and salad dressings 2 to 3 a day	1 tsp. oil or soft margarine 1 tsp. regular mayonnaise 1 Tb. low-fat mayonnaise 1 Tb. regular salad dressing 2 Tb. light salad dressing
Snacks and Sweets 5 a week	1 medium fruit 1 cup low-fat yogurt ½ cup low-fat ice cream or frozen yogurt ¾ cup pretzels 1 Tb. maple syrup, sugar, jelly, or jam ½ cup Jell-O 3 pieces hard candy 15 jelly beans

*The DASH diet doesn't distinguish between whole grains and refined grains, but results from other studies have indicated that whole grains are healthier.

DASH DIET—SAMPLE MENU	Amount	Amount of Sodium (mg)
Breakfast		
Cereals, shredded wheat	½ cup	2
Skim milk	1 cup	126
Orange juice	1 cup	5
Banana, raw	1 medium	1
Bread, 100% whole wheat	1 slice	149
Lunch		
Chicken salad	¾ cup	151
Whole wheat bread	2 slices	298
Dijon mustard	1 tsp.	125
Tomatoes, raw, fresh	2 large slices	6
Mixed cooked vegetables	1 cup	25
Fruit cocktail, juice pack	½ cup	5
Dinner		
Spicy baked cod	3 ounces	93
Beans, snap, green, cooked from frozen, without salt	1 cup	11
Potato, baked, with skin, without salt	1 large	15
Sour cream, low-fat	2 Tb.	30
Chives (or scallions)	1 Tb.	0
Fat-free natural cheddar cheese, shredded	3 Tb.	169
Tossed salad with mixed greens	1½ cups	25
Olive oil and vinegar dressing	2 Tb.	0
Snack		
Orange juice	½ cup	3
Almonds, dried, blanched, without salt	⅛ cup	3
Raisins, seedless	¼ cup	5
Yogurt, blended, fat-free with sugar	1 cup	103

The sample menu provides 2,010 calories, 5 servings of fruit, 7 servings of vegetables, 3 servings of dairy foods, 59 grams of fat, 13 grams of saturated fat, 121 milligrams of cholesterol, and 1,356 milligrams of sodium.

Source: National Heart, Lung and Blood Institute

Reducing Your Risk of Cancer

Even though you're more likely to die of heart disease, you're probably more afraid of cancer. And with good reason:

- With a heart attack, you may go quickly and painlessly. With cancer, you won't.
- Death rates from heart disease are half what they were in 1965. In contrast, death rates from cancer have declined only modestly in recent years, largely because of less smoking and better screening for colon cancer.
- You usually can determine your risk of heart disease by checking your cholesterol level, blood pressure, and whether you smoke. Cancer is tougher to predict and tougher to prevent.

At times, cancer seems indiscriminate, inexplicable, and unstoppable. Yet evidence suggests that you *can* eat your way to a lower risk.

We Can't Say It Often Enough: Eat More Fruits and Vegetables!

Experts estimate that 30 to 40 percent of cancers could be prevented by healthier diets and more exercise. Eating more fruits and vegetables alone could eliminate 20 percent of cancers, according to a major report published in 1997 by the World Cancer Research Fund (WCRF) and the American Institute for Cancer Research (AICR) titled *Food, Nutrition and the Prevention of Cancer: A Global Perspective.*

"It has become absolutely clear that a diet high in vegetables and/or fruit—that is, a diet high in plant foods—is associated with a lower risk of cancers at almost all sites," says John Potter, head of Cancer Prevention and Research at the Fred Hutchinson Cancer Research Center in Seattle, Washington. Potter chaired the panel that wrote the WCRF's 1997 report. "That's definitely not something that was terribly clear to us before the 1980s and 1990s," he points out.

The evidence is strongest that fruits and vegetables can cut the risk of cancers of the mouth, throat, esophagus, lung, stomach, colon, and rectum. Fewer studies have found a link with cancers of the breast and prostate.

It is not clear which components of fruits and vegetables are responsible for their ability to cut cancer risk. Is it the lycopene in tomatoes, the alpha-carotene in sweet potatoes, the isoflavones in soy, the sulforaphane in broccoli, the isothiocyanates in cauliflower, or any or all of dozens of other chemicals in plants that make them cancer fighters? Researchers don't know. But "even when we do understand, the simplest recommendation is still going to be to eat plenty of vegetables and fruit," sums up John Potter.

Why do plants have phytochemicals? "They're largely toxins that the plant uses to fight off predators—mostly insects," he explains. "When animals—and humans—eat the plants, the phytochemicals turn on enzymes that may allow us to detoxify other nasty things, including carcinogens."

The National Cancer Institute recommends eating five to nine servings of fruits and vegetables a day. (That's similar to the eight to ten servings in the blood-pressure-lowering DASH diet.) Unfortunately, it is tough to find fruits and vegetables at most restaurants. Chinese and other Asian restaurants and a few other ethnic cuisines offer a variety of vegetable-rich dishes (although they're often full of salt and calorie-dense oil). At most other restaurants, the vegetable will be iceberg lettuce, a slice of pallid tomato, a squeeze of ketchup, a baked potato, and a small side dish of overcooked green beans or carrots. And that's a shame, for as John Potter points out, "Eating vegetables and fruit that are well prepared and well presented is one of life's joys."

It's no coincidence that ethnic restaurants know how to make vegetable dishes taste good. "There's a wealth of experience around the world because almost all traditional diets are plant-based," says Walter Willett, chair of the Nutrition

Department of the Harvard School of Public Health. Yet many Italian, Mexican, and other ethnic restaurants have become so Americanized that the vegetables have been replaced by meat and cheese.

"In Asian and Mediterranean cuisines, cooking fruits and vegetables is an art form," says NYU's Marion Nestle. Perhaps that's why vegetable dishes persist in many of these restaurants.

Cutting Back on Meat and Fat

Meat consumption increases the risk of cancer, according to a growing body of research. "If eaten at all, limit intake of red meat to less than three ounces daily," advises the World Cancer Research Fund's 1997 report on diet and cancer.

The evidence that meat is linked to cancer is strongest for colon cancer. "Men who eat red meat as a main dish five or more times a week have four times the risk of colon cancer of men who eat red meat less than once a month," says Edward Giovannucci of Harvard Medical School. The results are similar for women.

Men who eat red meat frequently also have a higher risk of prostate cancer, which accounts for about a third of all cancers in American men. Of the 200,000 afflicted each year, 31,500 will die.

It is too early to tell whether it is the fat, the saturated fat, or something else in meat that promotes cancer. For this reason, the American Cancer Society advises people to reduce their intake of both meat and fat.

Down on the Farm

Increasing public concern about animal welfare has placed restaurant chains squarely in the bull's-eye of controversy. Most chickens and hogs are now being raised in concentrated "factory" farms, and cattle spend their last months in feedlots. These operations squeeze huge numbers of animals into small spaces. That generates awful odors, causes behavioral problems in the animals, facilitates the spread of diseases, and produces enormous volumes of manure, which may pollute local waterways. To help compensate for the effects of these inhumane conditions, farmers often feed antibiotics to healthy animals to increase growth rates and prevent diseases.

Advocates of humane treatment have persuaded McDonald's and several other fast-food chains to require the poultry farms that supply their restaurants to improve their practices. McDonald's, for instance, is requiring egg producers to provide 50 percent more space per hen, to stop withholding food and water to increase egg production, and to gradually phase out the practice of "debeaking," which can increase the level of *Salmonella* bacteria in the chickens. Another chain, T.G.I. Fridays, buys beef only from cattle that were not fed antibiotics. The American Medical Association, World Health Organization, and others have urged governments to ban the feeding of antibiotics to healthy animals because that practice increases the chances that humans will be infected with bacteria that are resistant to antibiotics.

Whole Grains: Not a Big Cancer Factor

The phytochemicals in whole grain breads and cereals may also help cut the risk of cancer, but the evidence for that is weaker than it is for fruits and vegetables. Also, whereas some studies had suggested that the fiber in whole grains offered protection from colon cancer, more recent and better studies have not supported that connection. However, fiber still appears to lower the risk of diabetes and heart disease, so bran cereals and whole wheat bread remain important to good health.

Fending off Diabetes

"America underestimates diabetes," Steve Smith of the American Diabetes Association recently told Congress. "It kills more Americans, afflicts more Americans, and costs more money than AIDS and breast cancer combined."

The statistics are shocking. Sixteen million Americans have diabetes, although a third of them don't know it. An additional 800,000 or more people are diagnosed with the disease each year. Diabetes is the seventh-leading cause of death in America. And because diabetes raises the risk of heart disease and stroke, most people with diabetes die of these illnesses. You could also end up blind, losing one or both feet, or on a dialysis machine. Even more troubling: What had been called adult-onset diabetes has become increasingly common in teenagers. Obscured by all that bad news is one crystal-clear fact: "At least 75 percent of the new cases of adult-onset diabetes can probably be prevented," says JoAnn Manson of Harvard Medical School and Brigham and Women's Hospital in Boston.

What Goes Wrong

Close to 95 percent of diabetics have non-insulin-dependent diabetes mellitus (NIDDM), which is also called type 2, or "adult-onset," diabetes. (The other form, insulin-dependent diabetes, strikes mostly young children and teens. It is really a different disease. When we say "diabetes" here, we are referring to type 2.)

Blood sugar, or blood glucose, is produced as we digest food. People with diabetes have trouble moving the sugar from their blood into the body's cells. During and after a meal, the pancreas secretes more insulin—the hormone that enables glucose to pass into the cells, where it is stored or used to produce energy. But sometimes a person's insulin loses its effectiveness, making it difficult to clear enough glucose out of the bloodstream. Some researchers think that obesity makes cells—or the insulin receptors on cells—resistant to the hormone. However, that may not be the full explanation, since many overweight people are not insulin-resistant yet many normal-weight people are. "We don't know exactly why this insulin resistance happens," says Norman Kaplan of the University of Texas Southwestern Medical Center in Dallas. "But it occurs more frequently in people who are overweight or physically inactive."

When high blood-sugar levels rise further, the pancreas "thinks" that more insulin can solve the problem and it reacts by churning out more. And, at least at first, that extra insulin forces blood-sugar levels back down to normal. But there's a cost. "If you have insulin resistance and are secreting lots of insulin to maintain your glucose levels near normal, you have a particularly dangerous form of LDL ("bad") cholesterol, as well as low HDL ("good") cholesterol, high triglycerides, and higher blood pressure," says Gerald Reaven, an endocrinologist who first identified the problem when at the Stanford University School of Medicine. "In other words, you have a whole cluster of abnormalities that increase your risk of coronary heart disease."

In some people, the pancreas may eventually lose the battle to supply enough insulin. If that happens, your blood glucose level *stays high* and you have diabetes.

"Unfortunately, by the time most people with diabetes are diagnosed, the disease has often progressed, and irreparable damage may have been done," says Harvard's JoAnn Manson. Diabetes increases the risk of heart disease, stroke, kidney failure, blindness, and nerve damage, which can lead to amputation.

Clearly, diabetes is a disease that you should be working to prevent. And for the vast majority of people, simple measures can be taken. The first two steps in keeping diabetes at bay are to exercise regularly and to lose weight or, better yet, to avoid weight gain in the first place.

Calorie Overload

"From 50 to 75 percent of the new cases of diabetes seem to be triggered by people weighing too much," according to JoAnn Manson. In a dozen studies that monitored tens of thousands of people for years, "being overweight increased the risk of developing diabetes in men and women more than tenfold."

Unfortunately, anyone trying to avoid weight gain and diabetes will find little help from restaurant menus. Restaurants serve large portions of tasty calorie-rich foods. That's a recipe for flab . . . and for diabetes.

"Americans are exposed to a toxic food environment," says Kelly Brownell, professor of psychology, epidemiology, and public health at Yale University. "Americans have unprecedented access to a poor diet—to high-calorie foods that are widely available, low in cost, heavily promoted, and good tasting." And much of that food is served in restaurants. (See Foods Highest in Calories, page 56, and Worst Snacks, page 59.)

"One of the first things people from other countries notice when they visit the United States is the large portions served in restaurants," says Brownell. "In most of the world, there's no such thing as a doggie bag."

In the United States, that doggie bag is one of the best strategies for dealing with the out-of-control serving sizes in restaurants. "Before you put the first fork in, think about how much you're going to eat and have them wrap up the rest for the next day," suggests Marion Nestle of New York University. It can pay off. Studies show that even modest weight loss can prevent diabetes. "Women and men cut their risk of developing diabetes by 30 percent over a two-year period just by losing ten pounds and keeping it off," says Rena Wing of the University of Pittsburgh.

There's no doubt that exercise and staying lean will both help cut the risk of diabetes. Exercise helps whether or not you are overweight, and staying lean helps whether or not you exercise. Either way, you come out ahead. The dishes listed in Foods Lowest in Saturated Fat and Calories (page 31) and Best Snacks (page 58) can help you.

Foods Highest in Calories

···

The average person needs only about 2,000 to 2,500 calories a day. Eating out makes it extremely easy to exceed that level. Some of the numbers in the table *under*estimate the calories because they don't include side dishes, appetizers, desserts, and drinks.

Item	Calories
Cheese fries with ranch dressing	3,010
Fried whole onion with dipping sauce	2,130
Orange (crispy) beef	1,770
Movie theater popcorn with "butter" (large)	1,640
Kung pao chicken	1,620
Sweet and sour pork	1,610
General Tso's chicken	1,600
The Cheesecake Factory Carrot Cake (1 slice)	1,560
Fettuccine Alfredo	1,500
House fried rice	1,480
Taco Bell Mucho Grande Nachos	1,320
Prime rib, untrimmed	1,280
Stuffed potato skins with sour cream	1,260
Spaghetti with meatballs	1,160
Fudge brownie sundae	1,130
Porterhouse steak, untrimmed	1,100
Fried calamari	1,040
Spaghetti with sausage	1,040
Burger King Double Whopper with Cheese	1,020
Buffalo wings with blue cheese dressing and celery sticks	1,010
McDonald's Vanilla Shake (large)	1,010

The Wrong—and Right—Calories

What you eat, not just how much you eat, may affect your risk of diabetes. A recent study found that women who ate larger quantities of refined, low-fiber carbohydrates like white bread and sugar had a higher risk of diabetes. Of course, those are precisely the kinds of carbohydrates that diners find in abundance on restaurant menus, where the vast majority of breads, pasta, and rice is refined. Restaurant desserts are laden with sugar or refined flour or both, and the most common beverages are, of course, sugar-laden soft drinks.

"Diets high in high-fiber foods like fruits, vegetables, and whole grains are associated with a lower risk of diabetes," says JoAnn Manson of Harvard University. Unfortunately, you really have to hunt through a restaurant menu to find meals that fit that description. "Healthy" or "light" menus are a good place to start. What's more, these menus are also lower in saturated fat and cholesterol.

People with diabetes should be especially careful to cut back on hamburgers, cheeseburgers, lasagna, pizza, beef tacos and cheese nachos, and other fatty cheese or meat dishes, as well as ice cream, cakes, cookies, pies, and other fatty sweets. This is critical, because the most common cause of death among diabetics is heart disease.

Best Snacks

································

These snacks don't load you down with calories and saturated fat. We list brand names, but sorbet is sorbet and fruit is fruit, no matter where you buy them.

	Calories	Total Fat (g)	Saturated Fat (g)
1. Au Bon Pain fresh fruit cup	90	1	0
2. Häagen-Dazs Sorbet (1 scoop)	120	0	0
3. Auntie Anne's Original Pretzel, no butter	340	1	0
4. Starbucks Cappuccino with skim milk or Caffè Latte (grande—16 oz.) *	140	1	1
5. Dunkin' Donuts Bagel with preserves	400	3	1
6. Au Bon Pain Low Fat Chocolate Cake or Low Fat Triple Berry Muffin *	280	4	1
7. McDonald's Garden McSalad Shaker with Fat Free Herb Vinaigrette Dressing	140	6	3

* Numbers are an average of the items listed.

Worst Snacks

■■■■■■■■■■■■■■■■■■■■■■■■■■■■■■■■

A snack is supposed to tide you over until lunch or dinner. Snacks like a 670-calorie pastry or a 1,000-calorie shake have enough calories to *be* dinner.

	Calories	Total Fat (g)	Saturated Fat (g)
1. Sbarro Sausage & Pepperoni Stuffed Pizza (1 slice)	880	44	*19*
2. McDonald's shake (large)	1,010	29	19
3. Au Bon Pain Almond Croissant	630	42	*18*
4. Burger King french fries (King size)	600	30	*16*
5. Starbucks White Chocolate Mocha with whole milk (venti—20 oz.)	600	25	15
6. Cinnabon	670	34	*14*
7. Dunkin' Donuts Bagel with cream cheese	540	22	*14*

Putting It All Together

A diet that is rich in fruits, vegetables, whole grains, and beans—
and low in meat, cheese, fried foods, egg yolks, and soft drinks—
can cut the risk of heart disease, stroke, obesity, diabetes, and
cancer. This book will guide you to the restaurant meals that can
protect your health without disappointing your taste buds. We've
highlighted some of your better choices with a Best Bite symbol
(✔). Those items tend to be lower in calories, fat, and especially
saturated fat.

The Lowdown on Nutrition Claims

What does it mean when a restaurant labels a dish "low-fat"?
Prior to May 1997, restaurants peppered their menus with terms
such as "light" and "heart-healthy" with impunity. Back then it
wasn't uncommon to find cases like the Washington, D.C., restaurant that labeled a brown rice terrine a "healthy choice" even
though it contained 48 grams (nine teaspoons) of fat—almost
two-thirds of a person's daily quota. But as a result of a lawsuit
filed by the Center for Science in the Public Interest (CSPI) and
Public Citizen, two nonprofit consumer-advocacy groups, restaurants must now adhere to the Food and Drug Administration's
(FDA) standards when making health and nutrition claims on
menus. These are the same guidelines that have applied to packaged foods since 1994, and they apply to every eating establish-
ment in the country, from mega-chains like Denny's to the tiny
hole-in-the-wall café in your neighborhood.

The Healthy Menu Lexicon

These claims commonly appear on menus:

Low-fat. Most foods may be labeled "low-fat" if a *standard* serving contains no more than 3 grams of fat. Main dishes can contain no more than 3 grams of fat per 3½ ounces of food. However, a restaurant's serving size often is three to four times the FDA's "standard" portion. For example, a restaurant may call its ice cream "low-fat" if it contains 3 grams of fat per *½-cup* serving (the FDA standard portion), but if it actually dishes out a *2-cup* serving, you'll get 12 grams of fat.

Fat-free. Items designated as fat-free must contain less than 0.5 grams of fat in a standard serving, so even large portions provide only small amounts of fat. They may still be high in calories.

Light. "Light" (or "lite") can mean many different things on the menu, but its meaning should be clearly conveyed. If "light" is used to signify fewer calories, fat, or sodium, the restaurant must provide information about those nutrients upon request. However, "light" can also refer to taste or texture, as in "light, fluffy waffles."

Healthy. A dish can be called "healthy" as long as it is low in fat and saturated fat and not high in cholesterol and sodium. However, there are no limits on the amounts of refined sugars or calories a "healthy" food may contain.

"Heart" claims. Claims like "heart-healthy" and "heart-smart" and heart symbols on menus imply that the food does not promote heart disease. Such foods must be low in fat, saturated fat, and cholesterol, and must not be high in sodium. Once again, there is no limit on sugar or calories.

Although restaurants are required to provide nutrition information upon request for any items for which they make health claims, they are not required to send samples to a lab for testing.

Data may be calculated using nutrient databases or recipes, neither of which may be as accurate as lab analyses.

Keep in mind that many restaurant owners may not be aware of the FDA's regulations. They may call their deep-fried chicken a "healthy choice" because it's prepared in "cholesterol-free vegetable oil." (All vegetable oil is cholesterol free. What's more, many restaurants say they use vegetable oil, when, in fact, they're using a solid, cholesterol-raising vegetable shortening.) Or perhaps a new chef at your local outlet of a big chain adds an extra handful of grated cheese to the company-prescribed and carefully analyzed recipe for a "light" entrée. Situations such as those are inevitable because the FDA and state and local health departments rarely police restaurant menus.

When CSPI sent "healthy" selections from several chain restaurants to a lab for analysis a few years ago, we found that the dishes were often higher in fat and calories than the restaurants claimed. However, they *were* usually still better than items from the regular menu. The bottom line: Order from the "healthy" or "light" menu, but be sure to ask questions if you're skeptical of the claims, and never take the nutrition numbers as gospel.

Safe and Healthy

Each year Americans eat nearly 50 billion meals in restaurants and school and work cafeterias. The overwhelming majority of those meals are perfectly safe. That fact, however, is small comfort to the thousands, or even millions, of diners who become sick from contaminated restaurant food each year. In fact, the most notorius food-poisoning episode in recent years occurred at fast-food restaurants in 1992. Ground beef used by Jack in the Box restaurants on the West Coast was contaminated with *Escherichia coli* O157:H7 bacteria and caused four children's deaths and hundreds of illnesses. That tragedy galvanized efforts—led by parents of the victims—to clean up the meat and poultry industries.

According to the federal Centers for Disease Control and Prevention (CDC), about 76 million food-related illnesses occur each year, 5,000 of them fatal and more than 300,000 of them requiring hospitalization. About half of all food-borne outbreaks (two or more illnesses linked to a single food source) have been traced to restaurants, delicatessens, and cafeterias.

Most food-borne illnesses are preventable. Restaurants can protect their patrons by taking such simple steps as thorough cooking, adequate refrigeration, and careful handling of raw and cooked foods. The Food and Drug Administration (FDA) spells out all these steps in detailed guidelines for restaurants. Unfortunately, the FDA does not have the legal authority to impose its standards nationwide. And even when state and local health agencies do adopt the federal standards, they frequently don't have the staff to enforce them.

A 1996 survey by the Center for Science in the Public Interest of 45 state and local health departments found that less than half of those agencies inspected restaurants twice a year, as recommended by the FDA. Also, only 16 percent of the agencies enforced the FDA's recommended cooking temperatures for pork, eggs, fish, and poultry. To its credit, the National Restaurant Association has been encouraging food-safety awareness within the industry. But although numerous restaurants seek to ensure safe meals, diners still have to be vigilant. These foods pose the biggest risks:

Chicken: *Campylobacter,* which infects as many as nine in ten chickens, is the most frequent cause of food poisoning. *Salmonella* contaminates roughly one in ten chickens. Both bacteria are readily killed if the bird is cooked properly. However, cross-contamination can spread germs from uncooked poultry to other foods via cutting boards and other work surfaces, cooking utensils, and employees' hands.

Eggs: *Salmonella* infects roughly one in 20,000 eggs and causes hundreds of thousands of illnesses each year. One in 20,000 may sound like long odds, but restaurants often pool dozens of eggs together in making dishes, thereby increasing the likelihood of contamination. Meringues and dishes like the Italian dessert tiramisu, eggs sunny-side up, and dressings that use raw egg are all suspect. When you are served (or prepare) fried eggs, make sure the whites are firm and the yolks have started to thicken. Dishes with cooked eggs are safe.

Beef: Undercooked ground beef is the most frequent source of *E. coli* O157:H7. That bug causes life-threatening illnesses in several hundred Americans annually. Heat kills *E. coli*, but simply cooking ground beef until it *appears* to be done (browned throughout) is not good enough. The safest, most reliable way to ensure that hamburgers are thoroughly cooked is to test them with a meat thermometer. Burgers are fully cooked and ready to eat when they have reached 160 degrees Fahrenheit. You can bet that few restaurants are taking temperatures. Obviously, you should avoid raw or undercooked ground beef, including rare or medium-rare hamburgers and steak tartare. Muscle meats like steak or prime rib cooked rare are much safer than ground beef, since any germs that might be present on the surface of the meat are killed during cooking. However, if a steak has been mechanically tenderized (pierced with needles to make it tender), a practice used by many steak chains, order it "medium" to be on the safe side.

Produce: Foodborne illnesses have been traced to lettuce, alfalfa sprouts, and unpasteurized apple juice, perhaps as a result of contamination through contact with animal waste. At home or at restaurants, all produce should be thoroughly washed under running water.

Shellfish: Raw shellfish cause the majority of seafood-related illnesses. In fact, about 60 percent of seafood-poisoning cases would be eliminated if clams, oysters, and mussels were thoroughly cooked. Raw sewage may contaminate shellfish with the Norwalk virus, which sickens about 100,000 people a year. Shellfish from the warm waters of the Gulf of Mexico are frequently contaminated with *Vibrio vulnificus*, a bacterium that kills up to 25 people each year. Don't eat Gulf Coast shellfish unless they are processed to eliminate harmful bacteria.

Fish: Ciguatera is a natural poison that sometimes occurs in barracuda, grouper, and red snapper in Florida, Hawaii, Puerto Rico, and the Virgin Islands. The most common cause of poisoning from eating fish is scombroid poisoning. It occurs when fresh tuna, mackerel, and mahimahi have been improperly refrigerated.

Illnesses picked up in restaurants may result from any food that has not been properly stored. *Clostridium perfringens* bacteria grow in cooked foods—especially meat dishes—that are not kept hot or cold enough. Symptoms may include nausea, vomiting, cramps, and diarrhea, all of which are classic indicators of food poisoning.

Food handlers and other restaurant employees can pass to customers viruses and bacteria such as Hepatitis A, *Shigella*, and *Staphylococcus aureus*. These germs are typically spread by infected workers who have not washed their hands thoroughly with hot soapy water before handling food.

Take-out food must be handled carefully too. The restaurant may prepare your order under the most sanitary conditions, but if you leave that carton of beef lo mein in your car for three hours while you run errands, you're asking for trouble. Hot foods should be eaten within two hours or refrigerated promptly. Food that has been stored in the refrigerator should be reheated to 165 degrees Fahrenheit or until hot and steaming. Cold foods should be held at 40 degrees Fahrenheit or colder.

Food poisoning usually stikes anywhere from two hours to two days after someone has eaten a contaminated food. However, some fish toxins work more swiftly, whereas some viruses may take over a month to cause problems. Those most vulnerable to food poisoning are young children, the elderly, pregnant women, people with compromised immune systems, and heavy users of prescription antacids (stomach acid helps to destroy bacteria). But anyone who experiences any of the following symptoms should call their doctor:

- Bloody diarrhea or pus in the stool, a symptom of an infection by *E. coli* O157:H7.
- Headache, stiff neck, and fever (together), which may be a sign of *Listeria monocytogenes* infection.
- A fever that lasts more than 24 hours.
- Faintness, rapid heart rate, or dizziness after sitting or suddenly standing up, when accompanied by nausea, vomiting, or diarrhea. Those are signs of dehydration, which could lead to kidney failure.
- Diarrhea that fails to subside after three days, which could lead to life-threatening dehydration.
- General weakness, numbness, or tingling, which could be a sign of botulism or seafood poisoning.

Always report food poisoning to your local health department. It is critical that you assist health officials so they can identify restaurants that need to be investigated and cleaned up. And remember, even chefs at the swankiest white-tablecloth restaurants can be careless. In addition to suspect foods, here are some other things to keep an eye out for:

- Hot food should be kept hot, cold food cold.
- Be suspicious of steam-table warming pans piled so high that the food cannot be kept hot all the way through or cold buffets in which bowls of food are resting in melted ice.
- Dish or silverware dirty? Ask for replacements.
- The restaurant should look clean. If you see insects or signs of rodents, tell the manager or your server and leave and call the health department!

Chapter 3

Rise and Dine: Breakfast

Back in the days when most Americans lived on farms, hearty breakfasts were a necessity. An abundant, nourishing morning meal supplied the energy required for a long day of physical labor. Today most of us no longer need such mammoth quantities of food, and we have less time to spend eating it. More often than not, breakfast has become a meal that we grab on the run and expect to fuel us until lunchtime at school or work.

Once the workweek winds down, breakfast becomes more relaxed and social. On weekends, many people take advantage of leisure time to indulge in a relaxing morning meal at home or in a restaurant. Although breakfast is the meal least frequently eaten outside the home, enjoying Sunday breakfast out is a tradition in many families.

And breakfast is no longer exclusively a morning meal. You can now eat that comforting American breakfast almost anytime. Every year Denny's sells 30 million Original Grand Slam breakfasts—two hotcakes, two eggs, two strips of bacon, and two sausage links—throughout the day. So it's not surprising that competing chains have risen to the challenge of creating their own not-just-for-breakfast versions. These days it's all too easy to find gargantuan high-fat, high-salt, high-cholesterol breakfasts available anytime, anywhere.

But we eat restaurant breakfasts at our own risk. The reality is that a typical breakfast—fatty, salty meat, eggs, cheese, butter, and margarine—is hard on the heart. And with chains like Denny's and IHOP (International House of Pancakes) featuring countless such meals, many consumers are indulging in hefty platters filled with the very foods they should be paring from their diets.

We tested popular breakfasts served at some of the country's largest family-style restaurant chains—Bakers Square, Big Boy, Bob Evans, Carrows, Cracker Barrel, Denny's, IHOP, Perkins, Shoney's, Village Inn, and Waffle House. Generally speaking, the breakfasts they serve are those traditional combinations of fatty meat, eggs, cheese, and margarine or butter. Cholesterol-laden eggs are not only served scrambled, fried, or as omelettes; they're also ingredients in the waffle, pancake, and French toast batters. You'll get a dose of saturated fat in the bacon and sausage, in the cheese melted in the omelettes, in the margarine or butter that's automatically slathered on everything, and in the shortening in which most of the foods are fried. Any one of those foods is bad news for your blood vessels—combine several on the same plate and you're headed for trouble.

The good news is that you *can* get a healthy breakfast at virtually every restaurant we visited. Most offer a variety of cereals, juice, fresh fruit, and unbuttered toast or English muffins. If cold cereal from a box sounds uninspiring, have a bowl of hot oatmeal with a little syrup and some banana slices. That makes for a filling, nutritious breakfast. Here are some other ways to start the day right.

The Dishes and the Data

We bought take-out portions of 12 popular main-dish breakfasts and breakfast side dishes at 17 midpriced family-style restaurants in Chicago, Denver, Los Angeles, and Washington, D.C. (For more on our methodology, see pages 12–14.)

Here are some of the most popular breakfast platters, with their main components, ranked from best to worst—that is, from least to most saturated fat.

Entrées and Platters

HOT OR COLD CEREAL
(210 calories and 5 grams of fat, 2 of them saturated)

This is the best breakfast you can get.

Typical Platter: Many restaurants offer a platter similar to Denny's Oatmeal N' Fixins, which consists of 2-percent reduced-fat milk, cereal, a cup of juice, a serving of fruit, and toast, a bagel, or an English muffin. If you get it with plain toast (ideally whole wheat), a bagel, or English muffin, and use preserves instead of butter or margarine, you could eat five of these breakfasts and still get less fat and saturated fat than you would from one ham and cheese omelette.

The Bottom Line: *You can't do better than this. But you could make sure that your cereal is low in sugar and made from whole grains (a cold one like Wheaties or shredded wheat, or a hot one like oatmeal) and your milk is 1-percent low-fat or fat-free (skim).*

SCRAMBLED EGGS
(290 calories and 13 grams of fat, 5 of them saturated)

Although two scrambled eggs contain only 13 grams of fat, 5 of them saturated, they'll cost you a day and half's cholesterol (440 milligrams). However, few people order just eggs; especially when, for a dollar or two more, you can add toast, hash browns, and bacon, sausage, or ham. But order an egg substitute, hash browns, and plain toast with preserves, and you've got a pretty decent breakfast—if you are served what you order. Judging by the cholesterol in the egg-substitute meals we analyzed, two of the nine

Customize Your Combo

········

Always feel free to ask if you can make substitutions on breakfast platters. If you request fresh fruit in place of the meat in a combo, most restaurants will be happy to oblige.

restaurants we visited served us regular eggs instead of the requested substitute.

Typical platter: As we've already noted, the Original Grand Slam (two eggs, two hotcakes, two strips of bacon, and two sausages), for as low as $2.99, is the best-selling menu item at Denny's, the nation's largest family restaurant chain. You can't beat this deal, which is why many other chains offer similar (but not as cheap) versions, among them IHOP's Rooty Tooty Fresh 'N Fruity. Carrows even throws in a side of hash browns or home fries with its Hearty Breakfast.

These feasts are a grand slam, all right—to your heart and hips. They contain more than 1,000 calories, at least three-quarters of a day's fat, saturated fat, and sodium, and nearly two days' cholesterol. Not even counting the cholesterol, that's as bad for your heart as two McDonald's Big Macs. If you want to remember that grand slam–type breakfasts have double everything, just think: double bypass.

The Bottom Line: *If you're at Denny's and don't feel like going the fruit-and-cereal route, order a Slim Slam. Elsewhere, request an egg substitute, hold the butter or margarine on your toast and pancakes, and see if you can replace sausage and bacon with fresh fruit. If you make all three changes, your meal will have 40 percent fewer calories.*

PANCAKES WITH SYRUP
(870 calories and 16 grams of fat, 6 of them saturated)
If you get a stack of four without the margarine and use a typical ¼-cup serving of syrup, you'll eat a decent, if large (870 calories), breakfast with only six grams of saturated fat and less than 100

milligrams of cholesterol. Consider cutting back on the syrup—or the number of pancakes—if you don't want to use up nearly half a day's calories at breakfast. If you forget to tell the kitchen to hold the margarine and your pancakes arrive with margarine oozing down the sides of the stack,

The Flip Side of Pancakes

In the pancake–French toast–waffle category, an order of pancakes with syrup has a third less fat than an order of French toast, and half the fat of a Belgian waffle with whipped topping and fruit.

the fat and saturated fat exceed what you would get in two full-fat hot dogs and you'll end up with about the same calories you would get in six hot dogs.

Typical Platter: Four pancakes with margarine or butter and syrup, with four strips of bacon or sausage links. Bacon boosts the calories to 1,040 and the saturated fat to three-quarters of your day's allowance. Sausage will bring it past a full day's worth.

The Bottom Line: Skip the margarine, bacon, and sausage. Use just two tablespoons of syrup or ask for light syrup, which has half the calories. You can also ask for a short stack (fewer than four). Chains like Perkins and some IHOPs list a short stack on their menus, and others may give you a smaller order if you ask.

FRENCH TOAST WITH SYRUP
(800 calories and 26 grams of fat, 8 of them saturated)

To make French toast, the cook dips bread in an egg and milk mixture and fries it in shortening. If you eat this meal, with the usual melted butter or margarine, the calories exceed 900 and the fat and saturated fat are equal to what you'd get from three McDonald's Egg McMuffins. Even without the butter or margarine, this dish has about 50 percent more fat and saturated fat than pancakes without margarine—and nearly three times the cholesterol.

Typical Platter: Three slices of French toast with butter or margarine or syrup, plus four strips of bacon or sausage links. At Denny's, it's two strips and two links. If you eat the four-link meal, you'll waddle out of the restaurant 1,300 calories heavier and with no room for more saturated fat until lunch tomorrow. To your arteries, it looks like three Dairy Queen Banana Splits.

The Bottom Line: *Ask your server if the kitchen can make French toast with an egg substitute and fat-free milk. Hold the butter and margarine, and use light syrup. If you use regular syrup, keep it down to two tablespoons.*

BISCUITS AND GRAVY
(580 calories and 31 grams of fat, 14 of them saturated)

Homey and satisfying as it may be, a biscuit smothered in milk gravy that's studded with sausage bits is no comfort to your heart.

Typical Platter: Some restaurants serve biscuits with two eggs, two strips of bacon, and two sausage links, giving the meal the fat and saturated fat content of a half-pound of Spam! Other restaurants team their biscuits and gravy with hash browns and four sausage links. To match the saturated fat, you'd have to put away seven Dunkin' Donuts Boston Kreme Donuts.

The Bottom Line: *Fuhgeddaboutit!*

BELGIAN WAFFLES
(900 calories and 32 grams of fat, 19 of them saturated)

Who would have guessed that a dressed-up seven-inch waffle could have 900 calories and more saturated fat than a 13-ounce rib eye steak? That's a Belgian waffle, loaded to the gills with whole milk, eggs, and butter in the batter and served with whipped topping.

Typical Platter: At most restaurants, a Belgian waffle stands alone.

The Bottom Line: *You can skip the whipped topping, but that will only help a little, since most of the fat and cholesterol are probably in the batter.*

HAM AND CHEESE OMELETTE
(510 calories and 39 grams of fat, 19 of them saturated)

Made of three eggs, two ounces of ham, and an ounce of cheese, this demurely folded omelette certainly doesn't take up as much room on the plate as some of the other breakfast bonanzas we've described. But eat one and you still take in a day's saturated fat. That's what you'd get in two corned beef sandwiches. Of course, the sandwiches wouldn't give you more than two days' worth of cholesterol (655 milligrams).

Typical Platter: Omelettes usually come with hash browns and toast. That's enough to saddle you with roughly 1,000 calories and to make the fat and saturated fat equal to three corned beef sandwiches.

The Bottom Line: *You can't win with this combination. Look for a cheeseless vegetable or "garden" omelette instead, and ask for egg whites only or an egg substitute. Spice things up with Tabasco or salsa.*

Ordering à la Carte

One good way to avoid "platter syndrome" is to create your own breakfast combination with side dishes. We've ranked the most common ones for you here, from best to worst—that is, from least to most saturated fat.

HAM
(100 calories and 3 grams of fat, 1 of them saturated)

A typical two-ounce serving is not as fatty as bacon or sausage. However, it contains 910 milligrams of sodium, which is more than one-third of your day's allowance.

HASH BROWNS (220 calories and 11 grams of fat, 3 of them saturated) **OR TOAST WITH MARGARINE** (260 calories and 12 grams of fat, 4 of them saturated)

Two slices of toast with margarine, the spread used by most restaurants, will do about as much damage as an order of hash browns. Each has about 11 grams of fat. And if the restaurant serves butter on its toast, 6 of the 11 grams of fat will be saturated. (That's a third of your day's quota.) Ask if the restaurant serves a *trans*-fat-free spread like Promise. A spokesperson for the makers of Promise says Carrows and Cracker Barrel are among the chains that use those margarines. Short of finding such a spread, use jelly or preserves.

BACON
(130 calories and 11 grams of fat, 4 of them saturated)

A typical four-strip (1 ounce) serving weighs in at 11 grams of fat, 4 of them saturated. The only reason its numbers are better than those of sausage is the small serving size. Ounce-for-ounce, Canadian bacon, which is available on some menus, has one-fifth the fat of regular bacon. However, the average restaurant serving size may be larger than that of regular bacon.

PANCAKES WITH MARGARINE AND SYRUP
(770 calories and 22 grams of fat, 9 of them saturated)

The calories in a three-pancake *side order* come to about a third of a day's worth! If you skip the margarine or butter and use just two tablespoons of syrup instead of the typical 4-tablespoon serving (¼ cup), you'll save nearly 200 calories.

SAUSAGE
(340 calories and 32 grams of fat, 13 of them saturated)

This is the worst side dish to order. In the breakfast meat hierarchy, a four-link order of sausage has ten times as much fat as ham (bacon is about in the middle). One side of sausage gives you about a half-day's quota of fat and saturated fat each. If your favorite restaurant serves sausage patties instead of links, one patty weighs roughly the same as two links. So, if you eat the typical two-patty serving, you're getting the fat of four links.

When Your Favorite Is Not on the List

Many popular breakfast-time baked goods—including muffins, sweet rolls, croissants, and scones—are discussed in chapter 15, Sweet Nothings: Pastry and Dessert, page 257, and in chapter 17, Shop Till You Drop: Mall Food, page 303. Breakfast sandwiches are included in chapter 16, On the Run: Fast-Food Restaurants, page 271.

Grits are a common regional dish we didn't analyze. If they are prepared and served without butter or margarine, grits are low in fat. But don't get the idea that grits are the equivalent of a bowl of oatmeal, which is made from whole grains. Because grits are a refined grain, they are the nutritional equivalent of white bread. As a result, you couldn't be getting the benefit of the fiber, vitamins, and minerals you would get in a whole grain cereal.

Breakfast Strategy

• **Order from the "healthy" or "light" section.** Some chains, like Perkins and Denny's, offer special "healthy" or "light" selections, which are almost always lower in calories and fat than the rest of the fare.

The Whole Truth

By law, restaurants that make nutritional claims must substantiate them and provide nutritional information upon request. However, because lab analysis isn't required and serving sizes may vary, the numbers supplied may not exactly match what you have been served.

Skillet-Style Breakfasts
●●

Many of the chains we surveyed offer skillet-style breakfasts that include home fries, eggs, bacon, sausage, cheese, etc. We didn't test these combinations, but according to the company, Denny's Big Texas Chicken Fajita Skillet has 1,220 calories, 70 grams of fat (19 of them saturated), and 1,820 milligrams of sodium. And that's if you don't touch the optional sour cream or guacamole. The Meat Lover's Skillet ups the ante with diced ham, bacon, and sausage. The result: 1,150 calories, 93 grams of fat, 26 grams of saturated fat, and 2,510 milligrams of sodium. Skillet? Skip it.

Denny's Slim Slam breakfast, for instance, is a hearty platter of Egg Beaters, lean grilled ham (instead of sausage or bacon), and hotcakes jazzed up with a fruity topping instead of butter or margarine. The company says this trim alternative to the Original Grand Slam clocks in at 600 calories, 12 grams of total fat—a mere 3 of them saturated—and 35 milligrams of cholesterol. (The Original Grand Slam platter has nearly twice the calories and five times more fat.) The chief caveat: It contains 1,760 milligrams of sodium.

● **Try an egg substitute.** Many restaurants offer egg whites, Egg Beaters, or other brands of egg substitutes as an alternative to whole eggs.

● **Fill up on fruit.** Order half a grapefruit, a melon slice, or a glass of juice with your breakfast. This is an easy way to have one of the five to nine servings of fruits and veggies you should eat every day, plus the fruit is delicious and filling. The National Cancer Institute counts one six-ounce glass of juice as a serving.

• **Choose whole wheat bread over white.** Ask your server if there are any whole wheat breads or bagels for toasting. Many places offer what they call "wheat" bread, which is as meaningful a description as "dairy" milk. It usually has only a touch of whole grains, embellished with caramel coloring. But some places do serve the real thing. For a topping, try preserves, honey, or a thin layer of tub margarine or light cream cheese (it's got half the fat of regular).

• **Nix the butter or margarine.** Be sure to tell your server to leave off the butter or margarine, since a large dollop is often added automatically in the kitchen to pan-

The Best Breakfast
••••••••••••••••••••••••••••

A hot or cold cereal platter with 1-percent low-fat milk and fresh fruit is hands down your best bet.

Juices
••••••••••••••••

Orange, grapefruit, apple, and tomato are the usual juices offered in most restaurants. Orange juice is the most nutritious. An eight-ounce glass has over a day's vitamin C and a fifth of a day's folic acid. Grapefruit juice isn't far behind. Apple juice ranks lowest, with nearly 10 percent of a day's potassium but little else, unless it is fortified with vitamin C. Tomato juice can be high in vitamin C, especially if it's fortified, and it also supplies a quarter of a day's vitamin A. Unfortunately, it is sky-high in sodium. Campbell's Tomato Juice, for instance, has 750 milligrams of sodium (nearly a third of a day's worth) in an eight-ounce glass. If you have the choice, fresh fruit has fewer calories and more nutrients than juice. Besides the sweet and sprightly flavor, it also provides fiber.

cakes, waffles, toast, and English muffins. If you do want some, ask for it on the side and use it judiciously.

• **Let a breakfast buffet work for you.** If your favorite restaurant offers a breakfast buffet, as Shoney's does, head for it. You probably won't find lower-fat meats like turkey bacon or veggie sausage, but you can help yourself to the cereal and fruit. If you choose wisely, it's easy to put together a healthful, hearty meal. Just put the blinders on when you pass the glistening sausages, bacon, sausage gravy, and corned beef hash.

Second-Best Breakfasts

Take eggs—or better yet, scrambled egg-substitute with ham (it's salty, but leaner than bacon or sausage)—unbuttered toast (whole wheat, we hope), and hash browns. Or you could get pancakes or French toast with ham. Skip the margarine and go easy on the syrup. They're not perfect breakfasts: You're still going to take in at least half a day's sodium—plus lots of empty calories from the syrup. But you could do a lot worse. Just don't think of it as breakfast. It's really the equivalent of dinner . . . a big dinner. And even if you pay extra for orange juice or a fruit cup, after a morning meal like this, you've got a lot of catching up to do if you're going to get five to nine servings of fruits and vegetables by bedtime.

n the following chart, the dishes that we analyzed are ranked from best to worst—that is, from least to most saturated fat in the entrée (not the full platter). Entrées and platters marked with a ✔ are Best Bites. Best Bites are relatively low in saturated fat.

Reminder

Recommended limits for a 2,000-calorie diet:

Total fat: 65 grams
Saturated fat: 20 grams
Cholesterol: 300 milligrams
Sodium: 2,400 milligrams

BREAKFASTS

Menu Item	Calories	Total Fat (g)	Saturated Fat (g)	Cholesterol (mg)	Sodium (mg)
ENTRÉES AND PLATTERS					
✔ **Hot or cold cereal** (about 1 cup) **with 2% reduced-fat milk** (⅔ cup)	210	5	2	10	380
✔ plus orange juice (1 cup), mixed fruit (¾ cup), and plain toast	600	7	3	10	660
✔ **Scrambled egg substitute** (2)	130	6	*2*	0	190
✔ plus mixed fruit (¾ cup) and 2 pancakes with syrup (2 Tb.)	710	15	*5*	45	1,180
✔ plus hash browns and plain toast	480	18	*6*	0	670
✔ plus hash browns, ham, and plain toast	580	22	*7*	50	1,580
Scrambled eggs (2)	290	13	*5*	440	180
plus hash browns and plain toast	650	25	*8*	440	660
plus hash browns, ham, and plain toast	740	28	*10*	490	1,570
plus hash browns and toast with margarine	770	35	*12*	445	780
plus hash browns, 4 strips of bacon, and toast with margarine	910	45	*16*	465	1,300
plus 2 pancakes with syrup and margarine, 2 sausage links, and 2 strips of bacon (Denny's Original Grand Slam–type platter)	1,010	49	*19*	525	1,770

BREAKFASTS (continued) Menu Item	Calories	Total Fat (g)	Saturated Fat (g)	Cholesterol (mg)	Sodium (mg)
plus hash browns, 4 sausage links, and toast with margarine	1,120	67	25	495	1,450
plus 3 pancakes with syrup and margarine, 3 sausage links, and 3 strips of bacon	1,570	73	28	785	2,660
Pancakes (4) with syrup (¼ cup)	870	16	6	95	1,960
plus ham (2 oz.)	970	20	8	140	2,870
plus bacon (2 strips)	940	22	8	105	2,220
plus sausage (2 links)	1,040	32	13	115	2,290
French toast (3 slices) with syrup (¼ cup)	800	26	8	250	730
plus ham (2 oz.)	900	30	10	300	1,650
plus bacon (2 strips)	870	32	10	260	1,000
plus sausage (2 links)	970	42	15	275	1,070
Pancakes (4) with syrup (¼ cup) and margarine	940	29	12	95	1,960
plus ham (2 oz.)	1,040	33	14	145	2,880
plus bacon (4 strips)	1,080	40	16	120	2,490
plus sausage (4 links)	1,290	62	25	145	2,630
French toast (3 slices) with syrup (¼ cup) and margarine	910	33	13	280	1,030
plus ham (2 oz.)	1,010	37	14	325	1,940
plus bacon (4 strips)	1,050	44	17	300	1,550
plus sausage (4 links)	1,260	65	26	325	1,700
Biscuits and gravy	580	31	14	35	1,800
plus 2 eggs, 2 sausage links, and 2 strips of bacon	1,110	65	27	510	2,580
plus hash browns and 4 sausage links	1,150	74	30	85	2,670

BREAKFASTS *(continued)*

Menu Item	Calories	Total Fat (g)	Saturated Fat (g)	Cholesterol (mg)	Sodium (mg)
Belgian waffle with fruit and whipped topping	900	32	*19*	240	1,160
plus ham (2 oz.)	1,000	35	*20*	285	2,070
plus bacon (2 strips)	970	37	*21*	250	1,420
plus sausage (2 links)	1,080	48	*25*	260	1,500
Ham and cheese omelette	510	39	*19*	650	1,200
plus hash browns and toast with margarine	990	61	*26*	655	1,790
SIDE DISHES					
Toast, plain (2 slices)	130	2	0	0	270
Ham (2 oz.)	100	3	*1*	50	910
Bacon (2 strips)	70	5	*2*	10	260
Hash browns (1 cup)	220	11	*3*	0	200
Bacon (4 strips)	130	11	*4*	20	530
Toast (2 slices) with margarine	260	12	*4*	5	390
Pancakes (3) with syrup (¼ cup)	720	12	*5*	70	1,480
Sausage (2 links)	170	16	*6*	25	330
Pancakes (3) with syrup (¼ cup) and margarine	770	22	*9*	75	1,490
Sausage (4 links)	340	32	*13*	50	670

Note: If you're served butter on your pancakes, French toast, or toast, you'll get more saturated fat. If you're served margarine, you may get slightly less. Numbers for cereal, milk, syrup, plain toast, mixed fruit, and orange juice are from USDA Nutrient Data Base for Standard Reference and manufacturers. Saturated fat numbers in *italics* include artery-clogging *trans* fat.

The numbers in the following Denny's chart are from the company. Saturated fat numbers do not include *trans* fat; if they did, the saturated fat numbers would be higher than those indicated. Most entrées come with a choice of bread, grits, and/or hashed browns (see Side Dishes below for numbers). The items are ranked from best to worst; that is, from least to most saturated fat. Entrées marked with a ✔ are Best Bites. Best Bites are relatively low in saturated fat.

DENNY'S

Menu Item	Calories	Total Fat (g)	Saturated Fat (g)	Cholesterol (mg)	Sodium (mg)
ENTRÉES					
✔ Oatmeal N' Fixins (oatmeal, milk, raisins, sliced banana, choice of bread, and a glass of juice)	460	6	3	10	90
✔ Slim Slam (Egg Beaters, grilled ham, and 2 hotcakes with fruit topping)	600	12	3	35	1,760
Ham & Cheddar Omelette	580	45	8	670	1,180
Eggs Benedict	700	46	11	515	1,720
Country-Fried Steak & Eggs	430	36	12	440	860
Ultimate Omelette	560	47	12	640	940
Veggie-Cheese Omelette	480	39	13	645	540
Original Grand Slam (2 hotcakes with margarine and syrup, 2 eggs, 2 bacon strips, and 2 sausage links)	1,030	60	16	460	2,380
Sirloin Steak & Eggs	620	49	18	570	630
Big Texas Chicken Fajita Skillet (country-fried potatoes, 2-egg omelette, grilled chicken breast, peppers, onions, cheddar, and salsa)	1,220	70	19	520	1,820
All American Slam (3 eggs and cheddar scrambled, 2 bacon strips, and 2 sausage links)	710	62	20	685	1,280

DENNY'S (continued)

Menu Item	Calories	Total Fat (g)	Saturated Fat (g)	Cholesterol (mg)	Sodium (mg)
Lumberjack Slam (grilled ham, 2 bacon strips, 2 sausage links, 2 eggs, and 3 hotcakes with margarine and syrup)	1,490	80	20	480	4,170
French Slam (French toast with powdered sugar, margarine, and syrup, 2 eggs, 2 bacon strips, and 2 sausage links)	1,260	81	22	775	1,570
Moons Over My Hammy (ham and egg sandwich with Swiss and American on grilled sourdough)	920	59	24	580	2,810
Farmer's Slam (3 scrambled eggs with crumbled sausage, hashed browns, peppers, onions, country gravy, cheddar, 2 hotcakes with margarine and syrup, 2 bacon strips, and 2 sausage links)	1,430	90	26	705	3,350
Meat Lover's Skillet (diced ham, bacon, and sausage over country-fried potatoes with cheddar and 2 eggs)	1,150	93	26	460	2,510
T-bone Steak & Eggs	990	77	31	655	1,000
Breakfast Dagwood (shaved ham, eggs, sausage, bacon, and 3 cheeses inside boule bread)	1,250	90	38	800	3,600
SIDE DISHES					
Grits (½ cup)	80	0	0	0	520
Toast, plain (1 slice)	90	1	0	0	170
Hash browns (¾ cup)	220	14	2	0	420

Chapter 4

Hold the Mayo:
Sandwich Shops

Sandwiches are virtually synonymous with "midday meal."
Fast, compact, and inexpensive, they also offer convenience and portability. Whether we eat one at an office or
school desk, a deli counter, restaurant or park bench, or
perched atop an I beam, sandwiches seem to fit perfectly into our
maxed-out schedules. But just as life has become more complex,
so too has the sandwich. Although Americans still love the classics like a BLT, PB&J, or tuna sandwich, we've also developed a
taste for the trendy combinations and sky-high stacked sandwiches made with unusual ingredients that now appear on restaurant menus. Both types of sandwiches are often nutritionally
deceiving. The most common ingredients—salty cured meat,
fatty cheese, or chunks of tuna or chicken suspended in full-fat
mayonnaise—can make these fast fill-ups a fattening proposition.
By the time you've crumpled the wrapping and brushed away the
crumbs, you may well have consumed as much fat, sodium, and
calories as you would have at a traditional sit-down meal.

Some of the basic sandwich ingredients are a problem, yet
they needn't be. Satisfying, lower-fat cold cuts, cheeses, and
mayonnaise are now standard in supermarkets. But for some reason, most sandwich shops and restaurants don't use them.
Restaurant owners, like many consumers, apparently just don't
know how nutritionally expensive a simple sandwich can be.
Even popular diet books frequently underreport the calories in
favorites like chicken-, tuna-, and egg-salad sandwiches.

Sandwich ingredients aren't the only problem; more trouble is served up alongside a sandwich. Add chips (extra fat), a pickle (extra salt), and a soda (extra sugar), and you've got more than a meal's worth of calories and fat.

The good news is that things may be improving. Subway, by far the nation's largest chain of sandwich shops, has a line of lower-fat subs that it advertises as "7 Subs with 6 Grams of Fat or Less." They put most of the sandwiches we tested to shame. Subway also now routinely makes its Classic Tuna and Classic Seafood & Crab salads with light mayo, and its Low Fat Chicken Salad is made with nonfat mayo. The lightened version of the tuna, for example, has one-third less fat and 25 percent fewer calories than the old recipe, according to numbers supplied by the company. (See Sub Plot, pages 95–96, for more about the chain's products.) Another national sandwich maker, Schlotzsky's Deli, has an entire line it calls Light & Flavorful. All but the Vegetarian (which comes with cheese) and the Santa Fe Chicken are low in saturated fat. All will run you only 350 calories for a small or about 500 for a regular (watch out—the large versions hit 1,000 calories each). (For more on Schlotzsky's Deli, see page 311.) And some Blimpie's outlets have light mayonnaise for customers who request it. If you're lucky, light mayonnaise may also be available at your favorite local deli; we found it at a number of those we surveyed.

The Dishes and the Data

We analyzed 12 of the most popular kinds of sandwiches purchased from 29 shops, including chains like Au Bon Pain, Schlotzsky's Deli, and Wall Street Deli, as well as independent delis, restaurants, and sandwich shops, in Chicago, Los Angeles, New York, and Washington, D.C. (For more information on our methodology, see pages 12–14.)

Here's the rundown on our deli dozen, ranked from best to worst—that is, from least to most saturated fat.

Amazingly, we found only one sandwich—turkey with mustard—that was truly low in fat, although it was high in sodium. A roast beef sandwich with mustard and a turkey sandwich with mayo were also Best Bites. And based on the numbers provided by the companies, 11 Subway subs and 7 Blimpie subs also earned a Best Bite designation.

Sandwiches

TURKEY BREAST WITH MUSTARD
(370 calories and 6 grams of fat, 2 of them saturated)
This was the only sandwich that was low in both saturated and total fat. It would have been an all-around winner if the restaurants had used turkey that wasn't so heavily salted. That sent the sodium soaring to 1,410 milligrams—more than half a day's worth.

If you get a turkey sandwich with a typical amount (about a tablespoon) of mayo, the fat triples from 6 to 19 grams. That boosts the calories to 470, which is on the high side for a sandwich.

The Bottom Line: This is your best choice, despite the high sodium. If you're lucky enough to find a deli that uses fresh instead of processed turkey, the sodium will be much lower.

ROAST BEEF WITH MUSTARD
(460 calories and 12 grams of fat, 4 of them saturated)
How could a red-meat sandwich take second place in any listing of healthful sandwiches? For one

> **Tasty Toppings**
> ••••••••••••••••••••
>
> For extra flavor, texture, and nutrition, ask to have sandwiches garnished with lettuce, tomato, onion, green pepper, cucumbers, and any other vegetables that are available.

thing, sandwich shops generally use lean beef. Beyond that, roast beef looks good when you consider that tuna, chicken, ham, and egg salads are made with vast amounts of mayonnaise.

Sandwich Caveat

....

Sandwiches containing red meat, even if they are low in fat, shouldn't be an everyday selection, since some researchers suspect that even lean beef, pork, or other red meat may increase the risk of colon and prostate cancer.

A one-tablespoon smear of mayonnaise instead of mustard doubles the total fat and boosts the calories by 100.

Roast beef was also the only sandwich we tested whose sodium stayed under 1,000 milligrams. Although that's not low—the bread alone contributes 400 to 500 milligrams —it was the best of the bunch.

The Bottom Line: *An excellent choice. If you don't like mustard, you can ask for light mayo or barbecue sauce instead.*

CHICKEN SALAD WITHOUT MAYO ON THE BREAD
(540 calories and 32 grams of fat, 6 of them saturated)

It wouldn't be chicken salad without mayo. At least ask them not to make things worse by putting mayo on the bread. If you don't, the sandwich could contain more calories (660) and fat (46 grams) than pot roast with mashed potatoes and gravy! Try to find a deli that makes its salads with light mayonnaise.

The Bottom Line: *Request less chicken salad and more lettuce, onion, and tomato. Or head to Subway—it offers a Low Fat Chicken Salad Sub.*

CORNED BEEF WITH MUSTARD
(500 calories and 20 grams of fat, 8 of them saturated)

As far as sodium goes, a corned beef sandwich is impossible to fix. The corning process involves curing the meat in brine and spices. A regular size sandwich has 1,920 milligrams—more than three-quarters of your daily maximum. If your deli piles on twice the customary amount of meat to create a "New York City"–style sandwich, you will easily consume more than 3,000 milligrams of sodium, along with three-quarters of a day's saturated fat. Want a pickle on the side? It's delicious, but just one spear will add another 400 milligrams of sodium to your meal.

The Bottom Line: *Skip it. You can't get rid of the sodium, and nearly half a day's saturated fat is no bargain either.*

TUNA SALAD WITHOUT MAYO ON THE BREAD
(720 calories and 43 grams of fat, 8 of them saturated)
If we had a nickel for every lunch-goer who thinks tuna salad is one of the healthier sandwich choices, we'd be rich enough to start a sandwich chain of our own. If you order a typical tuna salad sandwich, without mayo on the bread, you're consuming 720 calories, two-thirds of a day's fat, and half a day's sodium.

If you order a tuna salad sandwich "overstuffed" like they offer at the Carnegie Deli and Stage Deli, you're in for a whole day's fat and nearly 1,000 calories. That's pretty amazing when you consider that the fish starts out at a tiny fraction of that.

The Bottom Line: *If you can't convince your favorite deli to offer light mayonnaise, take your business to Subway—it does.*

HAM WITH MUSTARD
(560 calories and 27 grams of fat, 10 of them saturated)
If sandwich shops can order lean beef, why can't they also offer low-fat ham? Surely Oscar Mayer, Healthy Choice, and any number of other producers would be happy for the business. A typical ham sandwich has more than twice the fat of roast beef. And because ham is salted, you also get twice the sodium.

If you think that a ham sandwich is naked without the Swiss cheese, it's worth noting that you'll be adding a quarter of a day's saturated fat with a single 1-ounce slice of cheese.

The Bottom Line: *Forget this one if your sandwich shop doesn't offer low-fat ham. And encourage it to start offering more healthful ingredients.*

EGG SALAD WITHOUT MAYO ON THE BREAD
(550 calories and 31 grams of fat, 10 of them saturated)

The egg industry would have us believe that eggs are low in saturated fat. Although it's true that a single egg is close to low, an egg salad sandwich provides half a day's worth—as much as two McDonald's Egg McMuffins. And that's without any mayo on the bread.

If the saturated fat isn't enough to discourage you, consider the sandwich's 520 milligrams of cholesterol, which is almost two days' worth. Let the shop put mayo on the bread and your innocent-looking sandwich hits 660 calories—the equivalent of a Burger King Whopper.

The Bottom Line: *Encourage your deli person to lighten up by using fewer yolks and more whites, and by substituting light for full-fat mayonnaise.*

TURKEY CLUB
(740 calories and 34 grams of fat, 10 of them saturated)

The average six slices of bacon, as well as the mayonnaise, put this selection on a nutritional par with Wendy's Big Bacon Classic. If you're lucky, the turkey may be fresh and unsalted, which would cut down on sodium, but few shops offer it.

The Bottom Line: *Request more tomatoes and fewer slices of bacon—you'll be surprised how much flavor just a couple of strips provide. To cut calories, see if you can get light mayo.*

BACON, LETTUCE, AND TOMATO
(600 calories and 37 grams of fat, 12 of them saturated)

Bacon and mayonnaise again. You know what that means: more calories, fat, and sodium than a McDonald's Big Mac.

The Bottom Line: *Ask for light mayo and request only two strips of bacon and more tomatoes.*

VEGETARIAN
(750 calories and 40 grams of fat, 14 of them saturated)

It is heartbreaking—literally—that a sandwich that could be a nutritional gold mine is such a bust. Our samples packed as much fat and saturated fat as two McDonald's Quarter Pounders. The lettuce, sprouts, tomato, cucumber, and onion were fine. But the saturated fat in the 2 ounces of cheese outweighed the benefits, and the mayo-based dressing added extra calories.

Your favorite vegetarian sandwich may not always be a fat trap, however. Ask what's in it when you order.

The Bottom Line: Have the sandwich-maker hold all or all but one slice of cheese and skip the dressing, or use just a touch of it.

GRILLED CHEESE
(510 calories and 33 grams of fat, 17 of them saturated)

If only your mom had realized! The innocent-looking 3 ounces of cheese and lubricated bread aren't a melt; they're a meltdown. Nearly 90 percent of your day's quota of saturated fat sits in the gooey, golden square. That's about what you'd get in three glasses of whole milk.

The Bottom Line: It's bad news.

REUBEN
(920 calories and 50 grams of fat, 20 of them saturated)

Here we have 6 ounces of corned beef or pastrami, a couple of ounces each of cheese plus salty sauerkraut, and lots of Russian dressing between two pieces of rye bread, grilled. You'd get about the same amount of calories, fat, and saturated fat (and 1,280 milligrams less sodium) from a country fried steak dinner with mashed potatoes and gravy. Enough said.

The Bottom Line: There's no way to make this a healthful choice.

When Your Favorite Is Not on the List

Although we didn't analyze grilled chicken sandwiches, many of the shops we surveyed had them on the menu. Judging from the numbers fast-food chains publish for their grilled chicken sandwiches (see chart, page 284), this should be one of the better sandwich choices. Just make sure you're getting a chicken breast that's not covered with cheese or crunchy breading, and use none or just a small amount of the mayo and special sauces. With the exception of barbecue sauce, these sauces are usually fatty.

We covered several popular sandwiches in other chapters. For our analyses of bacon and cheese grilled chicken, see chapter 12, Where Everybody Knows Your Name: Dinner Houses, page 228; for patty melts, see chapter 13, Home away from Home: Family-style Restaurants, page 244. We didn't analyze shrimp/crab/seafood salad or ham salad, but we suspect they're

Philadelphia Story

The numbers for a Philly-style steak and cheese sandwich can vary from decent to downright awful. According to the company, Subway's six-inch Classic Steak & Cheese Sub has 13 grams of fat, 5 of which are saturated. Schlotzsky's Deli's and Blimpie's versions have at least twice that much. But our analysis of the Philly Cheese Steaks served in family-style restaurants (see page 242) turned up the most staggering numbers, averaging 35 grams of fat, 17 of them saturated, in a six-inch sandwich. And to think that some people call this a hero!

as fatty and salty as other mayo-based sandwiches. We also did not analyze tuna melts, but if you do the math—combine our numbers for plain tuna salad with those for a slice of American cheese—we bet you won't like the answer.

Many sandwich shops also offer garden salads. In theory, these can be a terrific choice; but some are nearly as bad as sandwiches. If they're loaded with cheese, eggs, or cold cuts, or come swimming in full-fat dressing, your seemingly light lunch may turn out to be far heavier than you thought. Chapter 13, on family-style restaurants explains why a chef salad entrée can be a big nutritional surprise (see page 243). For the lowdown on a chicken Caesar salad entrée and an Oriental chicken salad entrée, see Where Everybody Knows Your Name: Dinner Houses (pages 228 and 229). And you'll find our analysis of a Caesar side salad in chapter 11, Here's the Beef: Steak Houses (see page 223). For additional salads, see chapter 16, On the Run: Fast-Food Restaurants (page 271) and Mall Food (page 303).

Decoding a Deli Menu

We've been heaping ham on rye for years. So how can a sandwich that's everyone's idea of a light lunch turn out to be such bad news? The answer is that the sandwich-maker behind the counter doesn't build them the way you do at home. Sandwiches made at delis, take-out sandwich shops, and lunch counters can easily have twice the meat, cheese, or other filling as a homemade, brown-bag version. And the meat is also likely to be fattier than the brands we buy at the supermarket. On average, we found 5 ounces of sliced meat in our test sandwiches. A few places used 3 to 4, but they were balanced by those that used as much as half a pound! And these numbers do not pertain to the overstuffed or "New York–style" constructions popular at places like the famous Carnegie Deli or Stage Deli in New York City, where some sandwich fillings weighed in with more than 9 ounces of meat. Compare that to the 2-ounce serving size that the makers of packaged supermarket luncheon meats list as reasonable.

The average amount of mayo-based "salad" fillings (the tremendously popular tuna, chicken, and egg) was 6 ounces, or about three-quarters of a cup. Overstuffed versions weighed in at 9 ounces.

Plus, shops often spread about one 100-calorie tablespoon of full-fat mayonnaise on the bread before adding the tuna, egg, or chicken salad fillings, which are already full of it.

Sandwich Strategy

Because a sandwich is essentially defined by its filling, there often isn't much room for improvement. However, some general strategies can help a sandwich pass muster.

• **Get it your way.** Skip those plastic-wrapped, premade sandwiches at the deli counter and have yours made to order. That way you can get it exactly the way you want it.

• **Eat your veggies.** Ask for less meat or filling and more lettuce, tomatoes, onions, cucumber, or peppers. The deli guy may look at you like you're nuts, but he'll do it. You'll enjoy the extra crunch, and get the benefits of a small serving of vegetables.

• **Go for the grain.** Always order your sandwich on whole wheat bread. Many places offer you a choice; but, as far as nutritional value goes, "wheat" bread is virtually the same as white, as are rye, pumpernickel, and multigrain. Whole wheat contains the most fiber, vitamins, and minerals, much of which are removed when flour is refined. Your worst choice is a croissant, which is made with white flour *and* is high in fat.

• **Slash the sodium.** To keep the sodium down, avoid bacon, corned beef, and ham.

• **Do-it-yourself.** Make your own sandwich at the salad bar. Stuff a pita with fresh veggies, garbanzo beans, and light dressing or yogurt.

• **Cut back on cheese.** Ask for a vegetarian sandwich without the cheese, or with just one slice. Try hummus instead. Request a light dressing or sauce served on the side so you can use just a touch to moisten the filling.

• **Hold the mayo.** Try low-fat condiments like mustard, ketchup, or barbecue sauce.

Sub Plot

If a simple sandwich can be a nutritionist's nightmare, you're probably wondering about subs. They're not necessarily worse. Because you get more bread (unfortunately, Subway's wheat bread has more white flour than whole wheat) and less filling, subs—at least the six-inch ones from Subway and Blimpie—are often less fatty than regular sandwiches.

The nation's undisputed submeister, with about 15,000 outlets nationwide, is Subway. We applaud its "7 Subs with 6 Grams of Fat or Less" campaign. (All of the nutrition statistics cited in this section are from the company.) At Subway you can enjoy a six-inch Subway Club, Ham, Roast Beef, Roasted Chicken Breast, Turkey Breast, Turkey Breast & Ham, or Veggie Delite (with or without the cheese) with a clear conscience. The sodium numbers are higher than we'd like for everything but the Veggie Delite (500 milligrams without the cheese), but they're no worse than other sandwiches or fast-food fare. Some Subway shops offer a vegetarian Gardenburger or Garden Party Sub. The company wouldn't give us numbers for either one, but we suspect they'd qualify as Best Bites.

We have two other reasons to praise Subway. One is its switch to light mayonnaise. Although it's too fatty to be a Best Bite, as are a number of its other subs, Subway's six-inch Classic Tuna Sub has half the fat of a six-inch Blimpie Tuna Sub made with regular mayo. Subway's Low Fat Chicken Salad Sub is made with nonfat mayo and does get a Best Bite. Subway also gets points for prominently displaying nutrition information about some of its sandwiches right at the stores.

Blimpie, the nation's second-largest sub chain, with more than 2,000 outlets, has fat numbers similar to Subway's for its Turkey and Roast Beef subs. Its Grilled Chicken and meatless patty subs (Vegi, Grille, Mexi, and Chick Max) also qualify as Best Bites.

We don't want to give the impression that all offerings from a sub shop are a healthy choice, however. Blimpie says that its six-inch Italian Meatball sub packs 500 calories and 22 grams of fat, eight of them saturated. Subway's version is even worse. And top dishonors go to Blimpie's Cheese Trio because 12 of its 23 fat grams are saturated.

Sub Strategy

Here are some tips that will help you make a wise submarine choice:

- Overall, a six-inch sub usually has less fat than its sandwich counterpart. If you order a foot-long one, however, you'll have to double the numbers in our chart.
- As is true of regular sandwiches, turkey and roast beef subs are two of the least fatty, especially if you skip the cheese.

- Subway's Veggie Delite has much less fat than the other vegetarian sandwiches we tested because it has no cheese (unless you request it) and no mayo or avocado (like mayo, the avocado is rich in unsaturated fat, but it's high in calories). Subway's Ham Sub also has less fat. The chain apparently uses lower-fat ham (and less of it) than its competitors.
- Have them hold the mayo, oil, cheese, and salt, which are sometimes added automatically. Then experiment with adding mustard, light mayo, ketchup, or light salad dressing yourself.

Items in the following charts are ranked from best to worst—that is, from least to most saturated fat. Sandwiches and subs marked with a ✔ are Best Bites. Best Bites are relatively low in saturated fat.

Reminder

Recommended limits for a 2,000-calorie diet:

Total fat: 65 grams
Saturated fat: 20 grams
Cholesterol: 300 milligrams
Sodium: 2,400 milligrams

SANDWICHES

Menu Item	Calories	Total Fat (g)	Saturated Fat (g)	Cholesterol (mg)	Sodium (mg)
✔ Turkey with mustard (9 oz.)	370	6	*2*	75	1,410
✔ Roast beef with mustard (9 oz.)	460	12	*4*	115	990
✔ Turkey with mayo (9 oz.)	470	19	*4*	75	1,280
Roast beef with mayo (9 oz.)	560	24	*6*	120	850
Chicken salad without mayo on the bread (10 oz.)	540	32	*6*	90	1,140
Corned beef with mustard (9 oz.)	500	20	*8*	140	1,920
Tuna salad without mayo on the bread (11 oz.)	720	43	*8*	65	1,320
Chicken salad with mayo on the bread (10 oz.)	660	46	*8*	90	1,180
Overstuffed tuna salad with mayo on the bread (13 oz.)	980	63	*11*	95	1,310
Bacon, lettuce, and tomato (8 oz.)	600	37	*12*	60	1,560

SANDWICHES *(continued)* Menu Item	Calories	Total Fat (g)	Saturated Fat (g)	Cholesterol (mg)	Sodium (mg)
Overstuffed tuna salad with mayo on the bread (13 oz.)	860	50	*9*	90	1,270
Ham with mustard (9 oz.)	560	27	*10*	80	2,340
Egg salad without mayo on the bread (10 oz.)	550	31	*10*	520	1,110
Turkey club (13 oz.)	740	34	*10*	105	1,840
Tuna salad with mayo on the bread (11 oz.)	830	56	*10*	70	1,360
Ham with mayo (9 oz.)	670	40	*12*	85	2,200
Egg salad with mayo on the bread(10 oz.)	660	44	*12*	525	1,150
Overstuffed corned beef with mustard (13 oz.)	760	37	*14*	270	3,130
Vegetarian (12 oz.)	750	40	*14*	60	1,280
Grilled cheese (5 oz.)	510	33	*17*	70	1,540
Reuben (14 oz.)	920	50	*20*	230	3,270

All sandwiches except the Reuben were ordered on white bread.

Note: Saturated fat numbers in *italics* include artery-clogging *trans* fat. All cholesterol numbers are estimates. If sandwiches were analyzed with mustard, they were estimated with mayo and vice versa.

The numbers in the Blimpie and Subway Subs chart were provided by the companies and apply to subs made without the salt, cheese, oil, or mayo that many sub makers offer. Exception: numbers for Subway Classic Subs include optional salt, cheese, and oil. Saturated fat numbers do not include *trans* fat; if they did, the saturated fat numbers would be higher than those indicated.

BLIMPIE AND SUBWAY SUBS

Menu Item	Calories	Total Fat (g)	Saturated Fat (g)	Cholesterol (mg)	Sodium (mg)
BLIMPIE (weight of 6-inch subs)					
✔ Mexi Max (7 oz.)	390	5	1	0	1,000
✔ Grille Max (7 oz.)	410	6	1	5	820
✔ Vegi Max (9 oz.)	400	7	1	0	980
✔ Chick Max (7 oz.)	480	12	1	0.	1,290
✔ Turkey (9 oz.)	330	6	2	0	1,200
✔ Grilled Chicken (9 oz.)	400	9	2	30	950
✔ Roast Beef (9 oz.)	390	7	3	65	1,370
Club (9 oz.)	370	10	5	30	1,200
Best (9 oz.)	410	13	5	50	1,480
Chicken Caesar Wrap (12 oz.)	610	31	6	35	1,770
Ham & Swiss (9 oz.)	410	14	7	50	1,050
Zesty Italian Wrap (11 oz.)	530	22	7	45	1,850
South Western Wrap (11 oz.)	590	28	7	75	1,990
Ham, Salami, & Provolone (9 oz.)	480	20	8	55	1,370

BLIMPIE AND SUBWAY SUBS *(continued)*

Menu Item	Calories	Total Fat (g)	Saturated Fat (g)	Cholesterol (mg)	Sodium (mg)
SUBWAY (weight of 6-inch subs)					
Italian Meatball (8 oz.)	500	22	8	25	970
Tuna (10 oz.)	660	44	8	55	880
Cheese Trio (9 oz.)	490	23	12	55	1,130
✔ Veggie Delite, no cheese (6 oz.)	200	3	1	0	500
✔ Turkey Breast (8 oz.)	220	4	1	15	1,000
✔ Low Fat Chicken Salad (8 oz.)	250	4	1	20	1,100
✔ Roast Beef (8 oz.)	260	5	1	20	840
✔ Turkey Breast & Ham (8 oz.)	270	5	1	25	1,210
✔ Ham (8 oz.)	260	5	2	25	1,260
✔ Subway Club (9 oz.)	290	5	2	30	1,250
✔ Roasted Chicken Breast (8 oz.)	310	6	2	50	880
✔ Veggie Delite, with cheese (7 oz.)	240	7	3	10	700
✔ Asiago Caesar Chicken (9 oz.)	390	15	3	45	1,000
✔ Horseradish Roast Beef (8 oz.)	400	17	3	25	880
Honey Mustard Melt (9 oz.)	370	11	5	40	1,570
Classic Steak & Cheese (9 oz.)	360	13	5	35	1,200
Classic Subway Melt (9 oz.)	380	15	5	40	1,690
Classic Seafood & Crab (9 oz.)	380	16	5	25	1,270
Classic Tuna (9 oz.)	420	21	5	40	1,180
Southwest Steak & Cheese (9 oz.)	410	18	6	45	1,120

BLIMPIE AND SUBWAY SUBS (continued)

Menu Item	Calories	Total Fat (g)	Saturated Fat (g)	Cholesterol (mg)	Sodium (mg)
Classic Cold Cut Trio (9 oz.)	420	20	7	55	1,670
Classic BMT (9 oz.)	450	24	8	55	1,740
SUBWAY (weight of 6-inch subs)					
Classic Meatball (10 oz.)	500	25	10	55	1,350
EXTRAS					
Dill pickle (1 spear)	10	0	0	0	440
Mustard (1 Tb.)	20	1	0	0	190
Baked Lay's Potato Crisps	130	2	0	0	170
Mayonnaise (1 Tb.)	100	11	2	0	0
Potato chips (1½ oz.)	230	15	4	0	270
American cheese (1 oz.)	110	9	6	30	410

Note: Numbers for "Extras" are from USDA Nutrient Data Base for Standard Reference and manufacturers.

Chapter 5

Wok This Way: Chinese Restaurants

O f all the gifts from our immigrant heritage, the intro-
duction of new foods into the American repertoire is
among the most significant and enduring. Chinese is one
of our most popular choices of ethnic food—in part
because of the wide, pleasing variety of dishes, the informal
dining style, and the reasonable prices. Some people also favor
Chinese food because they perceive it to be among the most
nutritious of ethnic cuisines. A report written by the Food
Marketing Institute and *Prevention* magazine found that 52 percent of Americans believe that Chinese food is "more healthful"
than their usual diet. There's truth in that perception because
the Chinese diet, like that of so many immigrant groups, has
evolved from what was essentially a peasant diet that relied
heavily on grains, vegetables, fruits, and legumes. That tradition
continues today in most of China, where the rates of many cancers, heart disease, obesity, and diabetes are far below those in
the United States.

Unfortunately, the traditional healthful Chinese diet is not
what Americans eat in a typical Chinese restaurant. For example,
at a traditional Chinese restaurant in any area with a large
Chinese-American community, it's often obvious that the Chinese patrons don't order the same dishes that non-Asians choose.
While non-Asians are very likely to be scarfing down individual big glistening platters of deep-fried pork and pineapple or
orange (crispy) beef with few veggies, Chinese-Americans are

103

more likely to order a balanced variety of dishes—for instance, one steamed fish, one dish of braised greens, one stir-fried chicken—which they *share* among themselves.

It's important to know how to order wisely in a Chinese restaurant. And that's not always easy. The menus are filled with potential pitfalls. Who would guess, for example, that an order of house lo mein has as much sodium as a Large Domino's Hand Tossed Cheese Pizza? Or that an order of kung pao chicken packs nearly as many calories as four McDonald's Quarter Pounders? Or that moo shu pork socks you with as much cholesterol as a Denny's Original Grand Slam breakfast platter? And we're not talking about mall food-court counters or Chinese fast-food places (for information on those, see chapter 17, Shop Till You Drop: Mall Food, page 303). Our survey checked only midprice, high-volume restaurants in big cities, where the entrée prices typically ranged from $7 to $17.

East Meets West

We chose dishes for analysis after we called dozens of Chinese restaurants around the country and asked for the names of their most popular appetizers, soups, and main dishes. Then, for comparison, we added three additional dishes to our list of those to be analyzed. They were stir-fried vegetables, which we predicted would be a nutritional champion; Hunan tofu, a popular vegetarian entrée; and chicken chow mein, a veteran that's stood the test of time. In the final analysis, what we found would make your chopsticks splinter.

Fat for entrées ranged from a respectable 19 grams (Szechuan shrimp or stir-fried vegetables) to an outrageous 76 grams (kung pao chicken). And the calories ranged from 750 (stir-fried vegetables) to 1,800 (orange beef). Other than the

sweet and sour pork, the lowest-sodium dinner (stir-fried vegetables) still had over 2,100 milligrams—about your quota for the
day. The highest-sodium dish (house lo mein) clocked in at an
incredible 3,460 milligrams.

On the plus side, the amount of saturated fat was lower in
Chinese dishes than in most of the other dishes in all the cate-
gories we analyzed for this book. Only three dishes (moo shu
pork, sweet and sour pork, and kung pao chicken) climb over half
a day's limit; each had 13 grams. Most dishes had no more than
half a day's worth. However, many contained at least a day's cholesterol. For example, moo shu pork, which is made with eggs,
had a one-and-a-half-day supply per order.

The Lowdown on MSG
▪▪▪

Monosodium glutamate brings out the flavor of many foods
and is widely used by Chinese and other restaurants in soups,
sauces, and other foods. Although that may sound like a treat
for the taste buds, studies have shown that some people are
sensitive to MSG. Reactions include headache, nausea, weakness, and burning sensation in the back of the neck and fore-
arms. Some people complain of wheezing, changes in heart rate,
and difficulty breathing. Some people claim to be sensitive to
very small amounts of MSG, but no good studies have been done
to determine just how little MSG can cause a reaction in the
most sensitive people.

People who believe they are sensitive to MSG should ask
waiters if MSG—or "natural flavoring" or hydrolyzed vegetable
protein—is used. Foods such as Parmesan cheese and tomatoes
contain glutamate that occurs naturally, but no reactions to
those foods have been reported.

The Dishes and the Data

We bought dinner-size take-out portions of 15 Chinese menu staples from 20 midpriced, independently owned restaurants in San Francisco, Chicago, and Washington, D.C. (For more on our methodology, see pages 12–14.)

Since most Chinese restaurants are independently owned, their dishes lack the uniformity of those at chains, so preparation methods and ingredients may vary widely. For example, although it wasn't typical, we found that some San Francisco restaurants breaded and deep-fried their Szechuan shrimp, so we did not include those samples in our analyses. Bear in mind that a dish ordered at your neighborhood Chinese restaurant may not be identical to one with the same name ordered at a different restaurant. Still, our numbers will give you a ballpark idea of what you're getting. We've put an ingredient description of each dish in parentheses after the name; use it to see how your restaurant's version compares. Realize, too, that the numbers for each dish are for an entire dinner-size take-out order, which includes 1⅓ cups of rice. If you eat less, adjust the numbers accordingly.

Within each category, we've ranked the dishes from best to worst—that is, from least to most saturated fat. Note that we didn't test for *trans* fat, but we doubt that much is present, since Chinese restaurants typically fry in oil, not *trans*-laden shortening. We analyzed dishes without rice, then added nutrition information for 1⅓ cups of steamed rice to all items except egg rolls, hot and sour soup, house fried rice, and house lo mein.

Appetizers

HOT AND SOUR SOUP
(pork, tofu, and egg in broth; 110 calories and 4 grams of fat, 1 of them saturated)
If only you could remove the egg! That's what fills this 100-calorie cup of soup with half of your daily allowance of cholesterol.

But you can't, because most restaurants prepare their soups ahead of time. As a test, we called six restaurants to see if we could order the soup without egg, but only one said that we could. And you won't be able to remove the 1,090 milligrams of sodium per cup, or the MSG that's used in the soup stocks and sauces that are prepared ahead of time.

The Bottom Line: *There's little you can do to cut down on the sodium and MSG. And keep in mind that every ½ cup serving of fried noodles, which are often served as an accompaniment, will add about 150 calories to your soup.*

EGG ROLL
(minced vegetables and pork and shrimp wrapped in dough and deep-fried; 190 calories and 11 grams of fat, 1 of them saturated)

Surely no one will be surprised by the high fat content of this popular appetizer. Most of the fat comes from the oil-absorbent dough wrapper that surrounds a smidgen of filling. (What's a smidgen? It's about an ounce of veggies, a quarter ounce of pork, and a fifteenth of an ounce of shrimp in a typical roll.) The good news is that an egg roll doesn't have any cholesterol-laden egg!

The Bottom Line: *Your best bet in the appetizer category is to order lower-fat steamed vegetable dumplings. But if you just can't resist an egg roll, limit yourself to one. A typical order contains two.*

Entrées (Includes 1½ cups of steamed rice, except house lo mein and house fried rice)

SZECHUAN SHRIMP
(shrimp, stir-fried with vegetables in a spicy sauce; 930 calories and 19 grams of fat, 2 of them saturated)

This is one of the most healthful entrées you can have. Even though an average order contains more than a day's cholesterol, this dish was the lowest in saturated fat and close to the lowest in calories (although close to 1,000 calories is not low by any stretch of the imagination). Another plus: The dish is 40 percent vegetables. Strangely, one restaurant in Chicago added almost half a pound of *peanuts* to its version, which would have added nearly 100 grams of fat and 1,160 calories to the numbers. We didn't include any samples with nuts in our analyses, but this example shows why it pays to ask your server how a dish is prepared before you order it! Also, three restaurants in San Francisco breaded and deep-fried the shrimp. We excluded those from the analysis as well.

The Bottom Line: *This seafood entrée is one of your best choices. Just make sure the dish is made without nuts, and the shrimp are not breaded and deep-fried. If they're available, you could also try Szechuan scallops, which are lower in cholesterol.*

STIR-FRIED VEGETABLES
(sometimes called vegetarian delight or Buddha's delight. A mix of Chinese and seasonal vegetables like baby corn, bamboo shoots, broccoli, cabbage, carrots, mushrooms, snow peas, and water chestnuts; 750 calories and 19 grams of fat, 3 of them saturated)

Vegetables and sauce—you won't get much lower in saturated fat, and you sure can't beat zero cholesterol. You're not likely to do better than its 750 calories or 2,150 milligrams (yikes!) of sodium, either. But those nutrition numbers are just part of the story; don't forget the vitamins, minerals, and fiber you get when you fill up on veggies.

The Bottom Line: *An excellent choice.*

SHRIMP WITH GARLIC SAUCE
(shrimp, stir-fried with vegetables, usually including mushrooms, peppers, and water chestnuts; 950 calories and 27 grams of fat, 4 of them saturated)

Each order of shrimp has more than a day's cholesterol; on the other hand, it has only 4 grams of saturated fat, so it shouldn't raise your cholesterol as much as most restaurant meals. Most restaurants used nearly 6 ounces of shrimp, although one in Chicago used almost a pound. Scallops are lower in cholesterol and can easily step in for shrimp in this and many other Chinese dishes. Otherwise, shrimp with garlic sauce

> # It Pays
> # to Be Curious
> ....
> Always ask the server how a dish is prepared before placing your order.

is still a Best Bite. It isn't perfect, but only a few of the dishes we analyzed—like stir-fried vegetables or Hunan tofu—are in its class.

The Bottom Line: *This is a good choice. Cut the cholesterol by ordering scallops instead of shrimp.*

HUNAN TOFU
(sometimes called braised bean curd or braised tofu; tofu stir-fried in a spicy sauce, often served with scallions; 910 calories and 28 grams of fat, 4 of them saturated)

Although this wasn't one of the most popular dishes at the restaurants we surveyed, we wanted to see how much fat and sodium were in an entrée that's popular with vegetarians. It is low in saturated fat and has no cholesterol. A typical order contains a pound of tofu and very few veggies. The amount of vegetables varied from none (a restaurant in San Francisco) to a modest 2½ ounces (one in Chicago).

The Bottom Line: *A good dish, but one that's crying out to be mixed with an order of steamed or stir-fried vegetables.*

HOUSE LO MEIN
(some combination of chicken, shrimp, beef, or pork, stir-fried with soft noodles and vegetables; 1,060 calories and 36 grams of fat, 7 of them saturated)

With 70 percent noodles and 10 percent vegetables, this dish is relatively low in saturated fat. That's because most of the meat is chicken—half the restaurants used no beef or pork at all. Still, house lo mein has more than 1,000 calories and more salt than any other Chinese item we analyzed. The average 3,460 milligrams of sodium is almost 1½ days' worth!

The Bottom Line: *This choice is sodium city. You could mix it with an order of steamed unsalted vegetables.*

BEEF WITH BROCCOLI
(sliced beef stir-fried with broccoli in a brown sauce; 1,180 calories and 46 grams of fat, 9 of them saturated)

The average order of beef with broccoli was made with more than a half pound of meat; one Chicago restaurant packed in a full pound of beef! And with 3,150 milligrams of sodium per order, it is well over the recommended daily quota of 2,400 mg. The good news is that the average dish also included over half a pound of broccoli.

The Bottom Line: *Ask the restaurant to prepare this dish with half as much beef and twice as much broccoli as usual.*

CHICKEN CHOW MEIN
(chicken with Chinese vegetables like bean sprouts, carrots, Chinese cabbage, mushrooms, onions, and water chestnuts; 1,010 calories and 32 grams of fat, 10 of them saturated)

Fifty-five percent veggies and 30 percent chicken is our kind of dish. But forget about those fried noodles that are served to put on top. (We didn't include them in our analyses. Ditto for the non-fried lo mein noodles we were served in San Francisco restaurants. Each ½ cup serving adds 120 calories to your dish.)

The Bottom Line: *Enjoy this veggie and chicken combination, but if you can't resist temptation, ask the server to leave the fried noodles in the kitchen.*

Balancing Act
··················

Cut fat and calories by asking the kitchen to use twice as many vegetables and half as much meat as usual in your entrée.

HOUSE FRIED RICE
(some combination of chicken, shrimp, beef, or pork and egg, stir-fried with rice; 1,480 calories and 50 grams of fat, 10 of them saturated)

Get Steamed
••••••••••••••••••••
Whenever possible, order dumplings steamed rather than fried. And always opt for steamed rice in place of fried rice.

If you're watching your weight, think twice before ordering this 1,500-calorie dish. (Most people should eat only 2,000 calories in an entire day.) You probably don't think of cholesterol when you think of fried rice, but only moo shu pork has more. When we dissected the rice, it was clear why: an average of one egg per order. (One Chicago and one San Francisco restaurant used two eggs per order.) The rest of the cholesterol came from the combination of pork, beef, chicken, and shrimp—around a quarter of a pound in total.

The Bottom Line: *Some restaurants automatically serve house fried rice with entrées, especially at lunchtime. But as the numbers here show, you're better off with steamed rice.*

GENERAL TSO'S CHICKEN
(flour-coated chicken, stir-fried in a spicy sauce; 1,600 calories and 59 grams of fat, 11 of them saturated)

Although every version of General Tso's chicken we analyzed contained some veggies, most of the dish was little more than chicken, oil, and flour or batter. (Two Chicago restaurants batter-coated the chicken before frying it.) That's why it packs more than 1,600 calories. The general's 3,150 milligrams of sodium easily exceeds your 2,400 milligram daily limit.

The Bottom Line: *Order a dish that has unbreaded chicken like Szechuan chicken, chicken with vegetables, or chicken with garlic sauce.*

ORANGE (CRISPY) BEEF

(flour-coated beef, stir-fried in a spicy orange sauce; 1,770 calories and 66 grams of fat, 11 of them saturated)

Expect a huge amount of meat (three-quarters of a pound, on average) and a few veggies. Only one restaurant, in San Francisco, served the same amount of vegetables as beef. Eighty percent of the fat comes from the oil used to fry the beef. All told, you get 1,770 calories, more than a day's sodium, a day's fat and cholesterol, and half a day's saturated fat in one order.

The Bottom Line: *Order something else. If you must have a beef dish, opt for beef with broccoli, which has fewer calories and a lot more vegetables.*

MOO SHU PORK

(shredded pork stir-fried with vegetables and eggs, served with thin pancakes and hoisin sauce for wrapping; 1,230 calories and 64 grams of fat, 13 of them saturated)

There's no reason for moo shu pork to be this fatty. After all, the average order has three times more vegetables than pork. Some of the fat comes from the pork; some comes from the generous quantity of oil used in the stir-fry. The average order also contains 465 milligrams of cholesterol, which is about a day and a half's worth.

The Bottom Line: *Moo shu pork without the egg is a decent choice, but it can become a better one if you order moo shu vegetables without the egg instead. That should cut the saturated fat and cholesterol. To keep the sodium down, use a thin smear of hoisin sauce (260 milligrams of sodium per tablespoon) on the pancake.*

SWEET AND SOUR PORK

(batter-dipped, deep-fried pork stir-fried with pineapple and vegetables; 1,610 calories and 71 grams of fat, 13 of them saturated)

The best thing you can say about sweet and sour pork is that it's not loaded with sodium. In fact, at 820 milligrams, it was the only Chinese dish that clocked in under 2,000 milligrams! That's probably because much of its flavor comes from a load of sugar. There was a modest amount of vegetables, an average of about half a cup per order. This dish hits 1,600 calories and two-thirds of a day's saturated fat. The real problem here is the breading, which soaks up an incredible amount of oil. With the exception of an order from one restaurant in San Francisco, every batch of sweet and sour pork we analyzed contained more breading than pork!

The Bottom Line: *No amount of adjusting will make this good enough to eat. Skip it.*

KUNG PAO CHICKEN
(diced chicken stir-fried with peanuts in hot pepper sauce; 1,620 calories and 76 grams fat, 13 of them saturated)

Nuts. That's how a chicken dish could end up with 76 grams of fat, more than any dish we analyzed, and 1,620 calories. The average order contained nearly a quarter-pound (¾ cup) of peanuts. Two restaurants in Washington added more than a half pound each. That's 115 grams of fat—almost two days' allowance—and 1,360 calories. And where did 275 milligrams of cholesterol (almost an entire day's worth) come from? The average order had three-quarters of a pound of chicken. (One Chicago restaurant used a pound and a half.) Although most places included a decent amount of vegetables (5 to 12 ounces), two restaurants in Washington and one in San Francisco added only an ounce or so.

The Bottom Line: *You'd be better off ordering chicken chow mein, Szechuan chicken, or chicken with vegetables.*

Good Fortune
••••••••••••••••••

One fortune cookie has only 30 calories and no fat.

When Your Favorite Is Not on the List

The dishes we tested represent only a small sampling of what's on the average Chinese menu. "What about lemon chicken?" you ask. Or twice-cooked pork? Or beef with oyster sauce? Or pot sticker dumplings? Your best bet for sizing up a dish we haven't covered is to ask the server how it is prepared. Ask what the pot stickers are stuffed with and find out whether they're fried or steamed. Inquire if any vegetables are included in the beef with oyster sauce. We covered other popular dishes, like egg drop soup and orange chicken, in chapter 17, Shop Till You Drop: Mall Food, page 329.

Decoding a Chinese Menu

Understanding a few terms that commonly appear on menus at Chinese restaurants will enable you to make healthier choices:

• **Crispy** means fried. Typically, the ingredients are coated with breading or batter before frying.

• **Twice-cooked pork** may very well mean twice-*fried* pork. Although some restaurants boil the meat, then stir-fry it, some use an oil bath for both steps.

• Don't assume that a **tofu** dish will be low in fat, or even vegetarian. Tofu is sometimes deep-fried and often is served with pork or other meats.

Chinese Strategy

• **Look for a "light" menu.** Some Chinese restaurants offer a small selection of "light," "diet," or "low-cal and low-fat" items. Although the nutritional claims for them may not be exact, these dishes will generally be better for you than the rest of the menu.

Chinese Condiments

The three condiments most likely to be on your table at a Chinese restaurant are duck sauce (also known as plum sauce), hoisin, and soy sauce.

Duck sauce, a thick, sweet-and-sour concoction made from plums, apricots, sugar, and seasonings, is often served as a dipping sauce for egg rolls. It has the least sodium of the three sauces (100 milligrams per tablespoon). Second in the sodium hierarchy is **hoisin sauce** (260 milligrams per tablespoon), a thick, dark mixture of fermented soybean paste, garlic, sugar, chiles, and spices, which is primarily used as a glaze in cooking and also serves as a flavorful spread for the pancakes served with moo shu pork. You'll encounter the most sodium in a tablespoon of **soy sauce** (1,000 milligrams)—even a lite one (600 milligrams). There are always bottles of this sauce on the tables at Chinese restaurants, as it's used not only in cooking but also as a flavoring and dipping sauce at the table.

• **Ask for adjustments.** Speak up and request less oil, more vegetables and less meat, or fewer calorie-laden nuts. Most kitchens will be happy to accommodate special requests if they can. Also ask for no MSG, but keep in mind that in some restaurants the sauces are already prepared, so you may get MSG regardless of the waiter's promises. It's still worth asking, though, to send the restaurant a message that you'd prefer your food MSG-free.

• **Eat brown rice instead of white rice.** Whenever possible, it's a good idea to order brown rice instead of white. It's higher in fiber, magnesium, and vitamin B6, and it's the only rice that has vitamin E.

- **Choose healthy ingredients.** Make a habit of ordering vegetables, seafood, and poultry rather than red-meat dishes, especially if you are trying to eat less saturated fat and fewer calories.

- **Forget about deep-fried foods.** Opt for more healthful steamed, braised, or stir-fried foods instead of deep-fried choices.

- **Get steamed or stir-fried vegetables.** You can mix extra vegetables with an entrée and turn it into two (or more) lower-fat meals. Share these "stretched" dishes with friends at your table, or take home what's left for tomorrow's lunch or dinner.

- **Stick with steamed rather than fried rice.** You'll help keep cholesterol and calories to a minimum by ordering plain steamed rice with main courses. The fried version is usually made with eggs and meat or poultry.

- **Skip the fried noodles.** Ask the kitchen to hold the fried noodles that are often served with soup or chow mein. If you can't resist, sprinkle only a few of the noodles over your food.

- **Cut back on the nuts.** If you choose a dish that contains nuts—kung pao chicken, for instance—ask that the chef use fewer nuts to cut back on the calories.

- **Think fork, not spoon.** Sauces are a primary source of fat and sodium in Chinese food. You can leave more of the sauce behind on the serving plate by using your fork or chopsticks to transfer morsels of food into your rice bowl, then eating out of the bowl.

• **Ask for a doggie bag.** Most Chinese entrées have at least 1,000 calories. Take some home and you won't have to think about tomorrow's lunch.

The numbers in the following chart reflect what you'd get if you ate an *entire* dinner-size take-out order of each dish. Other than the egg roll, the hot and sour soup, house lo mein, and house fried rice, the numbers include a typical 1⅓ cups of steamed rice. Dishes are ranked from best to worst—that is, from least to most saturated fat. We didn't test for *trans* fat, but the saturated fat numbers wouldn't change much, since Chinese restaurants typically fry in oil, not *trans*-laden shortening. Entrées marked with a ✔ are Best Bites. Best Bites are relatively low in saturated fat and rich in vegetables.

Reminder

Recommended limits for a 2,000-calorie diet:

Total fat: 65 grams
Saturated fat: 20 grams
Cholesterol: 300 milligrams
Sodium: 2,400 milligrams

CHINESE FOODS Menu Item	Calories	Total Fat (g)	Saturated Fat (g)	Cholesterol (mg)	Sodium (mg)
APPETIZERS					
Hot and sour soup (1 cup)	110	4	1	130	1,090
Egg roll (1)	190	11	1	5	460
ENTRÉES (includes 1⅓ cups of rice, except house lo mein and house fried rice)					
✔ Szechuan shrimp (3½ cups)	930	19	2	335	2,460
✔ Stir-fried vegetables (4½ cups)	750	19	3	0	2,150

CHINESE FOODS (continued)

Menu Item	Calories	Total Fat (g)	Saturated Fat (g)	Cholesterol (mg)	Sodium (mg)
✔ Shrimp with garlic sauce (3½ cups)	950	27	4	305	2,950
✔ Hunan tofu (4½ cups)	910	28	4	0	2,320
House lo mein (4½ cups)	1,060	36	7	175	3,460
✔ Beef with broccoli (4 cups)	1,180	46	9	230	3,150
✔ Chicken chow mein (5 cups)	1,010	32	10	205	2,450
House fried rice (4½ cups)	1,480	50	10	345	2,680
General Tso's chicken (4½ cups)	1,600	59	11	340	3,150
Orange (crispy) beef (4½ cups)	1,770	66	11	295	3,140
Moo shu pork (4 cups)	1,230	64	13	465	2,590
Sweet and sour pork (3½ cups)	1,610	71	13	120	820
Kung pao chicken (4½ cups)	1,620	76	13	275	2,610

Use Your Noodle: Italian Restaurants

When it comes to ethnic eating in America, Italian food, together with Mexican and Chinese food, are what the restaurant industry calls the "Big Three." In addition to their popularity, these cuisines share something else—a loss of authenticity that with time has transformed some once-healthful traditional specialties into ones you should think twice about before ordering. The best way to enjoy a terrific Italian meal these days is to take your cues from the past.

The Italian food most Americans have grown up eating in restaurants has its roots in the cuisine of southern Italy, which is bolder, more highly seasoned, and has less meat, cheese, and cream sauce than northern fare. It evolved from traditional peasant food that made the best and most delicious use of inexpensive, readily available ingredients. Vegetables, including familiar favorites like tomato, eggplant, peppers, and artichoke, were served in season. Fresh seafood was caught and savored the same day. Sauces, whether fresh and uncooked or slow simmered until the flavors melted into one another, always included a splash of olive oil to add an extra dimension to the taste. Seasonings such as fresh basil, capers, oregano, lemon, and olives lent their zesty, lively flavors. Meat, expensive and far from abundant, was enjoyed on the occasional feast day or used in small quantities as a flavoring rather than as a main dish—a tradition that continues today in Italian home cooking. And flavorful cheeses were used sparingly but to great effect as a garnish rather than as the focus of a dish. From humble ingredients came a great cuisine. The Italian way of eating has become one of the world's most beloved.

Americans adore Italian food. It is a cuisine that wraps its arms around diners with bold, fresh flavors. Over the years, however, something has been lost in the translation. For many people, Italian food has become veal smothered in mozzarella, fettuccine coated with cream-and-cheese sauce, and lasagnas oozing with fatty meat and cheese. And our servings are far larger than is customary in Italy. Nothing could be further removed from the light, fresh preparations for which southern Italy is noted.

You can still find the basic components of low-fat, healthful eating in most Italian restaurants; you just need to choose carefully. If you opt for pasta with marinara, clam, or even meat sauce (forget the cream and cheese sauces) and add a salad of dark, leafy greens and fresh vegetables, you can have a delicious, healthy, and truly Italian meal.

The Dishes and the Data

We bought dinner-size take-out portions of 3 popular appetizers and 13 entrées from 21 midprice Italian restaurants in Chicago, New York, and San Francisco. (For more on our methodology, see pages 12–14.) We chose independent restaurants rather than chains like The Olive Garden because more than three-quarters of the country's Italian restaurants are independently owned. (However, The Olive Garden provides numbers on its healthy meals, which are found on a separate chart on page 133.) We didn't do pizza because it's more like fast food. It's covered in chapter 7, Any Way You Slice It: Pizzerias, page 135.

Within each category, we've listed the dishes from best to worst—that is, from least to most saturated fat. We did not test for *trans* fat; if we had, the saturated-fat numbers would be higher than those indicated.

Appetizers

FRIED CALAMARI
(1,040 calories and 70 grams of fat, 9 of them saturated)

Although most of the 1,000-plus calories and 70 grams of fat in an average 3-cup portion of fried calamari comes from the breading and deep frying, you can thank the squid itself for the whopping amount of cholesterol. The 925 milligrams of cholesterol in this dish are a three-day supply, or about what you'd get in a four-egg omelette. The restaurants told us that a portion serves just one, but even a half-portion is enough to make your arteries howl. When your appetizer packs 1,000 calories, your hips and paunch don't have a fighting chance.

The Bottom Line: *Don't order this unless you're dining out with a crowd of friends and can share the calorie and cholesterol burden.*

GARLIC BREAD
(820 calories and 40 grams of fat, 10 of them saturated)

Most restaurants consider an 8-ounce serving to be an order for one, so that's what our chart lists. But the equivalent of eight slices of Wonder bread seems extreme to us. The 40 grams of fat come from the olive oil (3 tablespoons) or butter (almost half a stick) and, in some restaurants, from the Parmesan cheese sprinkled on top.

The Bottom Line: *Order plain Italian bread instead and stop at one or two slices. If you're in a restaurant that brings olive oil to the table for dipping, dip lightly. Whether the olive oil is regular or extra-virgin, it will have 120 calories per tablespoon.*

ANTIPASTO
(630 calories and 47 grams of fat, 15 of them saturated)

Here's an appetizer that gives new meaning to the word *"Mangia!"* Its long list of components generally includes assorted meats like salami, mortadella, prosciutto, ham, and pepperoni; cheeses like provolone and mozzarella; and marinated vegetables, olives, hard-boiled eggs, lettuce, and tomato, all topped off with olive oil or other dressing. We estimate that if you eat the whole lolla-palooza (all 1½ pounds worth!) by yourself, you'll end up with three-quarters of the fat and saturated fat and all—or more—of the sodium you should eat in an entire day.

The Bottom Line: *Share the plate with three friends. Get the oil and vinegar or other dressing on the side and use just a touch. Ask the kitchen to go lightly on the meats and cheeses and heavy on vegetables, like peppers, olives, chickpeas, and kidney beans.*

Main Dishes

SPAGHETTI WITH MARINARA SAUCE
(850 calories and 17 grams of fat, 4 of them saturated)

Spaghetti with marinara (or just tomato) sauce is a winner be-cause it's low in saturated fat. The problem is that it's got 850 calories. It's the generous portion of pasta—3½ cups—that piles

---

Pillars of Salt
....

Italian restaurants are no different from others when it comes to sodium. It's nearly always a problem. You can replace a fatty dish with a lower-fat one, but no matter what you choose, chances are it's already been liberally salted or made with high-sodium sauces, meats, or cheeses. And there's virtually no way you can subtract the sodium. Most restaurant entrées have at least 1,500 milligrams, which makes it tough to stay below the recommended 2,400-milligram limit for the whole day.

the calories on. Then again, when it comes to restaurant meals, you could do a lot worse than 850 calories. And the tomato sauce is rich in lycopene, a carotenoid that may help cut the risk of prostate cancer. So overall, this one's a go.

The Bottom Line: *The best choice.*

LINGUINE WITH RED CLAM SAUCE
(890 calories and 23 grams of fat, 4 of them saturated)

This popular dish has only 4 grams of saturated fat. That's pretty hard to beat. But it serves up almost a day's sodium (2,180 milligrams). And, like other bountiful pasta dishes, the calories approach 900. Just make sure you start out with a salad (and light dressing) rather than half a loaf of garlic bread for an appetizer.

The Bottom Line: *A decent dish for seafood fans.*

LINGUINE WITH WHITE CLAM SAUCE
(910 calories and 29 grams of fat, 5 of them saturated)

The sauce for this Italian restaurant favorite, which is typically made with clams, olive oil, garlic, and sometimes white wine, has only 5 grams of saturated fat. It lacks some of the nutrients in its tomato-based counterpart, but it's a good alternative if you're looking for a change of pace from red sauce.

The Bottom Line: *A popular classic worth ordering.*

CHICKEN MARSALA
(460 calories and 25 grams of fat, 7 of them saturated; with a side order of spaghetti, 870 calories and 33 grams of fat, 9 of them saturated)

Surely the skinless chicken breasts or the mushrooms that are the basis of this relatively uncomplicated dish can't be to blame for all that fat? They're not. The sauce, which also has marsala wine in it, is made with butter or oil. And although the calories

(460) are far lower than any other Italian dish that we analyzed, most people get a side order of spaghetti to round out the meal. That would put its calories and saturated fat in line with a plate of spaghetti with meat sauce.

The Bottom Line: *Ask the kitchen to go easy on this rich sauce. If you're watching your weight, consider replacing the side of spaghetti with a side of vegetables or a salad (but only if you get light dressing).*

SPAGHETTI WITH MEAT SAUCE
(920 calories and 25 grams of fat, 7 of them saturated)

Often called Bolognese on menus, this meat and tomato sauce has nearly 50 percent more fat than marinara or tomato sauce. As restaurant dishes go, this one's not too fatty because the high proportion of pasta overwhelms the 3 to 4 ounces of greasy ground meat in the sauce.

The Bottom Line: *A satisfying choice for meat lovers who don't want to overdo it on the fat front.*

SPAGHETTI WITH SAUSAGE
(1,040 calories and 39 grams of fat, 10 of them saturated)

Because it contains three times more pasta than fatty Italian sausage (sometimes sliced into chunks, other times served as links), this dish is better for you than you might expect. Even so it'll cost you more than 1,000 calories and 2,400 milligrams of sodium.

The Bottom Line: *Order the sausage with marinara or tomato sauce rather than meat sauce.*

SPAGHETTI WITH MEATBALLS
(1,160 calories and 39 grams of fat, 10 of them saturated)

Between the meatballs and the meat sauce, you can expect a third more meat on your plate than you'd get by ordering spaghetti with meat sauce alone.

The Bottom Line: *No need to gild the lily by eating a meat sauce on meatballs. Do your arteries a favor and ask the kitchen to top the meatballs with a marinara meatless tomato sauce. Save half for tomorrow.*

CHEESE RAVIOLI
(620 calories and 26 grams of fat, 11 of them saturated)
Much of the saturated fat here comes from the 3 ounces of ricotta cheese filling in these square pillows of pasta served in marinara or tomato sauce. That's half a day's worth, but still one-third less than what you'd get in an order of cheese manicotti.

The Bottom Line: *A reasonable choice for people watching their weight, since it has about half the calories of a dish like spaghetti with meatballs.*

VEAL PARMIGIANA
(650 calories and 36 grams of fat, 12 of them saturated; with a side order of spaghetti, 1,060 calories and 44 grams of fat, 14 of them saturated)
You may think veal is heart-healthy, but think again. This entrée contains half of a day's fat, saturated fat, and cholesterol. Remember, anything *parmigiana* is going to be dipped in egg and milk, breaded, sautéed in oil or butter, topped with marinara sauce, and usually smothered with fatty melted cheese. Our average order was less than half veal; the rest was cheese and oil-soaked breading. Add a typical 1½ cup side order of spaghetti with marinara or tomato sauce, and the calories climb to over 1,000. (And all that is aside from the deplorable way in which most veal calves are raised.)

The Bottom Line: *Ask for veal parmigiana without the traditional mozzarella topping and you'll lose more than half the saturated fat.*

EGGPLANT PARMIGIANA
(800 calories and 54 grams of fat, 14 of them saturated; with a side order of spaghetti, 1,210 calories and 62 grams of fat, 14 of them saturated)

Did you think this vegetable dish was healthful? Would you just assume it's a better choice than veal parmigiana? Unfortunately, eggplant soaks up oil like a sponge. That's one reason the calories hit 800. A quarter of the fat here comes from the mozzarella cheese topping, the rest from the oil used to fry the breaded eggplant.

The Bottom Line: *Ask the kitchen to hold the mozzarella and you'll cut more than half the saturated fat.*

CHEESE MANICOTTI
(700 calories and 38 grams of fat, 17 of them saturated)

On average, we found almost half a pound of ricotta cheese stuffed inside and draped over the surface of these big tubes of pasta. That's enough to supply over three-quarters of your daily saturated fat quota. Our samples were served in marinara or tomato sauce, but some restaurants use béchamel, a creamy white sauce, which is even fattier.

The Bottom Line: *Skip the cheese topping and you'll avoid a quarter of the saturated fat.*

LASAGNA
(960 calories and 53 grams of fat, 21 of them saturated)

An average 2-cup serving of one of America's favorite Italian dishes charges you a day's saturated fat. That's what happens when you layer roughly a quarter pound of ground beef with one-third pound of ricotta and mozzarella cheese between wide, flat lasagna noodles. You'd have to eat two McDonald's Big Macs to get this much saturated fat.

The Bottom Line: *There's not much you can do to make this better, although skipping the melted cheese on top would certainly be a step in the right direction.*

FETTUCCINE ALFREDO
(1,500 calories and 97 grams of fat, 48 of them saturated)

This is truly a heart attack on a plate. A single serving of these sauce-drenched ribbons of pasta contains as much saturated fat as *two and a half pints* of Breyers Butter Pecan Ice Cream! What else would you expect from a dish loaded with cream, butter, Parmesan cheese, and, in a third of the restaurants we

Olive Gardening
■■■■■■■■■■■■■■■■■■■■■■■■■■■■■■■■■■■■■■■

Our survey of Italian food focused on independent operations because there's really only one heavyweight Italian restaurant chain—The Olive Garden, which has 460-plus outlets. (Its closest competitor, Romano's Macaroni Grill, has one-third as many restaurants.) Owned by Darden Restaurants, which also operates seafood-restaurant giant Red Lobster, The Olive Garden rang up $1.55 billion in sales in 2000. That's a lot of linguine!

On its menu, The Olive Garden designates four dinner entrées as "Garden Fare." The company says that those selections meet the FDA's guidelines for the definition of a low-fat main dish—that is, they contain no more than 30 percent of calories from fat and 3 grams of fat or less per 100 grams (3½ ounces) of food.

To its credit, The Olive Garden offers soup or salad with all entrées. (Its minestrone soup is the soup that is lowest in fat.) And its Chicken Giardino is one of the lowest-calorie restaurant entrées we've seen. The company provides nutrition information for its "Garden Fare" menu item on its Web site and on the menu, and we have included the numbers for dinner-size portions of these dishes in the chart on page 133. (Not shown are the numbers for the smaller portions of those entrées, which are on the lunch menu.)

visited, eggs? Fettuccine Alfredo's 48 grams of saturated fat are more than twice your daily limit. For the 97 grams of fat in a single serving of fettucine Alfredo, you could take total leave of your senses and gobble up an entire Domino's large Hand Tossed Pepperoni Pizza.

The Bottom Line: *If you are planning on ordering this, or its close relative spaghetti alla carbonara, make sure your cardiologist is on call.*

Decoding an Italian Menu

Understanding a few crucial terms that are common to Italian cooking (and menus) will enable you to make healthier choices at a restaurant.

Alfredo as part of a dish's name is the tipoff that it will be served with a very rich sauce made with cream, butter, cheese, and possibly eggs—in other words, it will be extremely high in fat. Equally high-fat **carbonara** (think spaghetti alla carbonara) refers to a pasta sauce made with cream, eggs, Parmesan cheese, and small bits of pancetta (Italian bacon).

Frito means "fried." **Frito misto** literally means "mixed fried" and is the name of a dish that usually consists of small pieces of batter-dipped, deep-fried meat or vegetables. **Frito misto di mare** is an assortment of seafood prepared in the same manner.

Griglia means "grilled." Although grilled dishes may not be fat-free, they are probably more healthful than other options.

Pancetta is Italian bacon. It is made from the same part of the pig as American-style bacon, but it is salted and lightly spiced rather than smoked. Pancetta is generally used in small quantities as a flavoring. As a result, the presence of pancetta probably won't appreciably increase a dish's fat and sodium content.

Parmigiana (or the term "alla parmigiana") denotes a dish in which a cutlet—usually veal, chicken, or eggplant—is dipped in a mixture of egg and milk, coated with bread crumbs, sautéed in oil or butter, and topped with marinara or tomato sauce. Quite often it is also smothered with a fatty blanket of mozzarella. Dishes alla parmigiana are usually high in calories and fat.

Pesto is an uncooked sauce traditionally made with fresh basil, garlic, pine nuts, Parmesan or pecorino cheese, and olive oil. It does not pose the same risk to your arteries as a cream sauce, but it's still high in calories.

Polenta is basically cornmeal mush. The cooked mixture of water and cornmeal is usually allowed to cool, then cut into pieces. Although you could easily make low-fat polenta at home, chances are restaurants add quite a bit of butter and cheese to theirs. Sometimes they also fry or sauté slices so they're crisp.

Primavera means "spring" in Italian. A primavera sauce traditionally contains a medley of fresh vegetables, ideally the tender young vegetables of spring. But be careful. Italian dishes made alla primavera ("springtime style") may not be as light and healthful as you expect. Instead of getting vegetables in a light marinara sauce, you might find them swimming in an ocean of fatty cream. Ask the server before you order.

Vitello is veal. Although certain cuts of veal are lean, restaurants frequently serve veal in fatty preparations. For veal **scaloppine,** thin slices of pounded veal are dredged in flour and sautéed in oil or butter. **Saltimbocca** is usually made by topping thin slices of veal with a slice of prosciutto and a sprinkling of sage, folding or rolling them together, then flouring the meat and sautéeing it in butter and/or oil. **Vitello tonnato** is a dish of sliced, cold, roasted veal topped with a sauce of puréed tuna, anchovies, capers, lemon juice, and olive oil.

Italian Strategy

• **Choose the right bread.** All breads are not equal. Garlic bread, for example, is five times higher in fat than plain Italian bread or breadsticks.

• **Start with soup or salad.** Fill up on a broth-based soup like minestrone or a side salad with light dressing before your main course. Healthful starters like these will make you feel full, so you will be less likely to overindulge on less healthful entrées.

• **Eat pasta.** What rice does for Chinese food and a big sub or hoagie roll does for a sandwich, pasta does for an Italian meal: It adds filling, low-fat volume and crowds out the saturated fat in your meal. Many Italian restaurants routinely add a side order of spaghetti with marinara or tomato sauce to nonpasta entrées. If you split this side order of pasta and a fatty splurge like eggplant parmigiana with a friend (or take half home for tomorrow), the 62 grams of fat is reduced to a more reasonable 31.

• **Select sauces wisely.** Order lean sauces with your pasta entrée. Choosing a marinara or tomato sauce, a red or white clam sauce, or a Bolognese sauce (made with a little ground beef) will help keep saturated fat levels admirably low. Steer clear of cream- and cheese-based sauces like Alfredo, which send the saturated fat soaring. And keep a sharp eye out on pesto. A tiny quarter-cup serving of Buitoni-brand pesto from the supermarket contains 24 grams of fat and 290 calories. Restaurant servings may well contain at least double that amount.

• **Eat your vegetables.** Veggies are an ideal choice as long as they aren't deep-fried. And Italian restaurants offer a range of vegetable options as side dishes, salads, and part of antipasti platters. Included on the menus of the restaurants whose food we analyzed were roasted or grilled portobello mushrooms, roasted red peppers, asparagus, spinach, broccoli, escarole, *insalata tricolore* (arugula, endive, and radicchio), green

---

Lighten Up!
••••••••••••••••

Always choose a light salad dressing. Every tablespoon of regular Italian dressing has nearly 100 calories.

beans, zucchini, and carrots. As always, be sure to ask the kitchen to go easy on the oil, serve the vinaigrette on the side, and hold the cheese.

• **Reduce the meat.** If you yearn for meatballs or sausage, ask that the meat be served with a marinara or tomato sauce, instead of meat sauce, to cut back on saturated fat and calories.

Count the Cheese
••••••••••••••••••••••••••

Many Italian restaurants offer diners freshly grated Parmesan cheese to sprinkle on their entrées. Add 2 grams of total fat and 1 gram of saturated fat for every tablespoon of Parmesan cheese you use. Use it to replace a thick layer of mozzarella and you come out ahead.

• **Control portions.** Italian restaurants are notorious for over-delivering, especially when it comes to pasta dishes. To protect your health from big servings that cry out *abbondanza* (abundance), be prepared to share with a friend, take leftovers home, or leave food on the plate.

Within each category, appetizers and entrées are ranked from best to worst—that is, from least to most saturated fat. We didn't test for *trans* fat. If we had, the saturated fat numbers would be higher than those indicated. Entrées marked with a ✔ are Best Bites. Best Bites are relatively low in saturated fat.

Reminder

Recommended limits for a 2,000-calorie diet:

Total fat: 65 grams
Saturated fat: 20 grams
Cholesterol: 300 milligrams
Sodium: 2,400 milligrams

ITALIAN DISHES

Menu Item	Calories	Total Fat (g)	Saturated Fat (g)	Cholesterol (mg)	Sodium (mg)
APPETIZERS AND SIDE DISHES					
✔ Spaghetti with marinara sauce (1½ cups)	410	8	2	15	700
Fried calamari (3 cups)	1,040	70	9	925	650
Garlic bread (8 oz.)	820	40	10	40	1,080
Antipasto (1½ lbs.)*	630	47	15	130	2,960
ENTRÉES					
✔ Spaghetti with marinara sauce (3½ cups)	850	17	4	30	1,450
✔ Linguine with red clam sauce (3 cups)	890	23	4	65	2,180
✔ Linguine with white clam sauce (3 cups)	910	29	5	110	1,880
✔ Chicken Marsala (10 oz.)	460	25	7	160	790
✔ with spaghetti with marinara sauce (1½ cups)	870	33	9	175	1,480
✔ Spaghetti with meat sauce (3 cups)	920	25	7	110	1,790
Spaghetti with sausage (2½ cups)	1,040	39	10	115	2,440
Spaghetti with meatballs (3½ cups)	1,160	39	10	165	2,210
Cheese ravioli (1½ cups)	620	26	11	115	1,290
Veal parmigiana (1½ cups)	650	36	12	210	1,350
with spaghetti with marinara sauce (1½ cups)	1,060	44	14	225	2,040

*The numbers for antipasto are estimates

ITALIAN DISHES *(continued)* Menu Item	Calories	Total Fat (g)	Saturated Fat (g)	Cholesterol (mg)	Sodium (mg)
Eggplant parmigiana (2½ cups)	800	54	14	170	1,300
with spaghetti with marinara sauce (1½ cups)	1,210	62	16	190	2,000
Cheese manicotti (1½ cups)	700	38	17	180	1,480
Lasagna (2 cups)	960	53	21	215	2,060
Fettuccine Alfredo (2½ cups)	1,500	97	48	420	1,030

All numbers have been provided by the company. Saturated-fat numbers do not include trans fat; if they did, some saturated fat numbers might be higher than those indicated. Within each category, appetizers and entrées are ranked from best to worst—that is, from least to most saturated fat. Entrées marked with a 4 are Best Bites. Best Bites are relatively low in saturated fat.

THE OLIVE "GARDEN FARE" DISHES Menu Item	Calories	Total Fat (g)	Saturated Fat (g)	Cholesterol (mg)	Sodium (mg)
APPETIZERS					
Minestrone soup	100	1	0	0	610
ENTRÉES (These numbers are for dinner-size entrées.)					
✔ Linguine alla Marinara	450	9	2	0	770
✔ Shrimp Primavera	630	13	2	275	1,220
✔ Chicken Giardino	460	8	3	60	1,180
✔ Cappellini Pomodoro	560	18	3	10	1,130

Chapter 7

Any Way You Slice It: Pizzerias

P izza has long been an American favorite, but in the past decade or so it has practically become a separate food group all its own. You can serve it to big kids and to little kids, to the meat-and-potatoes crowd, and to vegetarians. There's a pizza to suit every taste. You can order it with just cheese or pepperoni, or topped with everything from potatoes, pineapple, or pears to barbecue chicken, garlic shrimp, or roasted duck. (We even found a pizza topped with fried wontons!) Then there are the global touches, international accents like peanuts and sesame sauce, curry and chutney, or chilies and salsa. Even the crust rises above the ordinary—you can order a thin crust, hand-tossed crust, deep-dish crust, pan crust, stuffed crust, or practically no crust at all.

If you can't face cooking and don't feel like eating out, pizza is often the default. It's easy to see that pizza's greatest allure is that you can have it delivered right to your door. Plus, once the pie arrives, it serves more people for less money than virtually any other restaurant food.

According to *Restaurant Business,* we order 3 billion pies a year, most of them from the more than 60,000 pizzerias that operate out of strip malls and food courts and on Main Streets. And these pizza parlors are pervasive—one out of every six restaurants in the United State is a pizzeria. As a nation, we spend about $30 billion a year at pizza parlors, a figure that matches what we shell out at burger joints. (It's no coincidence that McDonald's now owns a pizza chain called Donatos.)

No one can dispute pizza's popularity, but when it comes to issues like health and nutrition, you'll typically hear at least two points of view. Many people consider pizza a junk food—period. On the other hand, some dietitians claim that pizza is a nutritious food because it has components from each of the four basic food groups. As American Dietetic Association spokesperson Connie Diekman explained to HealthScout News, an on-line consumer health site: "You get your grain in the crust; you get tomato sauce, which can count as your vegetable; a cheese, which is your dairy; and protein in many toppings."

Never mind that the typical serving of tomato sauce—about half a cup *per pizza*—isn't much "vegetable." The relevant question is: How many of our clogged arteries do we owe to this enormously popular Italian import? And, more to the point, is there any way to make pizza healthy?

Pizza Pitfalls

In reality, pizza can be healthful *or* junky, depending on how it's made. The greatest problem with pizza is saturated fat. And we're not just talking about the sausage, ground beef, or pepperoni toppings. Cheese is the prime culprit. And that's a problem, since to many people, pizza just isn't pizza without it.

Pizza has another drawback: It's high in salt. A typical two-slice serving of Domino's Hand Tossed Cheese Pizza has 880 milligrams of sodium, or one-third of a day's quota. And that's about as good as it gets. The same size serving of Papa John's Original Crust All the Meats Pizza approaches a full day's limit at 2,200 milligrams.

It pays to know what's in and on your pizza. Pizza makers range in size from large to small chains and also include independent local pizzerias, so it's not always easy for consumers to obtain nutrition information. But we found that the large chains such as Pizza Hut, Domino's, Little Caesars, and Papa John's have information on how much saturated fat, sodium, and other nutrients are in most of their pizzas, and they make the data available on their Web sites. Smaller, sit-down chains, such as California Pizza Kitchen and Pizzeria Uno, offer no numbers at all, nor do the thousands of independent local pizza parlors whose pies reflect regional preferences or a chef's whims rather than some national-chain formula.

The Dishes and the Data

To find out what big and not-so-big pizza makers are serving, we analyzed 15 popular types of pizzas purchased from 36 pizzerias in Chicago, Los Angeles, and Washington, D.C. The pizzerias ranged from major chains to smaller, sit-down chains, including Pizza Hut, Domino's, Little Caesars, Papa John's, California Pizza Kitchen, and Pizzeria Uno. (For more information on our methodology, see pages 12–14.)

The good news is that the nutritional numbers provided by the chains are pretty accurate (though, in some cases, companies serve less pizza than they advertise). The companies seem to have a good handle on what's between the crust and the mushrooms, especially considering that it's often a teenager who's the one sprinkling on the shredded cheese and green peppers. The bad news is that they're sprinkling on a lot more cheese than peppers. And that's a very real problem.

Here's a rundown of some of the most popular pizzas from some of the most popular chains. Just remember what you get depends on how much you eat. We ranked the pizzas from best to worst—that is, from least to most saturated fat.

Slice Size Matters

One slice is rarely enough, especially when chains like Pizza Hut cut most of their pies into 12 slices that each measure only 3½ inches at their widest.

How many slices is a *typical* serving? Since no one has good data for this, as a guide we used Pizza Hut's Personal Pan Cheese Pizza, which is meant to be eaten by one person. Since it weighs roughly 9 ounces, we calculated the number of whole slices of *cheese* pizza that came closest to 9 ounces. That gave us a serving size ranging from 2 to 4 slices each. In each case, the size was roughly one-quarter of a large (14-inch) pizza per person.

There were some exceptions. For California Pizza Kitchen, we used an entire pizza as a single serving because that's how it's usually served. And for Pizzeria Uno, we used half a pizza because the company's Web site says each regular pie serves two.

Obviously, no universal serving size applies to all people. So we have two charts, one showing pizza by the slice (so you can easily calculate your own typical serving) and the other by the typical serving.

DOMINO'S HAND TOSSED CHEESE PIZZA, MADE WITH "HALF THE CHEESE"

(2 slices have 480 calories and 12 grams of fat, 5 of them saturated)

Ironically, the pizza that's one of your best bets—a half-the-cheese pizza—doesn't officially exist on the menu at Domino's or any other chain. But Domino's cheese pizza is a good starting point because it has less saturated fat than most others. All you have to do is specify one adjustment when you order: Tell them you want only half the usual amount of cheese on your pizza. You'll need to make it very clear to the harried pizzeria order taker that you want half the usual cheese on *all* of your pizza, not the usual amount of cheese on only *half* of your pizza. It's a simple request for them to carry out.

Our "half-the-cheese" Domino's pizzas had anywhere from 15 percent to 75 percent less cheese than the chain's regular cheese pizzas. On average, that meant that a half-cheese serving had one-third less saturated fat. (Importantly, less cheese did not seem to make the pizza less enjoyable—after all, many people wouldn't be able to taste the difference between half-cheese and regular, especially if there were other toppings on it.) But even with less cheese, this pizza still leaves behind one-quarter of a day's saturated fat and sodium (800 milligrams) in a 2-slice serving. For pizza, that's not bad.

The Bottom Line: *If you keep it to two slices, this is one of your best choices.*

PIZZA HUT HAND TOSSED VEGGIE LOVER'S PIZZA
(3 slices have 550 calories and 14 grams of fat, 6 of them saturated)

As pizzas go, this is a good one. You get to savor a delicious mélange of onions, green peppers, mushrooms, tomatoes, and black olives. Even better, this tasty pizza is almost as low in saturated fat as a Domino's half-the-cheese pizza. That's because Pizza Hut adds less cheese to its Veggie Lover's pizzas than it does to regular cheese ones. (*Note:* Not all chains do this; see Domino's Hand Tossed Vegi Pizza.)

Although the chain's "pan" pizzas are its most popular, we decided to analyze the Hand Tossed Veggie Lover's since it had less fat than the Pan Veggie Lover's, according to the company. It's also worth remembering that regardless of type of crust, all of Pizza Hut's Veggie Lover's pizzas are consistently lowest in fat among Pizza Hut's pies. Thanks to those veggies, the Veggie Lover's pizzas are also highest in potentially beneficial phytochemicals and fiber. (Three slices had one-half of a cup of vegetables, not including tomato sauce.) Like most restaurant foods, the sodium in the pizza was a problem. Three slices have 1,420 milligrams of sodium, two-thirds of a day's worth.

The Bottom Line: *To cut the fat further, request half the cheese.*

DOMINO'S HAND TOSSED CHEESE PIZZA
(2 slices have 500 calories and 14 grams of fat, 8 of them saturated)

This is your typical ungussied-up cheese pizza. Eat 2 slices and you'll walk away with 500 calories and more than one-third of a day's worth of saturated fat and sodium.

The Bottom Line: *Any way you slice it, the best you can do here is order your pizza made with half the cheese so you end up with one-third less saturated fat.*

DOMINO'S HAND TOSSED VEGI PIZZA
(2 slices have 520 calories and 16 grams of fat, 8 of them saturated)

At Pizza Hut, a vegetable pizza has less saturated fat than a cheese pizza because the veggies replace some of the cheese. That's not so at Domino's, where the ingredients for its Vegi Pizza include onions, green peppers, mushrooms, olives . . . and *extra cheese.* Based on our analyses, however, the pizza makers at your local Domino's may not be that generous with the extra cheese. But why take a chance?

The Bottom Line: *Order all the vegetables you like, but make it very clear that you want less, not more, cheese on your Vegi Pizza.*

PAPA JOHN'S ORIGINAL CRUST CHEESE PIZZA
(2 slices have 560 calories and 20 grams of fat, 9 of them saturated)

Think of each Papa John's 2-slice serving as a Quarter Pounder plus another 150 calories. You'll also get a hefty 1,400 milligrams of sodium in those 2 slices—that's more than half a day's allowance.

The Bottom Line: *Order your pizza with half the cheese. Better yet, try Papa's Garden Special, which is flavorfully garnished with a combination of portobello mushrooms, onions, green peppers, and black olives.*

LITTLE CAESARS ROUND CHEESE PIZZA
(3 slices have 600 calories and 18 grams of fat, 10 of them saturated)

According to our analysis, equal amounts of Little Caesars Round Cheese Pizza and Papa John's Original Crust Cheese Pizza have about the same calorie and fat content, but both are better than Pizza Hut's Pan or Hand Tossed Cheese Pizza. To put this item in perspective, 3 slices are as bad for your waistline and heart as a corned beef sandwich from the deli.

The Bottom Line: *Do the right thing—order those slices with half the cheese.*

DOMINO'S HAND TOSSED PEPPERONI PIZZA
(2 slices have 560 calories and 20 grams of fat, 10 of them saturated)

Pepperoni is by far the most popular pizza topping. At Domino's, those thin rounds add an extra 60 calories, 2 grams of saturated fat, and 630 milligrams of sodium to a typical serving. If you think this pizza is a bargain, remember that 2 slices of pepperoni pizza are nearly the equivalent of two McDonald's Egg McMuffins. Still, the situation could be worse. Domino's also sells a Meatzza Pizza, which combines pepperoni, ham, sausage, and beef with extra cheese. It has 15 grams of saturated fat—50 percent more than the pepperoni pizza.

The Bottom Line: *If you must have meat on your pizza, your best bet is ham. According to Domino's, ham adds only about 30 calories and less than a gram of saturated fat to a 2-slice serving.*

DOMINO'S HAND TOSSED EXTRA CHEESE PIZZA
(2 slices have 560 calories and 20 grams of fat, 10 of them saturated)

It's no surprise that a sausage or a pepperoni pizza is fatty. But who would guess that ordering extra cheese on your pizza—but no meat—poses the same threat to your blood vessels? That's because the extra cheese pizza has as much saturated fat. It's not clear who orders extra cheese. Vegetarians who feel deprived because they don't eat meat? People who have to share a pizza with vegetarians? Or people who just can't get enough cheese? Whoever they are, it's a good bet that they mistakenly believe that the extra cheese isn't so bad.

The Bottom Line: *Never order an extra-cheese pizza. Instead, get into the habit of requesting only half the cheese on your usual cheese pizza. As a special treat, order a regular cheese pizza every once in a while—it may seem like an extra-cheese one.*

DOMINO'S HAND TOSSED ITALIAN SAUSAGE PIZZA
(2 slices have 600 calories and 22 grams of fat, 10 of them saturated)

Domino's sausage is no fattier than the pepperoni, and it's not as bad as the chain's bacon or beef toppings. But it's bad enough. Take a 2-slice serving of sausage pizza: How many of its 600 calories are going to end up as a spare tire where you least need it? How many of its 10 grams of saturated fat will take up residence in your arteries? A little sausage can add richness to a pasta, soup, or cassoulet. But adding sausage to a cheese-drenched pizza is overkill.

The Bottom Line: *If you can't live without sausage, at least order your pizza with half the usual amount of cheese.*

PIZZA HUT PAN CHEESE PIZZA
(3 slices have 630 calories and 27 grams of fat, 12 of them saturated)

This is the best-selling cheese pizza in America. Unfortunately, it is also one of the worst. A typical serving of this pizza has about one-third more saturated fat than a typical serving of cheese pizza at Domino's or Papa John's.

The Bottom Line: *Order your pizzas with half the cheese to trim the saturated fat.*

PIZZA HUT'S CHEESE PIZZAS

(Number of slices closest to 9 oz.)	Calories	Total Fat (g)	Saturated Fat (g)
Pan (3 slices)	630	27	*12*
Personal Pan (1 pizza)	630	28	12
Thin n' Crispy (3 slices)	540	24	14
Hand Tossed (3 slices)	650	27	14
The Big New Yorker (2 slices)	760	34	18
Stuffed Crust (2 slices)	890	38	20

Note: Saturated fat number in *italics* includes a small amount of artery-clogging *trans* fat.

PIZZA HUT PAN PEPPERONI PIZZA
(3 slices have 690 calories and 33 grams of fat, 13 of them saturated)

Think of each 3-slice serving of a Pizza Hut Pan Pepperoni Pizza as one and a half Swanson Hungry-Man Salisbury Steak dinners. And some folks don't stop at three. One of pizza's most convenient aspects is that it's often eaten family-style, which means different people can eat different amounts. But that convenience also means there's less portion control. It's not like unwrapping another burger—you can simply reach for another slice of pizza without realizing how many you've already eaten.

The Bottom Line: *If you like pepperoni, at least eat only two slices and add a salad to round out your meal.*

CALIFORNIA PIZZA KITCHEN ORIGINAL BBQ CHICKEN PIZZA
(1 pizza has 1,000 calories and 32 grams of fat, 14 of them saturated)

California Pizza Kitchen has traveled far beyond the borders of its namesake state. And its pizza, too, has ventured far afield from those pizza parlor warhorses—pepperoni, sausage, and mushrooms. You have to hunt hard to find an old standard among the more exotic choices such as Thai Chicken, Caramelized Pear & Gorgonzola, Grilled Garlic Shrimp, and Southwestern Chicken Burrito pizza. We analyzed only the top-seller, the Original BBQ Chicken Pizza, which is made with chicken, smoked gouda and mozzarella cheeses, sliced red onions, and cilantro. (Note that we analyzed the whole pizza because that is how the chain says it serves the pizza—one to a customer.)

If you ate equal amounts of the BBQ Chicken Pizza and Domino's, Pizza Hut's, or almost anyone's standard cheese pizza, the BBQ Chicken Pizza would have less saturated fat and fewer calories (although it's not quite as low as Domino's Hand Tossed half-the-cheese pizza or Pizza Hut's Hand Tossed Veggie Lover's). The problem is that many people eat the entire 14-ounce pizza, which weighs in at 1,000 calories, with three-quarters of a day's saturated fat.

Note: You can order any California Pizza Kitchen pizza with a crust made from "honey-wheat dough." It's only one-fourth whole wheat, but that's still more healthful for you than the usual white flour crust.

The Bottom Line: *Order your pizza with no cheese other than a sprinkling of Parmesan added before it goes into the pizza oven. (It will taste better than if you added it at the table.) Or split a pie and a Pizza Kitchen entrée-size salad (try the fat-free herb balsamic dressing). Or share a pizza and a simple pasta dish (steer clear of cream sauces and sausage on the pasta). If you're dining alone, have half the pizza wrapped to go.*

PIZZA HUT PAN ITALIAN SAUSAGE PIZZA
(3 slices have 750 calories and 39 grams of fat, 15 of them saturated)

At Pizza Hut, sausage is even fattier than pepperoni. Its extra fat pushes this doozy up to three-quarters of a day's worth of saturated fat and 750 calories. That's what happens when you layer a fatty meat over fatty cheese. Sure, some people crave meat. But they probably wouldn't order *four* Beef Soft Tacos at Taco Bell to satisfy that craving. That's about what you'll be getting if you eat 3 slices of this heartstopper.

The Bottom Line: *If you've got to have meat on your pizza, make it ham. Even pepperoni would be a better choice than sausage.*

PIZZA HUT STUFFED CRUST MEAT LOVER'S PIZZA
(2 slices have 830 calories and 42 grams of fat, 19 of them saturated)

The experts at Pizza Hut must sit around dreaming up new ways to cram fat and calories into their pizzas. They start with the brilliant Stuffed Crust concept. (You need cheese stuffed into a pizza crust like you need reverse liposuction to force more fat under your skin.) Then there's the "Meat Lover's" breakthrough. Pepperoni or sausage or ham or beef was enough to satisfy customers for decades—until Pizza Hut's marketing department ratcheted up the stakes. Why stop with just one meat when you can drown a pizza in pepperoni, sausage, ham, bacon, beef, and pork toppings? You'd be smart to avoid the entire "Lover's Line"—Pepperoni, Cheese, Sausage, and Meat—except for the Veggie Lover's. "Our Lover's Line pizzas pack on more of your favorite toppings!" boasts Pizza Hut's menu. They pack it on, all right—just where you need it least.

The Bottom Line: *There is no way to make this pizza healthful.*

PIZZERIA UNO CHICAGO CLASSIC
(4 slices have 1,500 calories and 74 grams of fat, 30 of them saturated)

The Chicago Classic is "the pizza that made us famous," proclaims Pizzeria Uno. "Extra sausage, extra cheese, extra tomato, extra crisp crust, and extra delicious." Extra dangerous is more like it. A "regular" pizza serves two, according to the company's Web site. Two teenage football players, maybe. How many people can shovel 1,500 calories and more than a day's saturated fat into their mouths and still stay upright? That's like eating *two* Pizza Hut Personal Pan Pizzas with Italian Sausage.

Pizzeria Uno says it invented the Deep Dish Pizza in Chicago in 1943. What a gift to humanity. This may explain why the Chicago Classics that we bought at Chicago-area Pizzeria Unos had nearly twice as much crust and meat as the pies we bought on the East and West coasts.

The Bottom Line: *Pizzeria Uno's Web site calls its pizzas "overfilled." That's what you'll be all right. Go to California Pizza Kitchen instead.*

Pizza Strategy

• **Order a half-the-cheese pizza.** This is an easy and tasty option at any pizzeria. Just be sure the server understands that you are requesting *half* the cheese on *all* of your pizza, not all the cheese on half of your pizza.

• **Request a no-cheese pizza.** Get over the notion that pizza isn't pizza unless it's smothered with cheese. Try ordering your pizza without any of the usual melted cheese. Instead, ask to have some Parmesan sprinkled over the sauce or a vegetable topping before the pizza goes into the oven. Another good option is California Pizza Kitchen's unusual but delicious Tricolore Salad Pizza. It's covered with arugula, radicchio, red-leaf lettuce, diced tomatoes, shaved Parmesan, and a vinaigrette dressing.

• **Avoid stuffed crust.** A cheese-stuffed crust is one of the fattiest types of crust.

• **Pick the right toppings.** Vegetables are your best bet because they're low in calories and rich in nutrients. Chicken and ham are also low in calories. Other meat toppings vary from chain to chain. But in general, pepperoni is leaner than pork, sausage, and beef.

• **Steer clear of combination pizzas.** More is definitely *much* more in these extravagantly unhealthy pizzas. They often have names like "supreme," "deluxe," "the works," or "extravaganzza."

• **Skip the extra cheese.** When you order a vegetable pizza, make sure that it doesn't come with the extra cheese that some chains automatically add.

• **Served with salad.** Smart eating is easier if you don't have a pizza-only meal. Pair a slice of pizza with a healthful side. Most sit-down pizza places now offer salads, soups, and some other decent choices. At home, even the least energetic cook can tear open a bag of salad greens or set out some baby carrots or sliced red or green pepper or cucumber with light ranch dressing as a dip. Or set out a plate of sliced melon such as honeydew, watermelon, or cantaloupe.

• **Beware of pizzeria sides.** You'd think that salad would be a good side dish to complement a pizza, but few take-out pizzerias offer it. Instead, they have extras like Buffalo wings, bread sticks, and cheesy bread. Just what you need to go with pizza crust and cheese—more bread and cheese! Each piece of cheesy bread from Domino's, for example, means another 140 calories and 2 grams of saturated fat. A typical order has 8 pieces, so 1 piece is the tip of the iceberg. Bread sticks aren't as fatty, but they still run more than 100 calories each. Wings are 50 calories a pop— but that's for less than an ounce of chicken, so the numbers add up quickly. It's fruit or vegetables, not bread or fried chicken, that you need to round out a pizza meal.

Reminder
Recommended limits for a 2,000-calorie diet:
Total fat: 65 grams
Saturated fat: 20 grams
Cholesterol: 300 milligrams
Sodium: 2,400 milligrams

The numbers in these charts were provided by the pizza chains, except for the 15 pizzas we had analyzed. Those are listed in **bold.** Pizzas are ranked from best to worst—that is, from least to most saturated fat. Those marked with a ✔ are Best Bites. Best Bites are relatively low in saturated fat when compared to their calorie content. That is, foods with more calories were allowed more saturated fat than those with fewer calories. Best Bites were given to typical servings of pizzas, not pizza by the slice. The Best Bites apply only if you eat the typical serving listed in the table. In other words, you can't eat unlimited quantities of any pizza even if it is a Best Bite.

The numbers in the first chart, By the Slice, are for 1 slice of most varieties of pizza. The numbers make pizza look good, but that's only because they're for 1 slice of a large pizza. What's more, a pizza may look good in this chart simply because it comes in small slices. For example, a slice from a pizza that's cut into 12 slices will be lower in calories and fat than a slice of that same pizza that's cut into 8 slices. But if you eat more of the smaller slices than the larger slices, you won't save any calories or fat. Use the chart on page 155 to find out what you'd get in a typical serving. If *your* typical serving is different, use this chart and multiply by the number of slices you eat.

In the Typical Serving chart, for each type of crust, we calculated a typical serving by estimating the number of slices of *cheese* pizza that came closest to weighing 9 ounces—the weight of a Pizza Hut Personal Pan Cheese Pizza. (We rounded up partial slices.) Then we used that number of slices as a serving for that crust, no matter how many toppings. Based on information from the companies, we used half a pizza for Pizzeria Uno and a whole pizza for California Pizza Kitchen.

BY THE SLICE **Pizza** (fraction of a pie; weight, if available)	Calories	Total Fat (g)	Saturated Fat (g)	Sodium (mg)
Little Caesars Deep Dish Cheese (1/12; 2 oz.)	140	5	2	280
California Pizza Kitchen Original BBQ Chicken (1/6; 2 oz.)	170	5	2	340
Pizza Hut Hand Tossed Veggie Lover's (1/12; 3 oz.)	180	5	2	470
Domino's Thin Crust Cheese (1/12; 3 oz.)	130	6	2	390
Domino's Thin Crust Ham (1/12)	140	6	2	490
Little Caesars Thin Crust Cheese (1/10; 3 oz.)	130	6	3	320
Pizza Hut Thin 'n Crispy Ham (1/12; 3 oz.)	150	6	3	550
Little Caesars Deep Dish Pepperoni (1/12; 3 oz.)	160	6	3	350
Pizza Hut Thin 'n Crispy Veggie Lover's (1/12; 4 oz.)	170	6	3	470
Pizza Hut Thin 'n Crispy Chicken Supreme (1/12; 4 oz.)	180	6	3	560
Little Caesars Round Cheese (1/10; 3 oz.)	200	6	3	330
Pizza Hut Hand Tossed Chicken Supreme (1/12; 4 oz.)	210	6	3	590
Domino's Hand Tossed Cheese, with half the cheese (1/6; 3 oz.)	240	6	3	400
Domino's Thin Crust Extra Cheese (1/12)	150	7	3	470
Little Caesars Round Pizza Veggie (1/10; 4 oz.)	190	7	3	500
Domino's Thin Crust Vegi (1/12)	160	8	3	490
Domino's Thin Crust Italian Sausage (1/12)	160	8	3	500
Domino's Thin Crust Deluxe (1/12)	160	8	3	510
Domino's Thin Crust Pepperoni (1/12)	160	8	3	510
Domino's Thin Crust Hawaiian (1/12)	160	8	3	540
Donatos Chicken Vegy Medley (1/8; 5 oz.)	240	10	3	750
Papa John's Original Crust Garden Special (1/8; 5 oz.)	280	10	3	710
Domino's Hand Tossed Cheese (1/8; 4 oz.)	250	7	4	440

BY THE SLICE (continued)

Pizza (fraction of a pie; weight, if available)

	Calories	Total Fat (g)	Saturated Fat (g)	Sodium (mg)
Pizza Hut Thin 'n Crispy Pepperoni (1/12; 3 oz.)	170	8	4	550
Little Caesars Round Pepperoni (1/10; 3 oz.)	200	8	4	460
Domino's Hand Tossed Vegi (1/8; 4 oz.)	260	8	4	480
Domino's Hand Tossed Ham (1/8)	270	8	4	690
Little Caesars Thin Crust Pepperoni (1/10; 2 oz.)	160	9	4	420
Domino's Thin Crust Beef (1/12)	160	9	4	490
Pizza Hut Pan Cheese (1/12; 3 oz.)	210	9	4	390
Domino's Thin Crust Bacon (1/12)	180	10	4	530
Domino's Thin Crust America's Favorite (1/12)	190	10	4	580
Domino's Thin Crust Extravaganzza (1/12)	190	10	4	620
Little Caesars Round Meatsa (1/10; 4 oz.)	220	10	4	570
Little Caesars Round Supreme (1/10; 4 oz.)	230	10	4	550
Pizza Hut Hand Tossed Pepperoni Lover's (1/12; 3 oz.)	230	10	4	570
Papa John's Original Crust Cheese (1/8; 4 oz.)	280	10	4	700
Pizza Hut Pan Pepperoni (1/12; 3 oz.)	230	11	4	540
Pizza Hut Pan Ham (1/12; 3 oz.)	240	11	4	550
Pizza Hut Pan Veggie Lover's (1/12; 4 oz.)	240	11	4	460
Pizza Hut Pan Chicken Supreme (1/12; 4 oz.)	240	11	4	530
Papa John's Thin Crust Garden Special (1/8; 4 oz.)	230	12	4	500
Papa John's Thin Crust Cheese (1/8; 3 oz.)	230	13	4	500
Pizza Hut Thin 'n Crispy Cheese (1/12; 3 oz.)	180	8	5	540
Pizza Hut Hand Tossed Cheese (1/12; 3 oz.)	220	9	5	590
Pizza Hut Hand Tossed Ham (1/12; 4 oz.)	240	9	5	730

BY THE SLICE *(continued)*

Pizza (fraction of a pie; weight, if available)	Calories	Total Fat (g)	Saturated Fat (g)	Sodium (mg)
Domino's Hand Tossed Extra Cheese (⅛; 4 oz.)	280	10	*5*	570
Domino's Hand Tossed Pepperoni (⅛; 4 oz.)	280	10	*5*	650
Pizza Hut Hand Tossed Supreme (1/12; 4 oz.)	240	11	5	660
Domino's Hand Tossed Italian Sausage (⅛; 4 oz.)	300	11	*5*	560
Domino's Hand Tossed Hawaiian (⅛)	310	11	5	770
Domino's Thin Crust Meatzza (1/12)	210	12	5	680
Pizza Hut Thin 'n Crispy Supreme (1/12; 4 oz.)	230	12	5	640
Pizza Hut Thin 'n Crispy Pepperoni Lover's (1/12; 3 oz.)	230	12	5	690
Pizza Hut Hand Tossed Pepperoni (1/12; 4 oz.)	250	12	5	720
Papa John's Original Crust Pepperoni (⅛; 5 oz.)	300	12	5	790
Domino's Hand Tossed Deluxe (⅛)	310	12	5	720
Pizza Hut Thin n' Crispy Pork (1/12; 3 oz.)	240	13	5	740
Pizza Hut Pan Italian Sausage (1/12; 3 oz.)	250	13	*5*	560
Pizza Hut Hand Tossed Super Supreme (1/12; 4 oz.)	260	13	5	770
Domino's Hand Tossed Beef (⅛)	310	13	5	690
Pizza Hut Thin 'n Crispy Super Supreme (1/12; 4 oz.)	250	14	5	760
Donatos Vegy (⅛; 6 oz.)	280	14	5	900
Papa John's Original Crust Sausage (⅛; 5 oz.)	320	14	5	880
Pizza Hut Pan Supreme (1/12; 4 oz.)	290	15	5	610
Pizza Hut Pan Pork (1/12; 4 oz.)	290	15	5	660
Donatos Hawaiian (⅛; 5 oz.)	310	15	5	890
Domino's Deep Dish Cheese (⅛; 5 oz.)	340	15	5	790
Papa John's Thin Crust Pepperoni (⅛; 3 oz.)	270	16	5	620

BY THE SLICE *(continued)*

Pizza (fraction of a pie; weight, if available)	Calories	Total Fat (g)	Saturated Fat (g)	Sodium (mg)
Pizza Hut Pan Super Supreme (1/12; 5 oz.)	310	16	5	710
Pizza Hut The Big New Yorker Ham (1/8; 6 oz.)	340	13	6	1,160
Pizza Hut Thin 'n Crispy Beef (1/12; 3 oz.)	240	14	6	680
Domino's Hand Tossed Bacon (1/8)	330	14	6	750
Pizza Hut Thin 'n Crispy Italian Sausage (1/12; 3 oz.)	260	15	6	730
Pizza Hut Hand Tossed Meat Lover's (1/12; 4 oz.)	290	15	6	820
Pizza Hut Hand Tossed Pork (1/12; 4 oz.)	290	15	6	830
Papa John's Original Crust The Works (1/8; 6 oz.)	340	15	6	940
Domino's Hand Tossed Extravaganzza (1/8)	350	15	6	890
Domino's Deep Dish Ham (1/8)	350	15	6	930
Pizza Hut Pan Beef (1/12; 4 oz.)	300	16	6	630
Pizza Hut Pan Pepperoni Lover's (1/1; 4 oz.)	300	16	6	690
Donatos Mariachi Beef (1/8; 5 oz.)	310	16	6	860
Papa John's Thin Crust Sausage (1/8; 4 oz.)	280	17	6	700
Pizza Hut Pan Meat Lover's (1/12; 4 oz.)	330	19	6	760
Pizza Hut The Big New Yorker Veggie Lovers' (1/8; 12 oz.)	450	22	6	1,340
Pizza Hut Hand Tossed Beef (1/12; 4 oz.)	300	15	7	800
Domino's Hand Tossed America's Favorite (1/8)	350	15	7	830
Pizza Hut Hand Tossed Italian Sausage (1/12; 4 oz.)	310	16	7	830
Pizza Hut The Big New Yorker Pepperoni (1/8; 6 oz.)	370	16	7	1,150
Pizza Hut Thin 'n Crispy Meat Lover's (1/12; 4 oz.)	280	17	7	830
Domino's Deep Dish Extra Cheese (1/8)	370	18	7	900
Pizzeria Uno Chicago Classic (1/8; 5 oz.)	380	18	7	730

BY THE SLICE *(continued)*

Pizza (fraction of a pie; weight, if available)	Calories	Total Fat (g)	Saturated Fat (g)	Sodium (mg)
Domino's Deep Dish Vegi (⅛)	380	18	7	930
Domino's Deep Dish Hawaiian (⅛)	390	18	7	1,020
Donatos Original Pepperoni (⅛; 4 oz.)	320	19	7	930
Domino's Deep Dish Deluxe (⅛)	390	19	7	960
Domino's Deep Dish Italian Sausage (⅛)	390	19	7	960
Domino's Deep Dish Pepperoni (⅛)	390	19	7	970
Papa John's Original Crust All the Meats (⅛; 6 oz.)	390	19	7	1,100
Papa John's Thin Crust The Works (⅛; 5 oz.)	320	20	7	870
Domino's Deep Dish Beef (⅛)	390	20	7	940
Domino's Hand Tossed Meatzza (⅛)	380	17	8	970
Pizza Hut Stuffed Crust Veggie Lover's (⅛; 7 oz.)	420	17	8	1,040
Pizza Hut Stuffed Crust Chicken Supreme (⅛; 7 oz.)	430	17	8	1,110
Donatos Serious Cheese (⅛; 4 oz.)	330	18	8	850
Domino's Deep Dish Bacon (⅛)	410	21	8	1,000
Donatos Classic Trio (⅛; 6 oz.)	360	22	8	960
Donatos Works (⅛; 6 oz.)	370	22	8	960
Donatos Founder's Favorite (⅛; 6 oz.)	380	22	8	1,350
Domino's Deep Dish Extravaganzza (⅛)	430	22	8	1,140
Pizza Hut The Big New Yorker Cheese (⅛; 6 oz.)	380	17	9	1,140
Pizza Hut Stuffed Crust Pepperoni (⅛; 6 oz.)	440	19	9	1,120
Domino's Deep Dish America's Favorite (⅛)	430	22	9	1,080
Papa John's Thin Crust All the Meats (⅛; 5 oz.)	390	26	9	1,050
Pizza Hut Stuffed Crust Cheese (⅛; 6 oz.)	450	19	10	1,090

BY THE SLICE *(continued)*

Pizza (fraction of a pie; weight, if available)

	Calories	Total Fat (g)	Saturated Fat (g)	Sodium (mg)
Pizza Hut Stuffed Crust Meat Lover's (⅛; 5 oz.)	420	21	*10*	1,330
Pizza Hut Stuffed Crust Pork (⅛; 6 oz.)	460	21	10	1,180
Pizza Hut Stuffed Crust Beef (⅛; 6 oz.)	470	22	10	1,140
Pizza Hut The Big New Yorker Supreme (⅛; 8 oz.)	450	23	10	1,350
Pizza Hut Stuffed Crust Italian Sausage (⅛; 6 oz.)	480	23	10	1,160
Domino's Deep Dish Meatzza (⅛)	460	24	10	1,220
Donatos Serious Meat (⅛; 6 oz.)	420	25	10	1,190
Pizza Hut The Big New Yorker Pork (⅛; 7 oz.)	470	25	10	1,470
Pizza Hut Stuffed Crust Supreme (⅛; 7 oz.)	490	23	11	1,230
Pizza Hut Stuffed Crust Super Supreme (⅛; 7 oz.)	510	25	11	1,370
Pizza Hut The Big New Yorker Beef (⅛; 7 oz.)	480	26	11	1,380
Pizza Hut Stuffed Crust Ham (⅛; 6 oz.)	400	22	12	1,190
Pizza Hut Stuffed Crust Pepperoni Lover's (⅛; 7 oz.)	530	26	13	1,410
Pizza Hut The Big New Yorker Sausage (⅛; 8 oz.)	570	33	14	1,620

Note: Saturated fat numbers in *italics* include a small amount of artery-clogging *trans* fat.

A TYPICAL SERVING

Pizza (typical serving; weight, if available)	Calories	Total Fat (g)	Saturated Fat (g)	Sodium (mg)
✔ Domino's Hand Tossed Cheese, with half the cheese (2 slices; 7 oz.)	480	12	5	800
✔ Pizza Hut Hand Tossed Veggie Lover's (3 slices; 9 oz.)	550	14	6	1,420
✔ Donatos Chicken Vegy Medley (2 slices; 10 oz.)	480	20	6	1,500
✔ Papa John's Original Crust Garden Special (2 slices; 11 oz.)	560	20	6	1,420
Domino's Hand Tossed Ham (2 slices)	540	16	7	1,380
Domino's Hand Tossed Cheese (2 slices; 7 oz.)	500	14	8	880
Domino's Hand Tossed Vegi (2 slices; 8 oz.)	520	16	8	960
Pizza Hut Thin n' Crispy Veggie Lover's (3 slices; 11 oz.)	510	18	8	1,410
Little Caesars Deep Dish Cheese (4 squares; 9 oz.)	560	20	8	1,120
Papa John's Original Crust Cheese (2 slices; 8 oz.)	560	20	9	1,440
Little Caesars Round Veggie (3 slices; 12 oz.)	570	21	9	1,500
Pizza Hut Personal Pan Ham (1 pizza; 9 oz.)	580	23	9	1,450
Pizza Hut Thin 'n Crispy Ham (3 slices; 8 oz.)	450	18	10	1,650
Pizza Hut Thin 'n Crispy Chicken Supreme (3 slices; 11 oz.)	540	18	10	1,680
Little Caesars Round Cheese (3 slices; 8 oz.)	600	18	10	990
Pizza Hut Hand Tossed Chicken Supreme (3 slices; 12 oz.)	630	19	10	1,770
Domino's Hand Tossed Pepperoni (2 slices; 7 oz.)	560	20	10	1,300
Domino's Hand Tossed Extra Cheese (2 slices; 8 oz.)	560	20	10	1,340
Domino's Hand Tossed Italian Sausage (2 slices; 8 oz.)	600	22	10	1,120
Domino's Hand Tossed Hawaiian (2 slices)	620	22	10	1,540
Papa John's Original Crust Pepperoni (2 slices; 9 oz.)	600	24	10	1,580
Domino's Hand Tossed Deluxe (2 slices)	610	24	10	1,440
Donatos Vegy (2 slices; 12 oz.)	560	28	10	1,800

A TYPICAL SERVING (continued)

PIZZA (typical serving; weight, if available)

	Calories	Total Fat (g)	Saturated Fat (g)	Sodium (mg)
Little Caesars Deep Dish Pepperoni (4 squares; 10 oz.)	640	28	10	1,400
Papa John's Original Crust Sausage (2 slices; 10 oz.)	640	28	10	1,760
Donatos Hawaiian (2 slices; 10 oz.)	620	30	10	1,780
Pizza Hut Thin 'n Crispy Pepperoni (3 slices; 8 oz.)	510	24	11	1,650
Little Caesars Round Pepperoni (3 slices; 9 oz.)	600	24	11	1,380
Domino's Hand Tossed Beef (2 slices)	620	26	11	1,380
Pizza Hut Personal Pan Pepperoni (1 pizza; 9 oz.)	620	28	11	1,430
Domino's Thin Crust Cheese (5 squares; 9 oz.)	640	28	11	1,950
Domino's Hand Tossed Bacon (2 slices)	660	28	11	1,500
Domino's Deep Dish Cheese (2 slices; 9 oz.)	680	30	11	1,580
Domino's Deep Dish Ham (2 slices)	710	31	11	1,870
Pizza Hut Pan Veggie Lover's (3 slices; 12 oz.)	720	33	11	1,380
Pizza Hut Pan Chicken Supreme (3 slices; 12 oz.)	720	33	11	1,590
Pizza Hut Pan Ham (3 slices; 10 oz.)	720	33	11	1,650
Pizza Hut The Big New Yorker Ham (2 slices; 12 oz.)	680	26	12	2,320
Pizza Hut Pan Cheese (3 slices; 8 oz.)	630	27	*12*	1,170
Pizza Hut Personal Pan Cheese (1 pizza; 9 oz.)	630	28	12	1,370
Little Caesars Round Meatsa (3 slices; 11 oz.)	660	30	12	1,710
Papa John's Original Crust The Works (2 slices; 11 oz.)	680	30	12	1,880
Pizza Hut Hand Tossed Pepperoni Lover's (3 slices; 10 oz.)	680	30	12	1,990
Little Caesars Round Supreme (3 slices; 12 oz.)	690	30	12	1,650
Domino's Thin Crust Ham (5 squares)	690	30	12	2,440
Domino's Hand Tossed Extravaganzza (2 slices)	700	30	12	1,780

A TYPICAL SERVING *(continued)*

PIZZA (typical serving; weight, if available)

	Calories	Total Fat (g)	Saturated Fat (g)	Sodium (mg)
Donatos Mariachi Beef (2 slices; 11 oz.)	610	32	12	1,720
Papa John's Thin Crust Garden Special (3 slices; 13 oz.)	680	36	12	1,490
Papa John's Thin Crust Cheese (3 slices; 10 oz.)	700	39	12	1,490
Pizza Hut The Big New Yorker Veggie Lovers (2 slices; 24 oz.)	900	44	12	2,680
Little Caesars Thin Crust Cheese (5 squares; 10 oz.)	650	30	13	1,600
Domino's Hand Tossed America's Favorite (2 slices)	700	30	13	1,660
Pizza Hut Pan Pepperoni (3 slices; 8 oz.)	690	33	*13*	1,620
Pizza Hut Personal Pan Pork (1 pizza; 10 oz.)	700	34	13	1,670
Pizza Hut Thin 'n Crispy Cheese (3 slices; 8 oz.)	540	24	14	1,620
Pizza Hut Hand Tossed Cheese (3 slices; 10 oz.)	650	27	14	1,770
Pizza Hut Hand Tossed Ham (3 slices; 11 oz.)	710	27	14	2,180
Pizza Hut The Big New Yorker Pepperoni (2 slices; 12 oz.)	740	32	14	2,300
California Pizza Kitchen Original BBQ Chicken (1 pizza; 14 oz.)	1,000	32	*14*	2,060
Pizza Hut Hand Tossed Supreme (3 slices; 12 oz.)	730	33	14	1,990
Pizza Hut Personal Pan Beef (1 pizza; 10 oz.)	710	35	14	1,580
Domino's Deep Dish Extra Cheese (2 slices)	740	35	14	1,800
Domino's Deep Dish Vegi (2 slices)	770	36	14	1,860
Domino's Deep Dish Hawaiian (2 slices)	780	36	14	2,040
Donatos Original Pepperoni (2 slices; 8 oz.)	640	38	14	1,850
Domino's Deep Dish Pepperoni (2 slices)	780	38	14	1,940
Papa John's Original Crust All the Meats (2 slices; 11 oz.)	780	38	14	2,200
Domino's Deep Dish Italian Sausage (2 slices)	790	38	14	1,920

A TYPICAL SERVING *(continued)*

PIZZA (typical serving; weight, if available)

	Calories	Total Fat (g)	Saturated Fat (g)	Sodium (mg)
Domino's Deep Dish Deluxe (2 slices)	790	38	14	1,930
Pizza Hut Personal Pan Italian Sausage (1 pizza; 10 oz.)	740	39	14	1,640
Domino's Hand Tossed Meatzza (2 slices)	760	34	15	1,940
Pizza Hut Pan Italian Sausage (3 slices; 9 oz.)	750	39	*15*	1,680
Domino's Deep Dish Beef (2 slices)	790	40	15	1,880
Papa John's Thin Crust Pepperoni (3 slices; 10 oz.)	800	48	15	1,860
Pizza Hut Stuffed Crust Veggie Lover's (2 slices; 14 oz.)	840	34	16	2,080
Pizza Hut Stuffed Crust Chicken Supreme (2 slices; 13 oz.)	860	34	16	2,220
Pizza Hut Hand Tossed Pepperoni (3 slices; 11 oz.)	760	35	16	2,150
Donatos Serious Cheese (2 slices; 8 oz.)	650	36	16	1,700
Pizza Hut Thin n' Crispy Supreme (3 slices; 11 oz.)	690	36	16	1,920
Pizza Hut Thin n' Crispy Pepperoni Lover's (3 slices; 9 oz.)	690	36	16	2,070
Domino's Thin Crust Extra Cheese (5 squares)	750	37	16	2,330
Domino's Thin Crust Vegi (5 squares)	780	38	16	2,430
Pizza Hut Hand Tossed Super Supreme (3 slices; 13 oz.)	790	38	16	2,310
Pizza Hut Thin n' Crispy Pork (3 slices; 10 oz.)	720	39	16	2,220
Pizza Hut Thin n' Crispy Super Supreme (3 slices; 12 oz.)	750	42	16	2,280
Domino's Deep Dish Bacon (2 slices)	830	43	16	2,000
Donatos Classic Trio (2 slices; 12 oz.)	720	44	16	1,920
Donatos Works (2 slices; 12 oz.)	740	44	16	1,920
Donatos Founder's Favorite (2 slices; 11 oz.)	760	44	16	2,700
Pizza Hut Pan Supreme (3 slices; 13 oz.)	870	45	16	1,830
Pizza Hut Pan Pork (3 slices; 12 oz.)	870	45	16	1,980

A TYPICAL SERVING *(continued)* PIZZA (typical serving; weight, if available)	Calories	Total Fat (g)	Saturated Fat (g)	Sodium (mg)
Pizza Hut Pan Super Supreme (3 slices; 14 oz.)	930	48	16	2,130
Domino's Thin Crust Hawaiian (5 squares)	810	38	17	2,720
Domino's Thin Crust Pepperoni (5 squares)	800	42	17	2,560
Domino's Thin Crust Italian Sausage (5 squares)	820	42	17	2,520
Domino's Thin Crust Deluxe (5 squares)	820	42	17	2,540
Domino's Deep Dish America's Favorite (2 slices)	850	44	17	2,160
Domino's Deep Dish Extravaganzza (2 slices)	870	45	17	2,270
Pizza Hut The Big New Yorker Cheese (2 slices; 12 oz.)	760	34	18	2,280
Pizza Hut Stuffed Crust Pepperoni (2 slices; 12 oz.)	880	38	18	2,230
Domino's Thin Crust Beef (5 squares)	820	44	18	2,470
Little Caesars Thin Crust Pepperoni (5 squares; 11 oz.)	800	45	18	2,100
Papa John's Thin Crust Sausage (3 slices; 12 oz.)	850	51	18	2,090
Pizza Hut Thin 'n Crispy Beef (3 slices; 10 oz.)	720	42	19	2,040
Pizza Hut Stuffed Crust Meat Lover's (2 slices; 10 oz.)	830	42	*19*	2,670
Pizza Hut Stuffed Crust Pork (2 slices; 12 oz.)	920	42	19	2,350
Pizza Hut Hand Tossed Pork (3 slices; 13 oz.)	870	44	19	2,500
Pizza Hut Thin n' Crispy Italian Sausage (3 slices; 10 oz.)	780	45	19	2,190
Pizza Hut Hand Tossed Meat Lover's (3 slices; 12 oz.)	870	46	19	2,450
Pizza Hut Pan Beef (3 slices; 12 oz.)	900	48	19	1,890
Pizza Hut Pan Pepperoni Lover's (3 slices; 12 oz.)	900	48	19	2,070
Domino's Thin Crust Bacon (5 squares)	890	49	19	2,660
Domino's Deep Dish Meatzza (2 slices)	910	49	19	2,440
Pizza Hut Pan Meat Lover's (3 slices; 13 oz.)	990	57	19	2,280

A TYPICAL SERVING (continued)

PIZZA (typical serving; weight, if available)

	Calories	Total Fat (g)	Saturated Fat (g)	Sodium (mg)
Pizza Hut Stuffed Crust Cheese (2 slices; 11 oz.)	890	38	20	2,180
Pizza Hut Stuffed Crust Beef (2 slices; 12 oz.)	930	44	20	2,270
Pizza Hut The Big New Yorker Supreme (2 slices; 16 oz.)	900	46	20	2,700
Donatos Serious Meat (2 slices; 11 oz.)	840	50	20	2,380
Pizza Hut The Big New Yorker Pork (2 slices; 15 oz.)	940	50	20	2,940
Pizza Hut Stuffed Crust Italian Sausage (2 slices; 11 oz.)	960	46	21	2,330
Pizza Hut Stuffed Crust Supreme (2 slices; 14 oz.)	970	46	21	2,450
Domino's Thin Crust Extravaganzza (5 squares)	950	52	21	3,120
Papa John's Thin Crust The Works (3 slices; 15 oz.)	970	60	21	2,610
Pizza Hut Hand Tossed Beef (3 slices; 13 oz.)	900	46	22	2,400
Pizza Hut Hand Tossed Italian Sausage (3 slices; 13 oz.)	930	49	22	2,480
Pizza Hut Stuffed Crust Super Supreme (2 slices; 14 oz.)	1,010	50	22	2,740
Pizza Hut Thin n' Crispy Meat Lover's (3 slices; 11 oz.)	840	51	22	2,490
Domino's Thin Crust America's Favorite (5 squares)	930	51	22	2,920
Pizza Hut The Big New Yorker Beef (2 slices; 15 oz.)	960	52	22	2,760
Pizza Hut Stuffed Crust Ham (2 slices; 11 oz.)	810	44	25	2,380
Pizza Hut Stuffed Crust Pepperoni Lover's (2 slices; 14 oz.)	1,050	52	25	2,830
Domino's Thin Crust Meatzza (5 squares)	1,030	59	25	3,400
Papa John's Thin Crust All the Meats (3 slices; 14 oz.)	1,180	78	27	3,150
Pizza Hut The Big New Yorker Sausage (2 slices; 16 oz.)	1,140	66	28	3,240
Pizzeria Uno Chicago Classic (½ pizza; 19 oz.)	1,500	74	*30*	2,940

Note: Saturated fat numbers in *italics* include a small amount of artery-clogging *trans* fat.

Chapter 8

Drop the Chalupa: Mexican Restaurants

Along with Italian and Chinese restaurants, Mexican restaurants are among the most popular eateries in America today. Their casual, convivial atmosphere, brightly colored festive decor, and flavorful food all appeal to a wide range of hungry eaters.

Mexican food evolved from a marriage of Spanish, Aztec, and other indigenous New World culinary traditions. It included the tomato, numerous varieties of beans and peppers, and the avocado, all flavorful ingredients that form the basis for what has traditionally been a healthful cuisine. But all is not what it seems.

The basic components of Mexican cooking—rice, beans, fresh vegetables, tomatoes, tortillas—are healthful enough. But after we analyzed some of the most popular dishes at Mexican restaurant chains like Chi-Chi's, El Torito, Don Pablo's, Chevys, and El Chico, we discovered that the standard traditional ingredients are all too often transmogrified into nutritional disasters by meat, cheese, sour cream, oil, and salt. The result is dishes that are a far cry from their humble, healthy origins.

We analyzed some of the most popular dishes served at these midpriced chain restaurants, as well as independents. Thousands of Americans visit such restaurants daily to ingest monster-size burritos and chimichangas dripping with cheese. You may be as surprised as we were to discover what they're actually made of and their nutritional values.

161

The Dishes and the Data

We bought take-out portions of 15 popular appetizers and main dishes at 19 midpriced Mexican restaurants in Chicago, Dallas, San Francisco, and Washington, D.C. The restaurants included some of the largest chains, such as Chi-Chi's, El Torito, Chevys, and Don Pablo's, as well as independents. (For more on our methodology, see pages 12–14.)

We obtained our numbers for the combination platters by adding together the lab results for their à la carte components. For guacamole and pico de gallo, we used the numbers that were given to us by a food-service supplier. For sour cream and tortilla chips, we used numbers from the USDA Nutrient Data Base for Standard Reference.

Nutritionally, the enchiladas, chimichangas, and most other entrées we tested are all pretty bad news. Most consist of a corn or white-flour tortilla stuffed with some combination of beans, cheese, beef, and chicken. The meat and cheese supply the saturated fat. Then the calories get a boost from the oil that's used to cook the tortillas. Add in the hefty side dishes (beans and rice) and rich condiments (sour cream and guacamole), and most platters end up with more than 1,500 calories. Some restaurants soften the tortillas by dipping them in hot oil. They deep-fry the tortillas for crispy tacos or taco salad shells. Likewise, once chimichangas are filled, the wrapped shells are submerged in boiling oil. Only the fajitas, burritos, and soft tacos escape an oil bath.

Because Mexican entrées are frequently served as part of a platter with accompanying side dishes and condiments, most notably refried beans, rice, sour cream, and guacamole, remember to total the numbers for each component on the plate, or check to see if your platter matches any of the ones we've listed.

Within each category we've ranked the dishes from best to worst—that is, from least to most saturated fat. We did not test for *trans* fat; if we had, the saturated fat numbers would probably be higher than those indicated.

Appetizers and Side Dishes

MEXICAN RICE
(230 calories and 4 grams of fat, 1 of them saturated)

The average three-quarter-cup serving of rice and bits of onion, tomato, and other vegetables is sautéed in a little oil or shortening before being cooked in sodium-laden chicken broth. This is much saltier than the steamed rice you get at a Chinese restaurant, but frankly Mexican-style rice is the least of your problems on a typical platter.

The Bottom Line: See if you can substitute a side salad for the rice on your platter.

TORTILLA CHIPS
(640 calories and 34 grams of fat, 6 of them saturated)

They're crunchy and fun, but the grease stain on the paper liner of the serving basket is the tip-off that there's trouble in every chip. The average basketful of chips contains 640 calories plus half your daily allowance of fat. Granted, most people share the chips (although some share two baskets), but even so, if you eat just a quarter of a basket (about 13 chips), you're 9 fat grams and 160 calories in the hole before you even place your order. And those automatic refills are hard to resist.

The Bottom Line: Ask your server to substitute some warm corn or flour tortillas to tear apart and dip into a bowl of salsa.

REFRIED BEANS
(also called *refritos;* 380 calories and 16 grams of fat, 7 of them saturated)

These refried beans start out as a healthy 1-cup serving of high-fiber, low-fat pinto beans. But by the time the chef is done, they're likely to contain enough lard, cheese, or bacon to use up a third of your day's allowance of saturated fat and sodium. That's the equivalent of six strips of bacon.

The Bottom Line: *Many restaurants offer cooked pinto or black beans that are not mashed and fried. At the small chain Acapulco they're called "charro beans." Chevys has them on the menu as* beans a la charra, *and at El Torito they're* frijoles de la olla. *(Chevys also has vegetarian black beans that are prepared without any additional fat or fatty ingredients.) But don't assume that these cooked beans are fat-free unless the menu says so. Still, they're a better choice than standard* refritos.

CHEESE QUESADILLA WITH SOUR CREAM, PICO DE GALLO, AND GUACAMOLE
(900 calories and 59 grams of fat, 24 of them saturated)

A 900-calorie Mexican grilled cheese sandwich is more like a (fattening) main dish than an appetizer. Cheese is sprinkled between two flat tortillas and then the tortillas are fried on a griddle. Like its gringo cousin, this dish is dangerously freighted with fat (13 teaspoons) and saturated fat (more than a day's worth). Even if you bypass the accompanying sour cream and guacamole, you'll still be eating a heart-heavy load of 680 calories, 40 grams of fat (17 of them saturated), and 1,100 milligrams of sodium.

The Bottom Line: *There's not much you can do to make this better. If you're at El Torito, order the grilled Chicken Quesadilla Lite, which is made with reduced-fat cheese and served with fat-free sour cream and fresh fruit. And with 530 calories, it's an entrée, not an hors d'oeuvre, so all you need is a salad to make it a meal.*

CHEESE NACHOS
(810 calories and 55 grams of fat, 25 of them saturated)

The average half-pound order contains nearly a quarter pound of cheese. Even split four ways as a shared appetizer, that's 200 calories and one-third of your day's limit of saturated fat—and you haven't even started your entrée.

The Bottom Line: *The quarter pound of cheese says it all.*

BEEF AND CHEESE NACHOS WITH SOUR CREAM AND GUACAMOLE
(1,360 calories and 89 grams of fat, 28 of them saturated)
This appetizer tops a 50-chip pile of greasy tortilla chips with a third of a pound of melted cheese and a quarter pound of ground beef—a staggering burden for your heart and the bathroom scale. Even without the sour cream and guacamole, this dish contains a day's saturated fat.

The Bottom Line: *This 1,360-calorie fiesta is worse than eating a half pound of Spam—before dinner. Order just about anything else.*

Entrées and Platters

The numbers following each dish are for a single piece of the entrée; in other words, one enchilada, one taco, one burrito, one chile relleno, one chimichanga, or one taco salad or the entire plate of fajitas with four flour tortillas. The numbers are also indicated for each typical platter, but if your favorite Mexican place serves a platter with a different number of items, you'll need to multiply accordingly.

CRISPY CHICKEN TACO
(220 calories and 11 grams of fat, 3 of them saturated, per taco)
Most restaurants serve two deep-fried corn tortillas each stuffed with 2 ounces of chicken, 2 ounces of lettuce and tomato, and a half-ounce of cheese. Half the restaurants we surveyed used dark-meat chicken, which is fattier than white.

Typical platter: Two tacos with refried beans and rice *(1,040 calories, and 42 grams of fat, 13 of them saturated)*.

The Bottom Line: *You can slash the fat and saturated fat in a taco platter by half if you order two tacos à la carte and skip the beans and rice. Still hungry? Replace the refritos with nonfried beans and have a salad instead of the rice.*

SOFT CHICKEN TACO
(210 calories and 11 grams of fat, 4 of them saturated, per taco)

A soft chicken taco has essentially the same ingredients as the crispy version except you're more likely to get a leaner, white-meat filling, which two-thirds of the restaurants we surveyed use. The soft flour tortilla has about as much fat as its deep-fried corn cousin—3 grams—but it is larger and, therefore, more filling.

Typical Platter: Two tacos with refried beans and rice *(1,020 calories, 43 grams of fat, 15 of them saturated)*

The Bottom Line: *See our advice for the Crispy Chicken Taco platter (above). If you're at Chi-Chi's, try the Low-Fat Chicken Soft Tacos served with Salsa Rice and steamed vegetables. At Acapulco, ask for Tacos al Carbon (served with charro beans and fresh vegetables) from the Healthy Dining Preparation menu.*

BEEF ENCHILADA
(320 calories and 19 grams of fat, 4 of them saturated, per enchilada)

Why does a beef enchilada have only one more gram of fat than its chicken counterpart? The average serving size of meat is small—1½ ounces. Steer clear of the meat chile sauce many restaurants serve on top of the enchiladas. It contains ground beef, which means the saturated fat numbers will be higher than for a simple red chile sauce.

Typical Platter: Two enchiladas with refried beans and rice *(1,250 calories and 58 grams of fat, 16 of them saturated)*

The Bottom Line: Order just one enchilada (or take one home) to save 320 calories. Order a salad instead of rice and nonfried beans instead of regular to make it a healthful meal.

CHICKEN FAJITAS
(840 calories and 24 grams of fat, 5 of them saturated)

On average, these fajitas were made with 6 ounces of sliced, marinated skinless chicken breast sautéed with 4 ounces of onions and green peppers and served with four flour tortillas. Although a few other à la carte entrées have less saturated fat, fajitas are the only dishes in Mexican restaurants we found that give you a decent serving of vegetables. Our only caveat is the high sodium level—1,530 milligrams.

Typical Platter: Four fajitas with refried beans, rice, sour cream, and guacamole and four flour tortillas *(1,660 calories and 63 grams of fat, 19 of them saturated)*

The Bottom Line: This is by far your best choice at a Mexican restaurant, if you pass on the sides, which cuts the calories in half. If you think that won't fill you up, replace the rice and refried beans with nonfried beans and a salad.

CHICKEN ENCHILADA
(330 calories and 18 grams of fat, 6 of them saturated, per enchilada)

Chicken in an oil-dipped corn tortilla has a little more saturated fat than a beef enchilada—probably because of its sour cream sauce. Its nutrient profile is similar to that of a McDonald's cheeseburger.

Typical Platter: Two enchiladas with refried beans and rice *(1,260 calories, 57 grams of fat, 19 of them saturated)*

The Bottom Line: *Order your chicken enchilada with red chile sauce instead of fatty sour-cream sauce. If you're near a Chi-Chi's or Acapulco, you're in luck. Both offer a lighter version of chicken enchiladas. At Acapulco they're called Enchiladas Rancheras on the Healthy Dining Preparation menu; at Chi-Chi's look for Low-Fat Chicken Enchiladas.*

CHEESE ENCHILADA
(370 calories and 24 grams of fat, 7 of them saturated, per enchilada)

This oil-dipped corn tortilla has more than 2 ounces of cheese in its filling and topping. And sometimes it is covered in meat chile sauce (which contains fat) instead of red chile sauce (which is fat-free). It has almost twice the saturated fat of a beef enchilada.

Typical Platter: Two enchiladas with refried beans and rice *(1,530 calories and 68 grams of fat, 22 of them saturated)*

The Bottom Line: *If it's an enchilada you want, you're better off ordering beef or chicken. Hold the cream sauce; top with red chile sauce instead.*

CHICKEN BURRITO
(720 calories and 29 grams of fat, 8 of them saturated)

Expect a flour tortilla wrapped around 4 ounces of chicken and 2 ounces of refried beans, then topped with cheese and sauce. Usually you'll be served a red chile or ranchero (tomatoes, onions, hot green peppers) sauce on the dish, although some places serve a green chile sauce. One-third of the restaurants we surveyed used chunks of grilled white meat; others used a mix of shredded white meat and fattier dark meat. Still, a chicken burrito has 25 percent less fat and nearly 40 percent less saturated fat than its beef counterpart, and a tad less sodium.

Typical Platter: One burrito with refried beans, rice, sour cream, and guacamole *(1,530 calories and 68 grams of fat, 22 of them saturated)*

The Bottom Line: *If you're eating in a place like El Torito, which offers a chicken Sonora Burrito Lite, get that. Otherwise, order the burrito à la carte and consider it a 700+ calorie whole meal. If you want to order the whole platter, take half home for tomorrow.*

CHILE RELLENO
(490 calories and 38 grams of fat, 11 of them saturated, per chile relleno)

This cheese-stuffed, batter-coated, deep-fried pepper is topped with cheese and red chile sauce. You may find it *delicioso,* but *one* contains as much saturated fat as 10 strips of bacon. What a thing to do to a vegetable!

Typical Platter: Two chilies with refried beans and rice *(1,580 calories and 96 grams of fat, 30 of them saturated)*

The Bottom Line: *The entire platter has the saturated fat of 27 strips of bacon. Nothing will make this better for you. If you want a vegetarian entrée, you'll be much better off with vegetable fajitas.*

BEEF BURRITO
(830 calories and 40 grams of fat, 13 of them saturated)

Wrap a quarter pound of beef and some refried beans in a flour tortilla and top it with cheese. You'll get 830 calories and the saturated fat of three hot dogs, along with 1,970 milligrams of sodium, the highest sodium level of all the Mexican entrées we tested. You'll also consume twice the calories and 85 percent more saturated fat than a 9-ounce Burrito Supreme from Taco Bell. With sides included, you're talking 1,600 calories.

Typical Platter: One burrito with refried beans, rice, sour cream, and guacamole *(1,640 calories and 79 grams of fat, 28 of them saturated)*

The Bottom Line: *Skip it.*

BEEF CHIMICHANGA
(800 calories and 47 grams of fat, 13 of them saturated)

A beanless beef burrito is fatty enough. Deep-fry it and no one will be surprised to get 800 calories and enough fat and sodium to fulfill about two-thirds of your daily allowance of each. Then come the sides, to the tune of an additional 800 calories.

Typical Platter: One chimichanga with refried beans, rice, sour cream, and guacamole *(1,610 calories and 86 grams of fat, 27 of them saturated)*

The Bottom Line: *Forget about this dish. The platter provides more than 1½ teaspoons of salt (more than you should get in a whole day!). If it's beef you're after, order one beef enchilada with nonfried beans and a salad.*

TACO SALAD WITH SOUR CREAM AND GUACAMOLE
(1,100 calories and 71 grams of fat, 20 of them saturated)

Calling this dish a salad is a real stretch. The ingredients are basically those of a beef taco—plus extra lettuce—and yet you'll consume your day's quota of fat and saturated fat and 1,100 calories—not including the full-fat salad dressing that a third of the restaurants served with it.

The Bottom Line: *Bypass this fat-filled version and look for a lighter alternative. For example, Acapulco offers the Tostada Grande—a baked shell filled with chicken, nonfried beans, lettuce, and tomatoes tossed with fat-free herb dressing.*

According to the company, it contains only 440 calories, 16 grams of fat, and 580 milligrams of sodium.

When Your Favorite Is Not on the List

Although we analyzed only chicken fajitas in this chapter, we take a look at steak fajitas in chapter 12, Where Everybody Knows Your Name: Dinner Houses (see page 223). (If you compare them, be aware that the steak fajitas numbers don't include rice and beans as part of the meal.) That's also where you'll find the scoop on a bowl of chili. We didn't analyze shrimp, vegetable, or portobello mushroom fajitas, but they're also a good bet.

Although we didn't analyze beef tacos, the versions served at sit-down restaurants probably don't differ much from what's served at fast-food Mexican chains. At Taco Bell, the biggest Mexican chain, a crispy beef taco weighs in at 210 calories, 12 grams of fat (4 of them saturated) and 330 milligrams of sodium. Its Beef Soft Taco provides 210 calories, 10 grams of fat (4 of them saturated), and 570 milligrams of sodium. For more information about Taco Bell's menu items, check out chapter 16, On the Run: Fast-Food Restaurants, page 271.

Fish tacos, already popular in California, are working their way across the country, according to industry trade magazine *Restaurant Business.* Chains like Chevys, Acapulco, and Una Mas have jumped on the bandwagon with grilled fish tacos. They may be comparable to grilled chicken, if you watch the sides and garnishes carefully. Some restaurants batter their fish first, which means you're stuck with more fat than grilled chicken or fish. Consult with your server before ordering.

Many restaurants offer tortilla soup, which is vegetables in beef or chicken broth, topped with tortilla strips. If you eat just a few of the crunchy strips, this option doesn't look too bad—but tell the kitchen to hold the melted jack cheese that some places add. Or get the "light" or "healthy" versions of soups available on the special menus at places like Acapulco.

The fajita salads now offered by some restaurants sound better than they are. Although chicken fajitas were one of our better entrée choices, and supplementing their ingredients with greens sounds ideal, restaurants also pile on cheese and sometimes fried tortilla strips, guacamole, sour cream, and other high-fat trimmings. The salad may even be served in a fried tortilla shell bowl.

For information about other Mexican dishes we did not analyze, ask your server how they're prepared before you order.

Decoding the Mexican Menu

Understanding a few crucial terms that are common to Mexican-style menus will enable you to make healthier choices at a restaurant.

Al carbón means "grilled" and usually describes chicken or beef preparations.

A **chalupa** is a boat-shaped corn tortilla that has been deep-fried and filled with meat—either beef, pork, or chicken—vegetables, cheese, or a combination of these ingredients. It's definitely not a wise choice for healthful eaters.

Charra or **charro beans** are usually pinto beans that have been cooked and seasoned but not mashed and fried into *refritos*. They may be fat-free or cooked with bacon or some other fat. Ask your server how they're prepared. Even if they have some added fat, they're still bound to be better for you than *refritos*.

Chile con queso is chili-spiked melted cheese, usually used as a dip for nachos. We didn't need to test it to know that the cheese-chip combo will be hard on your arteries.

Any dish that's described as **"crispy"** is inevitably a deep-fried one.

Pico de gallo is a flavorful raw relish made from fresh tomatoes, onions, and hot peppers and flavored with seasonings that may include lime juice and cilantro. Versatile and vibrant in flavor, it is a great way to add flavor and a few nutrients to your entrée without adding fat.

Fat-free **ranchero sauce** is usually made from fresh tomatoes, onions, and hot peppers. Some restaurants top enchiladas with it.

Fat-free **red chile sauce** is similar in consistency and color to marinara sauce but is made with mild red peppers, not tomatoes.

Sopaipillas are deep-fried, puffy, pillow-shaped pastries that are drizzled with honey and served as a dessert. They are far from good for you—save them to share with a friend.

Tamales are little oblong packages of corn dough and fat filled with finely chopped and seasoned pork, chicken, or beef that is wrapped in corn husks for steaming.

Tomatillo sauce, which has little or no fat, is made of chopped tomatillos, hot green peppers, and cilantro. Also called **green salsa** or **salsa verde**, it is sometimes used on enchiladas and burritos.

Mexican Strategy

• **Look for special menus.** If the restaurant has "light" or "healthy" selections, choose from those. An increasing number of Mexican restaurant chains are featuring healthier versions of their specialties on a separate part of their menus.

• **Nibble on tortillas instead of greasy chips.** Don't even think of letting the server set that basket of tempting greasy chips on your table. Instead ask for warm tortillas and dip them in salsa.

• **Make abundant use of Mexican condiments and seasonings.**
Fresh and dried chiles, pico de gallo, tomatillo sauce (sometimes
called green salsa or salsa verde), fresh cilantro and fresh limes,
and other seasonings that typify classic Mexican cuisine add
wonderful flavor and no fat.

• **Substitute salsas for sour cream and cheese.** Order dishes
without sour cream or cheese, then garnish them at the table
with ranchero sauce, red chile sauce, salsas, or pico de gallo.

• **Avoid deep-fried dishes.** Eating chimichangas, chile rellenos,
or specialty salads served in crispy fried tortilla shells is a losing
proposition.

• **Skip the typical side dishes.** If the restaurant does not offer
nonfried beans and reduced-fat sour cream, you're better off
without them. The fat in guacamole isn't saturated, but a typical
¼-cup serving does add about 100 calories. You know whether
you can afford all or some of them.

• **Look for healthful alternatives.** If the restaurant offers selections such as whole-wheat tortillas, brown rice, or reduced-fat
cheese or salad dressing, by all means order them instead of the
usual fare.

• **Avoid red meat.** When it comes to entrées, stick with chicken,
vegetable, or shrimp fajitas and simple grilled fish or chicken
dishes. Or for an inexpensive meal, just order black beans and
rice, a side salad, and a warm tortilla with salsa.

• **Build your own burrito.** Many Mexican restaurants are happy
to substitute or omit some ingredients to create a burrito to your
specifications. Ask for chicken or nonfried beans instead of beef
and salsa or pico de gallo instead of cheese and sour cream. You'll
skip most of the fat, but not the flavor.

How Mexican Stacks Up to Italian and Chinese Food

Can't decide between the Szechuan Palace, the Spaghetti Garden, and El Taco Rancho? You'll probably have the fewest healthy options at the ranch.

All three ethnic cuisines can be sources of hidden fat and sodium. But the standard repertoire of Mexican-American restaurants relies too heavily on cheese, meat, sour cream, deep-fat frying, and other fat- and salt-rich elements to give you much room to maneuver. Italian and Chinese menus generally offer a variety of dishes, like spaghetti or stir-fried vegetables and seafood, that rarely exceed half a day's saturated fat.

In contrast, none of the Mexican platters we looked at used up fewer than 1,000 calories—several were closer to 1,500—and none used less than half a day's allowance of fat and saturated fat. Most blew your whole day's quota. The refried beans, sour cream, and guacamole—always popular components of a Mexican meal— saw to that.

If you want to use up only half a day's fat, you'll likely do better with grilled chicken or fish that isn't served in a cream or cheese sauce. But if you're yearning for one of the typical tortilla entrées, get the chicken, shrimp, or vegetable fajitas, two chicken tacos, or one beef enchilada. And whatever you order, eat the accompaniments sparingly—a couple of tablespoons to garnish your entrée, rather than everything crowded onto your plate—or ask your server for charro beans, pico de gallo, and reduced-fat sour cream. The more we ask for these healthier foods, the greater the odds that the restaurants will get the message.

What Is Fresh Mex?

As burritos seem to get bigger and too many entrées rely on the deep-fat fryer to make us happy, there's one trend in Mexican cooking that we'd like to encourage—Health Mex or Fresh Mex. It's slowly but surely lightening things up on Mexican menus.

Chevys, for example, offers a departure from the usual creamy, meaty, cheese-laden choices. It features a variety of grilled fajitas, like the traditional favorites made with chicken, shrimp, and steak, and sometimes offers more inventive ones with portobello mushrooms and salmon. Acapulco now offers several entrées on its Healthy Dining Preparation menus, like Enchiladas Rancheras, Garden Tostada, and Tacos la Carbon. At El Torito the lite menu features dishes like Chicken Quesadilla Lite, Sonora Burrito Lite, and Chicken Fajita Lite.

The trend toward downsizing calories on Mexican menus appears strongest on the West Coast, especially in the fast-food segment. Rubio's Baja Grill, a popular California-based chain with restaurants in the Southwest and Northwest, has a Health Mex menu of chicken and grilled fish tacos and burritos that the company claims range from just 3 to 13 grams of fat. Nearly half the menu at Una Mas, a northern-California chain, meets the American Heart Association's guidelines that limit dishes to less than 30 percent of their calories from fat. The chain also offers to substitute whole wheat for regular tortillas at no extra charge.

We welcome those steps forward on the nutrition front, but our wish list for a Mexican menu makeover doesn't stop with grilled fish and more veggies. We're still waiting for restaurants to routinely offer the reduced-fat sour cream, nonfried beans, and baked tortilla chips that consumers can so readily buy at a supermarket but can't order off a restaurant menu. In the meantime, Health Mex is a great step in the right direction.

We've ranked appetizers, side dishes, and entrées (not the full platters) from best to worst—that is, from least to most saturated fat. We didn't test for *trans* fat; if we had, the saturated fat numbers would be higher than those indicated. A typical ¼ cup serving of guacamole contains about 100 calories.

Reminder
Recommended limits for a 2,000-calorie diet:
Total fat: 65 grams
Saturated fat: 20 grams
Cholesterol: 300 milligrams
Sodium: 2,400 milligrams

Entrées marked with a ✔ are Best Bites. Best Bites are relatively low in saturated fat.

MEXICAN DISHES

Menu Item	Calories	Total Fat (g)	Saturated Fat (g)	Cholesterol (mg)	Sodium (mg)
APPETIZERS AND SIDE DISHES					
Mexican rice (6 oz., ¾ cup)	230	4	1	5	820
Tortilla chips (4½ oz., 50 chips)	640	34	6	0	680
Refried beans (8 oz., 1 cup)	380	16	7	15	790
Cheese quesadillas with sour cream, pico de gallo, and guacamole (11½ oz.)	900	59	24	105	1,630
Cheese nachos (7 oz.)	810	55	25	115	880
Beef and cheese nachos with sour cream and guacamole (19 oz.)	1,360	89	28	210	2,430
ENTRÉES AND PLATTERS					
✔ Crispy chicken taco (5 oz.)	220	11	3	50	360
two tacos with refried beans and rice	1,040	42	13	120	2,320
✔ Soft chicken taco (6 oz.)	210	11	4	65	550
two tacos with refried beans and rice	1,020	43	15	145	2,700
✔ Beef enchilada (5½ oz.)	320	19	4	55	640
two enchiladas with refried beans and rice	1,250	58	16	130	2,880

MEXICAN DISHES (continued)

Menu Item	Calories	Total Fat (g)	Saturated Fat (g)	Cholesterol (mg)	Sodium (mg)
✔ Chicken fajitas and flour tortillas (17½ oz.)	840	24	5	140	1,530
with refried beans, rice, sour cream, and guacamole	1,660	63	19	180	3,660
Chicken enchilada (6 oz.)	330	18	6	85	620
two enchiladas with refried beans and rice	1,260	57	19	190	2,850
Cheese enchilada (5 oz.)	370	24	7	60	630
two enchiladas with refried beans and rice	1,350	68	22	135	2,880
Chicken burrito (14½ oz.)	720	29	8	115	1,740
with refried beans, rice, sour cream, and guacamole	1,530	68	22	150	3,690
Chile relleno (8½ oz.)	490	38	11	135	870
two chile rellenos with refried beans and rice	1,580	96	30	290	3,350
Beef burrito (14 oz.)	830	40	13	125	1,970
with refried beans, rice, sour cream, and guacamole	1,640	79	28	165	3,290
Beef chimichanga (10 oz.)	800	47	13	100	1,680
with refried beans, rice, sour cream, and guacamol	1,610	86	27	140	3,630
Taco salad with sour cream and guacamole (21 oz.)	1,100	71	20	125	1,850

Chapter 9

Acropolis Now:
Greek Restaurants

A merican diners are already steady customers at restaurants the industry calls the "Big Three"—Italian, Mexican, and Chinese—but there is growing interest in many other ethnic cuisines as well. Greek food is a good example. It's now so solidly ensconced in the second tier of popular ethnic food choices that a 1999 survey by the National Restaurant Association revealed that more than half of the respondents indicated they eat Greek food occasionally or frequently.

Like its neighbor Italy, Greece has a rich and fascinating culinary history grounded in thousands of years of farming and seafaring. Like other Mediterranean cuisines, traditional Greek cooking has been influenced by its Turkish, Lebanese, and Balkan neighbors. For centuries, vegetables, grains, herbs, and olives have been the staple ingredients. Delicious use is made of dairy products like yogurt, feta, and other cheeses; fish, squid, and other seafood; and ground and grilled meats, especially beef and lamb. However, the Greeks traditionally used meat and cheese as flavoring elements in dishes, so they were not eaten in large portions.

Everyone knows that burgers, french fries, nachos, and doughnuts are fatty foods. But what about souvlaki, gyros, spanakopita, and baklava? A few Greek specialties, including chicken, lamb, or pork souvlaki, are on a nutritional par with the most healthful meals at Italian-, Chinese-, or American-style restaurants. Unfortunately, some other choices are more "grease" than "Greece." A typical entrée of stuffed grape leaves or spinach pie, for instance, has more saturated fat than a McDonald's Big Mac. And a gyro or an order of moussaka has twice as much.

As Greek specialties become increasingly available at a widening range of places from sit-down restaurants to mall food courts and airports, it becomes important to know which dishes are good for you and which spell trouble for your heart or hips. Our findings here will point you in the right directions.

The Dishes and the Data

We bought dinner-size take-out portions of six popular entrées, one sandwich, one side dish, and one dessert from nine Greek

The Greek Way of Eating

The landmark Seven Countries diet and heart disease study, begun just after World War II and lasting about two decades, studied men from the Greek island of Crete, who had a remarkably low rate of heart disease. Why so low? First of all, the traditional Greek diet consisted largely of fresh vegetables, grains, and olive oil, with just a *smattering* of seafood, meat, and cheese. As a consequence, the men of Crete got a low 8 percent of their calories from saturated fat. Clearly, they weren't sitting down to a big plate of spanakopita every day. Second, they weren't actually *sitting down* very much, so they weren't overweight. They were much more active than Americans—or Greeks, for that matter—are today. In a nutshell, the men had healthy hearts because they ate large quantities of the foods that were good for them, only small quantities of those that weren't, and they were physically active. Then as now, good habits equal good health.

restaurants in Chicago, Los Angeles, and Washington, D.C. (For more on our methodology, see pages 12-14.)

Within each category we've ranked the dishes from best to worst; that is, from least to most saturated fat.

Entrées

CHICKEN SOUVLAKI
(260 calories and 8 grams of fat, 2 of them saturated)

Whether it's called souvlaki in Greece or shish kebab in the Middle East, this dish is usually the same: marinated chunks of chicken (or lamb, beef, or pork) threaded on a skewer with vegetables, then broiled or grilled and served over rice. Of all the Greek main dishes we tested, this was the clear winner. A typical order of chicken souvlaki contains only 260 calories, 8 grams of fat (2 of them saturated), and 370 milligrams of sodium. Best of all, the skewers generally yield about two-thirds of a cup of vegetables, not counting the usual side dishes like carrots and green beans. When you add the 1½ cups of rice, the numbers climb to just 500 calories and 14 grams of fat, 5 of them saturated. That's about the same as a grilled chicken breast entrée with vegetables and a baked potato. Although the souvlaki's 1,050 milligrams of sodium are nearly half a day's worth, not many restaurant meals do better.

The Bottom Line: *Clearly your best choice.*

LAMB OR PORK SOUVLAKI
(310 calories and 11 grams of fat, 4 of them saturated)

If it's red meat you're seeking, you can't beat lamb or pork kebabs. On the skewers you'll find only 310 calories and 11 grams of fat, 4 of them saturated. If you add 1½ cups of rice, the numbers rise to 550 calories and 18 grams of fat of which 7 are saturated. Sodium, again, is an unfortunate 1,230 milligrams. Still, restaurant meals with meat just don't get any leaner than this. Only a handful of the meat dishes we've tested from other types of restaurants even come close to these numbers. They were spaghetti with meat sauce (not meatballs); a trimmed sirloin steak with salad and a baked potato; and pot roast with vegetables, mashed potatoes, and gravy.

The Bottom Line: *This is one of the leanest meat-based restaurant meals you can order.*

SPANAKOPITA
(410 calories and 24 grams of fat, 12 of which are saturated)

This flaky spinach pie originated in northwestern Greece, according to Diane Kochilas, author of *The Food and Wine of Greece*. Spanakopita is made of paper-thin layers of delicate phyllo dough that have been basted with melted butter and filled with a mixture of spinach, feta cheese, oil, and egg. Despite the fact that spinach is loaded with vitamins and phytochemicals, a modest-sized entrée portion is as bad for your blood vessels as a Burger King Whopper. The pastry is light and flaky, but the 410 calories and 12 grams of saturated fat—more than half a day's worth—may leave you feeling heavy and sluggish. If you add the rice, potatoes, or other vegetables often served on the side, the numbers will go up. The spinach in this pie is certainly a plus, but it doesn't cancel out the effects of the saturated fat.

The Bottom Line: *Split spanakopita and an order of souvlaki with a friend, and get some extra veggies on the side.*

GREEK SALAD
(390 calories and 30 grams of fat, 12 of which are saturated)

It's painful to criticize salads! They're largely vegetables, after all—low-cal, low-fat, crisp and crunchy, and full of the phytochemicals, fiber, and vitamins we all need in abundance. But this Greek restaurant classic, typically made with romaine or iceberg lettuce, cubes of feta, olives, onion slices, tomatoes, cucumber, pepperoncini (pickled hot peppers), and sometimes anchovies, could be far better. The 30 grams of fat, 12 of them saturated, in a typical entrée-size Greek salad put it closer to a McDonald's Quarter Pounder with Cheese than a salad. Most of the saturated fat comes from the salty, strongly flavored feta. The 3 tablespoons of dressing added roughly 250 calories. On average, the salads we analyzed had 4½ tablespoons, or 1½ ounces, of feta. Some had just 1½ tablespoons, but others had as much as 8. The cheese also helps boost the sodium level to over 1,000 milligrams. The olives, dressing, and hot peppers also add to the sodium figure.

The Bottom Line: *You can easily turn this dish into a winner. Ask for the feta cheese and dressing on the side, and use only a tablespoon or two of each. And remember that a little strong-flavored feta goes a long way.*

MEAT-AND-RICE DOLMADES
(540 calories and 32 grams of fat, 15 of them saturated)

Dolmades, which are stuffed grape leaves. are the Greek equivalent of stuffed cabbage. The leaves are rolled around a filling of either meat and rice (typically served as an entrée) or rice and herbs (usually served cold as a *meze,* or appetizer). They're often drizzled with *avgolemono,* a traditional egg and lemon sauce. We analyzed only entrée-size portions (four rolls) of meat-and-rice dolmades. While the ground beef or lamb filling and sauce supply the fat (32 grams, 15 of them saturated), the leaves probably account for much of the sodium here. Grape leaves are traditionally cured in brine—a mixture of water and salt—to prepare them for stuffing. Even if the chef rinses the leaves well before using them, the brine could explain why this dish's sodium hits 1,470 milligrams.

The Bottom Line: *You'll get less saturated fat if you order rice-stuffed dolmades rather than meat-and-rice ones.*

GYRO
(760 calories and 44 grams of fat, 20 of them saturated)

A gyro (pronounced *"YEAR-oh"*) is a pita bread sandwich stuffed with meat, a quarter-cup of *tzatziki* (a sauce made with yogurt, garlic, oil, and cucumber), about ⅔ cup of lettuce, tomato, and onion, and sometimes a little feta. To make a gyro, restaurants roast a molded mixture of compressed, seasoned beef and lamb, bread crumbs, and onions on a vertical spit, then carve off thin slices of the meat for the sandwich.The slices are skinny, but the meat is fatty. We typically found 5 ounces of meat per sandwich, although one restaurant served as little as 2 ounces, and two of the three Chicago eateries piled on at least 10 ounces! All told, this Greek sandwich delivers a third of a day's calories, two-thirds of a day's total fat, and an entire day's saturated fat and sodium.

The Bottom Line: *There's no way to make this a healthful choice. Instead, get a lamb or pork souvlaki sandwich, which is made with chunks of leaner meat.*

MOUSSAKA
(830 calories and 48 grams of fat, 25 of them saturated)

Anyone who has eaten moussaka, one of the most familiar Greek specialties, knows that by no stretch of the imagination is it wholesome or low-fat. We're talking about a casserole of fatty ground beef or lamb layered with eggplant slices, which are usually fried; the whole thing is topped off with a béchamel sauce made of butter, egg yolks, and milk. You may have guessed it wasn't good for you, but you probably wouldn't have figured on the 830 calories and the hefty 48 grams of fat. And that doesn't include the accompanying rice, potatoes, or vegetables. A plate of moussaka contains more than an entire day's saturated fat allowance (25 grams), and the bad news doesn't end there. The average 2,010 milligrams of sodium per serving is just short of your 2,400-milligram daily limit.

The Bottom Line: *There's not much you can do to make this better. The only viable strategy is to share an order with one* *or two friends and fill up the rest of your plate with rice and vegetables.*

Dessert

BAKLAVA
(550 calories and 21 grams of fat, 5 of them saturated)

One glance at a recipe for baklava and your arteries may start to harden, but there's actually less cause for alarm than you might expect. Each tissue-thin layer of phyllo dough is brushed with melted butter and sprinkled with chopped nuts. The whole layered stack is baked until golden brown, then drenched with a syrup of honey, sugar, and lemon juice. What pastry could possibly be worse? For starters, a croissant, a Cinnabon, a scone, and a Danish are all worse for you. Those pastries can have as much as three times more saturated fat than a typical serving of baklava. What's surprising is that brushing melted butter on the dough evidently delivers only 2 teaspoons of butter (5 grams of saturated fat). That's not to suggest that baklava is a health food. The calories hit 550, the total fat climbs to 21 grams, and last but not least, there are the 8 teaspoons of sugar. Still, for a restaurant dessert, you could do far worse.

The Bottom Line: *Split this sweet treat with a friend.*

Decoding Greek and Middle Eastern Specialties

We've shared the results of our analyses of some of the popular Greek dishes on restaurant menus. Now here's a quick look at some other Greek specialties that we did not send to the laboratory, along with some Middle Eastern ones that are sometimes on the menu with Greek ones at some sit-down restaurants, mall eateries, airports, and other locations.

Avgolemono soup, also called egg and lemon soup, is chicken stock that's been simmered with rice, then thickened with egg yolks or whole eggs and flavored with fresh lemon juice. Just what you need—more egg yolks in your diet. (A thicker version of avgolemono without the rice is traditionally used as a sauce for Greek and Middle Eastern dishes.) We estimate that indulging in a 1-cup serving of this tangy soup will sock you with about half your daily quota of cholesterol.

A **falafel** sandwich is made of cooked chickpeas (garbanzo beans) which are mashed and seasoned with cumin, cayenne, and other spices, shaped into little balls or patties, deep-fried, and then stuffed into pita bread along with lettuce, tomatoes, cucumbers, and tahini (sesame seed paste) or yogurt dressing. Although the sandwich provides a decent amount of fiber, the frying oil does make it high in calories.

Hummus and **baba ghanouj** are creamy Middle Eastern spreads meant to be scooped up with wedges of pita. Hummus is made from chickpeas, tahini, garlic, olive oil, lemon juice, and other seasonings. Two tablespoons of grocery store hummus have just 50 calories and 4 grams of fat, nearly all of it unsaturated. The restaurant version may differ, since olive oil is often drizzled over the plate. *Baba ghanouj* is made from puréed eggplant, tahini, garlic, lemon juice, and olive oil. It, too, is rock-bottom low in saturated fat and makes an excellent filling or dip for pita bread. But don't go overboard. The olive oil hikes the calories with each dip.

Greek *keftedes* or ***kefte*** (also known as *kofte* in Turkey) are small seasoned patties of ground lamb or beef that are made in a variety of shapes in Greece and throughout the Middle East. Sometimes they are molded around skewers for grilling as *kefte kebob* or shaped into fingers or flat patties and fried in oil. They might also be partially grilled, then baked and served with a tomato sauce or other topping. When you're talking ground beef or lamb, you're talking saturated fat, which means trouble for your arteries. You can't see it . . . and you can't trim it away. If it's skewers you want, you're better off with leaner Greek chicken, lamb, or pork souvlaki.

Pastitsio is a Greek main-course baked casserole that's similar to moussaka. It's put together with alternating layers of spaghetti (or ziti) and a tomato-meat sauce (usually made with lamb or beef), then topped with a heavy coating of béchamel sauce and a sprinkling of Parmesan cheese. Eat a modest portion and we estimate that you'll use up a day's worth of saturated fat and more than a day's limit of cholesterol. Think of it as an order of lasagna with an egg on top.

Tabbouleh is the Middle Eastern name for a delightful salad that's generously filled with steamed cracked wheat (bulgar), chopped parsley and tomatoes, mint, lemon juice, garlic, scallions, and a little olive oil. Traditionally it's scooped up with lettuce leaves or pieces of pita bread. This excellent appetizer or side dish is very low in saturated fat and, if made from whole grain wheat, is high in fiber.

Greek Strategy

• **Think twice before ordering.** Although many popular Greek specialties can arrive at the table with more saturated fat than a fast-food burger, you do have some good options. Chicken, lamb, or pork souvlaki is just as good for you as the most healthful meals in Italian, Chinese, and American-style restaurants.

• **Split portions.** Cut the calorie count and the fat by sharing a fatty entrée (like spanakopita or dolmades) with a friend.

• **Hold the cheese.** When ordering a salad, ask to have the cheese (and the dressing) served on the side, then use just a tablespoon of each. Greek cheeses like feta are quite strong in flavor, so a little goes a long way.

• **Think lean.** Opt for specialties made with whole pieces of lamb, pork, or beef (kebabs), rather than fattier ground meat (like moussaka, pastitsio, or *keftedes*) or gyro meat, which is a sausage-like mixture of beef and lamb.

Within each category, dishes are ranked from best to worst—that is, from least to most saturated fat. Entrées and platters marked with a ✔ are Best Bites. Best Bites are relatively low in saturated fat.

Reminder

Recommended limits for a 2,000-calorie diet:
Total fat: 65 grams
Saturated fat: 20 grams
Cholesterol: 300 milligrams
Sodium: 2,400 milligrams

GREEK FOODS

Menu Item	Calories	Total Fat (g)	Saturated Fat (g)	Cholesterol (mg)	Sodium (mg)
ENTRÉES					
✔ Chicken souvlaki (kebab) (7 oz.)	260	8	*2*	145	370
✔ plus rice (13 oz.)	500	14	*5*	155	1,050
✔ Lamb or pork souvlaki (kebab) (8 oz.)	310	11	*4*	165	550
✔ plus rice (13 oz.)	550	18	*7*	175	1,230
Spanakopita (spinach pie) (8 oz.)	410	24	*12*	95	730
Greek salad (3½ cups) with dressing	390	30	*12*	25	1,060
Meat-and-rice dolmades (stuffed grape leaves) (4 pieces; 12 oz.)	540	32	*15*	120	1,470
Gyro (pita sandwich with meat) (12 oz.)	760	44	*20*	95	2,390
Moussaka (ground beef and eggplant casserole) (12 oz.)	830	48	*25*	140	2,010
SIDE DISH					
Greek rice (1½ cups)	240	7	*3*	10	680
DESSERT					
Baklava (honey and nut pastry) (5 oz.)*	550	21	*5*	15	N/A

*Contains 32 grams (8 tsp.) of sugar

N/A=number not available

Note: Saturated fat numbers in *italics* include artery-clogging *trans* fat.

Chapter 10

Catch of the Day: Seafood Restaurants

F ish has always been one of America's richest and most bountiful edible resources. Historically, wherever there was water, Americans harvested seafood—from Maine lobsters and Louisiana catfish to Maryland crabs and Wisconsin lake trout. And we've traditionally enjoyed and celebrated seafood at fish boils in the Midwest, church fish fries in the South, and clambakes on the East Coast.

But until recently, unless you lived near the source, access to fresh seafood was pretty limited or very expensive. Seafood often meant mysterious frozen fish sticks and unappetizing rectangular slabs of frozen fillets. Happily, all that has changed. Improved transportation now makes it possible for fresh fish to glisten in almost every supermarket (some even have live lobsters scuttling around in tanks), and advanced flash-freezing techniques ensure that even frozen seafood can be tasty. Eating delicious fish or shellfish at home or in a restaurant has never been easier.

By and large, fish are good for us. Most seafood—cod, flounder, haddock, Pacific halibut, ocean perch, orange roughy, pollock, sole, shrimp, scallops, crabs, and clams—is a nutritional bonanza, exceptionally low in fat, and loaded with B vitamins, iron, zinc, selenium, and copper. Salmon, catfish, bluefin tuna, swordfish, and rainbow trout, although somewhat fattier, are nevertheless also low in saturated fat and are a source of omega-3 fats, which may also prevent strokes caused by blood clots (see page 192). These fats appear to prevent abnormal heart rhythms that can lead to sudden cardiac arrest.

Other welcome news is that most seafood meals have less sodium than a typical Chinese, Italian, or Mexican spread. According to the U.S. Department of Agriculture, only a few kinds of shellfish, like Alaska king crab, are naturally high in salt. A 3-ounce serving of unseasoned Alaska king crab has about 900 milligrams of sodium. But you'd have to go out of your way to come anywhere near that figure with another seafood choice—provided your seafood doesn't come with a salty sauce, breading, or batter. So if you order carefully, you can get what's next to impossible at most other kinds of restaurants (with the exception of steak houses): meals that aren't loaded with sodium.

As for cholesterol, most seafood (except for shrimp) has about the same amount as chicken, turkey, pork, or beef. The difference is that all seafood—shrimp included—is so low in saturated fat that it won't raise your *blood* cholesterol as much as other meats.

Seafood has a healthy reputation, and we wanted to find out if the most popular dishes at midpriced seafood houses—places like Red Lobster and Landry's Seafood House, as well as smaller chains and independents—deserved it. We're relieved to say that lower-fat and lower-sodium options abound. Seafood restaurants offer plenty of healthy choices: Have your fish broiled, baked, blackened, grilled, or steamed. Seafood is a great choice, as long as you don't order it fried, stuffed, or smothered with cream, cheese, butter, or tartar sauce. In fact, seafood is almost a freebie—even if the chef uses a little butter or margarine to lubricate the grill or the pan.

Sorting Out the Sides

Many restaurants offer fish dinners with a choice of green salad, coleslaw, or a vegetable of the day, along with potato or rice. If you order simple sides like an unbuttered baked potato, a salad dressed with vinegar or lemon juice, and an unbuttered roll along with a broiled lean fish entrée, you've got a filling and delicious meal for around 600 calories. That's low for an entire restaurant meal. It will have less fat than the lowest-fat Chinese or Italian dishes like Szechuan shrimp and spaghetti with marinara sauce. What's more, the whole meal has less than one-third the fat of an ordinary deli tuna salad sandwich.

Does a naked baked potato, a lemon-juiced salad, and a dry roll sound a trifle... stark? If so, you can use a tablespoon of sour cream on the potato, a tablespoon or two of light dressing on your salad, and a pat of butter or margarine on your roll. You'll still be at about 20 grams of fat, which is terrific for a restaurant meal, plus the sodium stays at about 1,000 milligrams. But if you use the full quarter-cup serving of sour cream and the two pats of butter that are often served on a baked potato, you might as well have gotten french fries. Choose rice pilaf instead of the potato and you'll keep the fat to a minimum, although the sodium soars (770 milligrams in a one-cup order).

On the salad front, a 2-cup side salad with 4 tablespoons of light dressing adds only 90 calories to your meal. But get that salad with the typical 4 tablespoons of regular dressing and it will contain 300 calories (and almost half a day's fat). That's three times fattier than a typical half cup of coleslaw.

What if your favorite fish house serves biscuits instead of bread or rolls? Think of a biscuit as a salted dinner roll that leaves the kitchen with a pat of butter, which, of course, only gets worse if you add more butter. Our advice is to skip the biscuit.

Trans Fat Transgression

We're pleased to report that you'll encounter few bad surprises at most seafood restaurants. You already know what the fattiest menu items are: seafood swimming in butter, cheese, or cream

Fishing for Omegas

Nearly half a million Americans will die of a heart attack this year. That's about one every minute.

Roughly half of those people will suffer a myocardial infarction due to clogged arteries. The other half will suffer a "sudden cardiac death"—that is, they'll die within an hour after the heart attack begins. In most cases, the heart stops beating because the electrical impulses that control its rhythm go awry (arrhythmia). More than half of the victims have no history of heart disease.

Relatively little is known about how to prevent sudden cardiac death. The omega-3 fats in salmon and other fatty fish may be a help. When animals are fed diets rich in fish oil instead of other fats, they are less likely to suffer arrythmia.

Fish oil may also protect humans. The Physicians' Health Study, for example, followed more than 20,000 men for 11 years. The men who reported eating fish at least once a week were half as likely to die of sudden death over the next decade as the men who reported eating fish less than once a month.

Other studies suggest that fish oil may also help prevent blood clots, which would lower the risk of both heart attacks and strokes. In one study, women who ate seafood two to four times a week had about half the risk of strokes caused by blood clots compared to women who ate seafood less than once a month.

In some studies, the risk was lower in people who ate one serving of fatty fish (about 1½ grams of omega-3 fats) a week.

Fish (6 oz. cooked, unless specified)	Fat (g)	Omega-3 Fats (g)
Salmon, Atlantic, farmed	21	3.7
Salmon, Atlantic, wild	14	3.1
Sardines, in sardine oil (3 oz.)	13	2.8

Fish (6 oz. cooked, unless specified)	Fat (g)	Omega-3 Fats (g)
Salmon, coho, farmed	14	2.2
Trout, rainbow, farmed	12	2.0
Salmon, coho, wild	7	1.8
Herring (3 oz.)	13	1.5
Swordfish	9	1.4
Oysters (3 oz.)	4	1.1
Pollock	2	0.9
Flounder or sole	3	0.9
Rockfish	3	0.8
Halibut	5	0.8
Sardines, in vegetable oil (3 oz.)	10	0.8
Tuna, white, canned in water (3 oz.)	3	0.7
Scallops	2	0.6
Tuna, fresh	2	0.5
Haddock	2	0.4
Fish sticks (6)	21	0.4
Cod	1	0.4
Crab, Dungeness (3 oz.)	1	0.3
Shrimp (3 oz.)	1	0.3
Catfish, farmed	14	0.3
Tuna, light, canned in water (3 oz.)	1	0.2
Clams (3 oz.)	2	0.2
Lobster (3 oz.)	1	0.1

Source: USDA and (for sardines in sardine oil) the *American Journal of Clinical Nutrition* 66 (1997):1029S.

sauce, and breaded or batter-dipped, deep-fried dishes. But you may not know that the fat many seafood houses use for frying is worse than lard. The problem is those nasty *trans* fats that help make margarine and shortenings more solid than oils. As we discussed in chapter 2 (see pages 27–30), they'll raise your cholesterol about as much as saturated fats do. When the staff at several Red Lobster restaurants told us that their frying fat was a solid soaplike block at room temperature, we sent our fried items off to be analyzed for *trans* fat. The results showed that the amount of *trans* roughly equaled the amount of saturated fat, which means it doubled the artery-clogging fat in fried items.

The 39 grams of saturated plus *trans* fat in a typical fried seafood platter (including fries, coleslaw, two biscuits, and tartar sauce) propels it into the ranks of the infamous fettuccine Alfredo, cheese fries with ranch dressing, and movie theater popcorn.

Many restaurants use partially hydrogenated *liquid* shortening. That means that although their fried foods have less *trans* fat than the dishes at Red Lobster, they will still have more than foods cooked in regular vegetable oil (the kind you use at home). It means their numbers are somewhat better than our averages; Red Lobster's are worse.

The Dishes and the Data

We bought take-out portions of 14 popular appetizers, side dishes, and entrées at 32 midpriced seafood restaurants, including the 670-restaurant Red Lobster chain, small regional chains like Landry's Seafood House, Legal Sea Foods, Rusty Pelican, and Weathervane, as well as several independent restaurants, in Boston, Chicago, Los Angeles, Seattle, and Washington, D.C. (For more on our methodology, see pages 12–14.)

We didn't analyze popular steamed seafood dishes like lobster or crab because those numbers are readily available from the USDA. Keep in mind, however, that the numbers in our table for steamed items don't include the salt and other seasonings a chef might add to the pot, or the melted butter usually served alongside

Within each category we've ranked the dishes from best to worst; that is, from least to most saturated fat.

Appetizer

NEW ENGLAND CLAM CHOWDER
(250 calories and 7 grams of fat, 2 of them saturated)
Expect to find about 2 ounces of clams in that 1½-cup bowl of creamy soup. If a restaurant makes its chowder with cream or butter, which many do, the fat content could be higher than our average sample. As for sodium, even though clams are low in sodium, the salty soup will blow almost two-thirds of your day's allotment before you even touch your main course. This chowder has far more sodium than the crackers served with it.

The Bottom Line: *Tomato-based Manhattan clam chowder, has less fat and fewer calories (although it does have much more sodium).*

Entrées

BROILED OR GRILLED SCALLOPS
(150 calories and 3 grams of fat, 1 of them saturated)
Wow, is this delicious entrée low in fat! But the sodium in a typical 6-ounce serving was so high—almost 1,000 milligrams—that it appears some chefs add far too much salt when they marinate or season the scallops.

The Bottom Line: *To keep the sodium level of your entire meal in check, get a baked potato with a tablespoon of sour cream and a salad dressed with oil and vinegar.*

BROILED LOW-FAT FISH
(210 calories and 5 grams of fat, 1 of them saturated)

This nutritionally wise choice can be made with any lean, white-fleshed fish like haddock, cod, scrod (baby cod), sole, flounder, Pacific halibut, ocean perch, and pollock. You won't find a better entrée.

The Bottom Line: *Order your broiled fish with a side salad and a baked potato with a tablespoon of sour cream and you've got a nearly perfect meal. Although it's not really necessary, you could trim the fat even more—to a puny 2 grams per 6-ounce serving—by asking to have the fish broiled "dry" (without any butter or margarine).*

SHRIMP SCAMPI
(150 calories and 5 grams of fat, 2 of them saturated)

The low numbers for this deliciously garlicky broiled entrée don't include most of its buttery sauce because you can improve this dish right at the table. Simply fork up each shrimp as you go, and leave the fatty sauce behind. If the restaurant normally serves scampi over pasta or rice, ask to have them arranged on the side of the plate instead, so the mound of starch won't get soaked with the fatty sauce.

The Bottom Line: *A succulent, satisfying choice.*

BLACKENED CATFISH
(300 calories and 15 grams of fat, 3 of them saturated)

This popular Cajun classic is another dish you can relish. Although a 6-ounce fillet is twice as salty as plain broiled fish, it's still pretty good compared to most restaurant entrées. Almost all of the fat here comes from the fish, not the wonderful seasonings that form the blackened crust, so there's very little saturated fat.

The Bottom Line: *A flavorful, nearly flawless main course.*

BROILED SALMON
(420 calories and 21 grams of fat, 4 of them saturated)

The restaurants we surveyed were more generous with their salmon than with other fish—the average portion size was half a pound. The hefty portion and salmon's higher fat content boosted the calories above a low-fat fish, but don't let it stop you from digging in. Most of the fat is unsaturated, so it should help lower your cholesterol. What's more, salmon is the best source of omega-3 fats, so it should help prevent heart attacks. And salmon is less likely to have contaminants than fatty fish like bluefish or lake trout because salmon spend most of their lives in relatively clean waters. And as any fish lover knows, salmon's flavor is in a class of its own.

The Bottom Line: *Sit back and enjoy.*

BAKED STUFFED SHRIMP
(470 calories and 30 grams of fat, 6 of them saturated)

Shrimp is so naturally low in fat that you might think a little stuffing won't hurt, but think again. On average, you'll be getting two-thirds stuffing and one-third shrimp! All that buttery, stuffing-studded seafood adds up to nearly 500 calories and a day's cholesterol, but the saturated fat is still low compared to most restaurant dishes.

The Bottom Line: *Not a disaster, but broiled or grilled shrimp is much better.*

FRIED FISH
(520 calories and 24 grams of fat, 8 of them saturated)

Ponder this: A 9-ounce fried fillet has more than twice the calories and sodium and five times the fat of an order of broiled fish And the saturated fat eats up almost half your daily limit. If you use all four tablespoons of the tartar sauce that most restaurants serve with fried fish, the fat doubles and the calories climb by 300. Plus, more than a third of your entrée will be breading or batter, which is where much of the fat is.

The Bottom Line: *Do the math, then place your order for broiled, grilled, or blackened fish.*

FRIED SHRIMP
(510 calories and 26 grams of fat, 10 of them saturated)

An average 7-ounce order, about 14 shrimp, contains a day's cholesterol. But unlike grilled or broiled shrimp, the shortening-soaked breading or batter supplies half a day's saturated fat.

The Bottom Line: *Want to slash the fat by about 90 percent? Order your shrimp unbreaded and steamed or grilled. Not only is this healthier, you'll actually be able to savor the flavor of the shrimp!*

FRIED CLAMS
(830 calories and 47 grams of fat, 19 of them saturated)

You might as well just eat fried breading; it's that simple. Most 8-ounce restaurant orders contain only a smidgen of clams. One restaurant sold us less than an ounce of clams covered with 9 ounces of breading. You'd expect an entire day's saturated fat from a steak house, not a seafood restaurant. Dip the clams in a typical serving of tartar sauce, and you'll end up consuming as much fat as three large orders of McDonald's French Fries, along with more than 1,000 calories.

The Bottom Line: *If you want clams, have them prepared so that you can taste them. Many restaurants offer steamers and chowder. Either would be healthier.*

FRIED SEAFOOD COMBO
(970 calories and 50 grams of fat, 19 of them saturated)

Eat a pound of fried fish, shrimp, clams, and scallops and you can kiss your daily saturated fat budget good-bye. This platter also contains a day's cholesterol, three-quarters of a day's sodium, and half a day's calories. Use 4 tablespoons of tartar sauce and the fat equals that in 30 McDonald's Chicken McNuggets. Add the traditional fries, coleslaw, and biscuits with butter, and you'll down a staggering 130 grams of fat, 39 of which are saturated (two days' limit); more than a day's cholesterol; and nearly two days' sodium.

The Bottom Line: *If you care about your health, avoid this fried fish festival on a platter—it won a spot on our Ten of the Worst Restaurant Meals list (see page 39). Choose instead one of the grilled or broiled seafood combos featured on seafood restaurant menus.*

SEAFOOD CASSEROLE
(640 calories and 43 grams of fat, 21 of them saturated)

You'll find this dish under various names on restaurant menus: Newburg, Thermidor, Alfredo, au gratin. Typically, it's a combination of crab, shrimp, and scallops in a cream or cheese sauce. An average 12-ounce portion contains over a day's cholesterol and saturated fat and more than half a day's sodium.

The Bottom Line: *This casserole's rich sauce literally buries the lean, sweet seafood. Why order a dish with so little fish flavor, when you could enjoy a healthier, more flavorful entrée such as broiled scallops or grilled shrimp?*

When Your Favorite Is Not on the List

Restaurants are constantly exploring new varieties of fish as market shortages drive up the prices of popular species. If your favorite is not mentioned here, keep in mind that when looking for healthier options, it's more important to pay attention to the cooking technique and the sauce that accompanies a dish than to the fat content of a particular fish.

Decoding a Seafood Restaurant Menu

Most seafood menus are refreshingly straightforward, so there should be few culinary mysteries to solve and very little guesswork.

Typically, a menu entry will identify the fish species and the manner in which it is prepared. For example: "Farm-Raised Blackened Catfish," "Salmon Fillet Grilled with Lemon Butter," or "Mussels Steamed in Garlic and White Wine."

You'll find that even the descriptive names of unhealthful dishes can be pretty straightforward and revealing. For example if "Scallops Wrapped in Bacon," "Grilled Grouper with Coconut Milk Sauce," and "Halibut Topped with Salsa and Melted Jack Cheese" are on the menu, you can tell at a glance they're going to be loaded with saturated fat.

When the menu is not specific enough, ask the server to describe a dish in greater detail. Even something that sounds as

Overfished Species

●●●

It's easy to feast on a delicious and healthful seafood dinner and overlook a sad reality. Seafood's surge in popularity, coupled with high-tech methods of search and capture, have put many varieties of seafood in danger of depletion and possibly even extinction. According to the Natural Resources Defense Council, about 70 percent of the world's commercially important marine fish population is in trouble. Does that mean we must give up this magnificent food? Not entirely, but we should keep in mind that some species—like shark, North Atlantic swordfish, Atlantic cod, sturgeon, and black sea bass—have been overfished. Until responsible fishing policies can be implemented worldwide, avoid these.

pristine as a salad of cold, poached shrimp and scallops may come to the table drowning in full-fat dressing that you could easily get on the side. You'll never know if you don't ask.

Seafood Strategy

• **Women who are or may become pregnant, nursing mothers, and young children should avoid fish that may be contaminated with toxic chemicals.** Mercury, which can affect the brain, is a special risk in swordfish, shark, king mackerel, tilefish, and fresh tuna steaks. PCBs and dioxins, which may cause cancer, are likeliest to contaminate bluefish, as well as lake trout and other inland freshwater fish.

• **Pick a low-fat preparation method.** Order seafood broiled, baked, grilled, blackened, or steamed.

• **Beware of breading and batter.** Avoid high-fat breaded or deep-fried entrées, which have at least double the calories of grilled or broiled seafood. Your fish will have more flavor, too, since there'll be no breading barrier between the fish and your taste buds.

• **Hold the fries.** Have the kitchen hold the fries and substitute a baked potato garnished with one tablespoon of sour cream. Fries may be slightly lower in fat and calories at a seafood restaurant than at a steak house or dinner house, simply because some are cut thicker. (The thinner the fry, the more surface area it's got and the more fat it absorbs.) Still, you're better off eating a baked potato.

• **Seek out healthy sides.** Skip the coleslaw. Opt instead for a green salad tossed with light dressing, lemon juice, or vinegar. And order a vegetable side dish whenever possible.

• **Bye-bye biscuits.** Dinner rolls have less fat and sodium.

Contamination Concerns

Government inspectors are stationed at every slaughterhouse and visit every beef-, pork-, and poultry-processing plant every day. But no similar system is in place for the seafood industry, and even plant inspections may occur no more than once a year or less. The risk of contamination is unsettling. Here's some information that can help you avoid an encounter with tainted fish.

Chemical Contaminants

Because harmful chemicals accumulate in a fish's fat, your safest choices are lean fish like cod, flounder, haddock, Pacific halibut, ocean perch, pollock, and sole. In general, catfish and salmon (except those caught in the Great Lakes) are also fine.

Bacteria and Viruses

Be warned that you eat raw shellfish such as oysters and clams at your peril. Raw shellfish—particularly those harvested from Gulf of Mexico waters—account for the majority of seafood-poisoning cases. They can also contain bacteria or viruses that cause hepatitis or gastroenteritis. If you are elderly or pregnant, or have cancer, diabetes, kidney or liver problems, or a compromised immune system, then you are at greatest risk.

Mercury

Mercury is a highly toxic substance that can contaminate seafood. Don't eat swordfish, shark, king mackerel, white or golden snapper, or fresh tuna steaks more than once a week. Women who are or could become pregnant in the next year, nursing mothers, and young children should avoid these fish entirely and limit their consumption of canned tuna. This will lessen their exposure to mercury, a contaminant that may raise the risk of cerebral palsy, learning disabilities, and other problems in infants and young children. For serious recreational fishermen, high mercury exposure can result in numbness and loss of coordination, as well as hearing and vision problems.

Natural Toxins

Ciguatera and scombroid poisoning are caused by natural toxins in finfish. Ciguatera poisoning is linked to consumption of barracuda, grouper, amberjack, and snapper from tropical or subtropical waters, primarily in the Caribbean, Florida, and Hawaii. Ciguatera causes unique symptoms, such as "hot-cold inversion" (a symptom in which hot coffee feels cold and ice cream feels hot). Scombroid poisoning can occur when fresh tuna, mackerel, bluefish, and mahimahi are not kept constantly cold. Scombroid can cause severe diarrhea, vomiting, difficulty swallowing, and rash with itching.

Bluefish Blues

Bluefish are large, fatty, and migratory. Each of these characteristics increases the odds that the fish is contaminated, often by PCBs. PCBs may cause cancer and also contribute to learning problems in children. Bluefish are also the fish most likely to contain the carcinogen dioxin. Lake trout and other inland freshwater fish can suffer from the same two problems. The less of all these fish you eat, the better. Women who could become pregnant are advised to avoid them altogether.

Within each category we ranked the dishes from best to worst— that is, from least to most saturated fat. Items marked with a ✔ are Best Bites. Best Bites are relatively low in saturated fat.

Reminder

Recommended limits for a 2,000-calorie diet:

Total fat: 65 grams
Saturated fat: 20 grams
Cholesterol: 300 milligrams
Sodium: 2,400 milligrams

SEAFOOD

Menu Item	Calories	Total Fat (g)	Saturated Fat (g)	Cholesterol (mg)	Sodium (mg)
APPETIZERS					
✔ Steamed shrimp (¼ lb. unpeeled—3 oz. peeled)	80	1	0	165	190
✔ Steamed clams (½ lb. with shells—3 oz. shelled)	130	2	0	55	100
New England clam chowder (1½ cups)	250	7	2	50	1,430
ENTRÉES					
✔ Steamed lobster (1⅛ lb. with shell—3 oz. shelled)	80	1	0	60	320
✔ Steamed Alaska king crab (¼ lb. with shells—3 oz. shelled)	80	1	0	45	910
✔ Broiled or grilled scallops (6 oz.)	150	3	1	65	990
✔ Broiled low-fat fish (cod, haddock, etc.) (6 oz.)	210	5	1	125	360
✔ plus tossed salad with light Italian dressing (4 Tb.) and baked potato with sour cream (1 Tb.) and a dinner roll with butter (1 pat)	730	21	7	145	1,070
✔ Shrimp scampi (4 oz.)	150	5	2	230	550
✔ Blackened catfish (6 oz.)	300	15	3	130	700
✔ Broiled salmon (8 oz.)	420	21	4	155	340

SEAFOOD *(continued)* Menu Item	Calories	Total Fat (g)	Saturated Fat (g)	Cholesterol (mg)	Sodium (mg)
Baked stuffed shrimp (8 oz.)	470	30	6	285	1,040
Fried fish (9 oz.)	520	24	8	145	840
Fried shrimp (7 oz.)	510	26	10	280	970
Fried clams (8 oz.)	830	47	19	65	1,660
Fried seafood combo (14 oz.)	970	50	19	295	1,920
plus tartar sauce (4 Tb.) and french fries, coleslaw, and biscuits (2) with butter (2 pats)	2,170	130	39	360	4,390
Seafood casserole (12 oz.)	640	43	21	320	1,470
SIDE DISHES					
Tossed salad, without dressing (2 cups)	30	1	0	0	20
Dinner roll	90	1	0	0	150
Tossed salad with 4 Tb. light Italian dressing	90	7	1	5	490
Coleslaw (½ cup)	100	8	1	10	210
Baked potato with 1 Tb. sour cream	310	3	2	5	30
Rice pilaf (1 cup)	260	5	2	10	770
Biscuit	150	6	2	5	350
Dinner roll with 1 pat butter	120	6	3	10	190
Biscuit with 1 pat butter	180	11	4	15	390
Tossed salad with 4 Tb. regular Italian salad dressing	300	29	4	0	480
French fries (2 cups)	420	18	7	5	760
Baked potato with 4 Tb. sour cream and 2 pats butter	470	20	12	45	140

SEAFOOD (continued) Menu Item	Calories	Total Fat (g)	Saturated Fat (g)	Cholesterol (mg)	Sodium (mg)
CONDIMENTS					
Tartar sauce (1 Tb.)	80	8	1	5	180
Sour cream (1 Tb.)	30	3	2	5	10
Butter (1 pat)	40	4	3	10	40

Note: Numbers for steamed seafood, baked potato, tossed salad, dinner roll, butter, sour cream, Italian dressing, and tartar sauce are from the USDA Nutrient Database for Standard Reference. Numbers for steamed lobster, crab, shrimp, and clams do not include any added butter, salt, or other seasonings. Saturated fat numbers in *italics* include artery-clogging *trans* fat.

Chapter 11

Here's the Beef: Steak Houses

P erhaps no meal is considered as all-American as meat and potatoes, and no meat is as highly desired as beef. From the roast beef and Yorkshire pudding served by gracious colonial hostesses on the East Coast to the hearty stews cooked over open fires by early American settlers on the western frontier, beef has long been the centerpiece of the American table. As one mid-century frontier newspaper declared, "We are essentially a hungry beef-eating people." The statement was quite true, of course, but it was not until after 1877 that beef finally became widely available.

That year, Gustavus F. Swift helped to revolutionize the American diet by inaugurating the first refrigerated train cars. This enabled freshly butchered meat to be transported from the Chicago stockyards to other regions of the country, making meat accessible to anyone who could afford it. In no time at all, the national appetite for beef was satisfied, and red meat was firmly established as America's main dish. Today this country's predilection for red meat is echoed in the virile voice-over and references to cowboy country in the Beef Board's commercials that tout the meat as: "Beef. It's What's for Dinner."

Despite the warnings over the past several decades about the risks of eating too much red meat, many Americans still crave the taste—whether ground, grilled, smothered with ketchup on a bun, or broiled to sizzling perfection. And while some people may be preparing red meat at home less often, we seek it more and more when we dine out.

When people hanker after a slab of beef these days, they often head to restaurants like Outback, Lone Star, and LongHorn, all midpriced, publike chain steak houses where the lively atmosphere is just as important as the sirloin. The explosive growth of industry leader Outback in the early-1990s—with its beefed-up Australian decor, a menu studded with Down-Under slang, and a now-famous trademarked Bloomin' Onion—set the stage for a stream of imitators. Today diners can rustle up a steak at Lone Star, a make-believe western saloon where the floors are strewn with peanuts and the servers occasionally burst into dance. They can soak up country-and-western atmosphere at LongHorn. And they can sit in a wilderness of animated moose, buffalo, and dancing trees at Bugaboo Creek.

Selecting a Steak

Don't mosey into a steak house until you know which cuts are leanest. Both a sirloin steak and a filet mignon put all the other beef choices to shame. Every other cut we tested flunked the fat test and showed us how steak got its reputation as a heartbreaker. If you choose a New York strip or T-bone, for instance, you'll use up about a day's worth of saturated fat, even if you carefully trim all of the fat from the edges. A trimmed porterhouse steak or prime rib contains almost two days' saturated fat. Eat them untrimmed, and these cuts will cost you even more.

Other Types of Steak Houses

Keep in mind that our findings, which came from analyses of food at midpriced steak houses, may not hold true for budget-priced places, where serving sizes may be smaller or the steaks are cut and trimmed differently. And our numbers certainly won't apply to high-end cigar-and-single-malt-whiskey steak restaurants, where the beef is usually fattier Prime and the portions are bigger. Chicago's Chop House, for example, serves a porterhouse that weighs a gargantuan 64 ounces—4 pounds—and is sometimes accompanied by a monster 1-pound baked potato.

Where the Beef Is

According to *Restaurant Business,* an industry periodical, traffic at casual steak houses has increased 80 percent since 1993. Diners want their beef in big portions and boldly presented in what they call "high-concept venues." You can enjoy your high-concept entertainment—and your steak—if you're willing to choose carefully. Steak can be decent or disastrous, but an occasional steak doesn't have to do in your diet. You can ride into the sunset satisfied—but not saturated—if you know what you're doing.

Strangely enough, the biggest problem we found at steak houses wasn't the steak. It was all those rootin'-tootin' appetizers. Fanciful starters are fun-food concoctions—and a major attraction at steak houses. However, they're more about novelty than nutrition, and they deliver colossal amounts of the very things you should be eating less of. For example, even if you split an order of cheese fries with ranch dressing with a friend, you'll still be getting 1,500 calories and more fat than an untrimmed 16-ounce slab of prime rib.

The Dishes and the Data

We bought take-out portions of 15 popular appetizers, entrées, and side dishes at 26 steak houses. Restaurants included casual chains like Bugaboo Creek, Damon's, Hungry Hunter, Lone Star, LongHorn, Outback, Steak and Ale, Stuart Anderson's, and Tony Roma's, plus some smaller chains and independents in Chicago, Columbus (Ohio), Las Vegas, and Washington, D.C. (For more on our methodology, see pages 12–14.)

The weights given for the steaks refer to *uncooked* meat (except for prime rib), since that's how the steaks are described on restaurant menus. The cooked meat, of course, will be several ounces lighter. We analyzed all meat untrimmed because that's the way it's served. But we also calculated numbers for steaks and chops trimmed of visible fat because that's the way we advise you to eat them. To do that, we followed one of the U.S. Department of Agriculture's protocols for trimming meat. We asked laboratory technicians to cut off—with scalpels—all the fat around the edges of, but not inside, the meat. Some people also trim the fat that's inside their steaks. On the other hand, most people aren't as careful as technicians. So on balance, our trimming probably approximates what you'll do with a steak knife and fork. If you trim every speck of fat off the outside and inside of a steak, you'll get less fat than our "trimmed" numbers reflect.

Within each category we've ranked the trimmed meats and other foods from best to worst; that is, from least to most saturated fat.

Appetizers

FRIED WHOLE ONION
without dipping sauce (1,690 calories and 116 grams of fat, 44 of them saturated), **with dipping sauce** (2,130 calories and 163 grams of fat, 57 of them saturated)

Outback calls it a Bloomin' Onion, but several other steak-house chains also offer a batter-dipped, deep-fried whole onion cut to open like a flower and served with a creamy dipping sauce. Lone Star serves a similar creation called a Texas Rose. If you only eat *half*—without the sauce—you'll consume about a day's fat and saturated fat, more than half a day's sodium, and more than 800 calories. That's like whetting your appetite with two McDonald's Quarter Pounders all by your lonesome! Using half a serving of the dipping sauce would tack on a McDonald's Baked Apple Pie.

The Bottom Line: *The battered onion is a bomb.*

CHEESE FRIES
without ranch dressing (2,380 calories and 151 grams of fat, 79 of them saturated), with ranch dressing (3,010 calories and 217 grams of fat, 91 of them saturated)

Picture this: more than a pound of french fries smothered in a third of a pound of melted cheese, sprinkled with the equivalent of four strips of crumbled bacon, served with ranch dressing. Eat this whole pile of food with the dressing and you'll swallow over 3,000 calories, three days' fat, and more than all the artery-hardening fat you should eat in *four* entire days. Even if you share it with a friend—or two or three—the numbers are still staggering. A single order of cheese fries is worse than any of the steak *platters* we analyzed. In fact, cheese fries are worse than *anything* we've ever analyzed. That includes both fettuccine Alfredo and a large bucket of movie theater popcorn popped in highly saturated coconut oil and topped with ersatz "butter."

The Bottom Line: *Make this better? You must be joking.*

Entrées

BARBECUE CHICKEN BREAST
(280 calories and 5 grams of fat, 2 of them saturated)

As usual, chicken breast tops the list of lower-fat entrées. (Its only competition is grilled fish.) Our testing found that the barbecue sauce was salty but not fatty. To create a 700-calorie dinner with a mere 11 grams of fat, order your chicken with smart side dishes like a house salad with two tablespoons of light dressing and a baked potato with a tablespoon of sour cream. The calories drop to 550 if you replace the potato with the vegetable of the day, which is usually seasoned broccoli, cauliflower, and carrots. You can also cut the sodium by about 200 milligrams if you ask for a potato that hasn't been rolled in salt before it was baked. That's why baked potatoes at steak houses have more sodium than the spuds you get at some restaurants.

The Bottom Line: *Hands down, this is your best choice at a steak house. If you want to cut back on the sodium, ask for the barbecue sauce on the side and use just a tablespoon.*

SIRLOIN STEAK
(390 calories and 15 grams of fat, 8 of them saturated)
Luckily, one of the most popular steaks is also one of the leanest. Only round steak has less fat than sirloin. What's more, casual steak houses serve Choice-grade meat, which has less fat than the heavily marbled Prime that upscale establishments like Morton's of Chicago and Ruth's Chris serve. Accompany your 12-ounce sirloin with wisely chosen side dishes and you'll have consumed just half a day's saturated fat. Of course, that won't be as low fat as a chicken breast platter, but by steak-house standards it could be a lot worse. Just remember that adding higher-calorie sides like a Caesar salad and a buttered baked potato will triple the fat to a day's worth.

The Bottom Line: *This is your best bet on the red-meat front. You could trim the meat if you want, but sirloin usually has too little to do you much harm.*

FILET MIGNON
(350 calories and 18 grams of fat, 9 of them saturated)
This cut of beef from the tenderloin is small (*mignon* means "cute" in French). A 9-ounce filet mignon has only a tad more fat

than a 12-ounce sirloin. After cooking, it ends up at 6½ ounces, which is double the government's recommended 3-ounce serving for meat. However, compared to most steak-house offerings, that's a downright dainty serving. You can get by with just 800 calories for a whole meal if you stick with the right side dishes. But if you choose a Caesar salad and a buttered baked potato, they would ratchet up the calories to 1,060. Note that our numbers here apply to a plain filet only, not a stuffed version like the one on the menu at Steak and Ale.

The Bottom Line: *Filet mignon is a good steak-house choice as long as you skip the bacon that Lone Star and some other restaurants automatically wrap around their filets.*

PORK CHOPS
(480 calories and 26 grams of fat, 11 of them saturated)
We're not buying into those ads that tout pork as "the other white meat." Pork *tenderloin* may be as lean as a skinless chicken or turkey breast, but even trimmed, the pork chops served at steak houses have five times the fat of barbecue chicken. Think of *each* untrimmed chop—most restaurants serve two—as the equivalent of a McDonald's Quarter Pounder. Cutting all the fat off the edges of both chops brings their saturated down from three-quarters to a half-day's allotment.

The Bottom Line: *Eat only one trimmed chop accompanied by smart sides. Ask for a doggie bag so you can take the second chop home for a meal the next day.*

RIB EYE STEAK
(550 calories and 30 grams of fat, 16 of them saturated)
Did you know you could eat *two* 12-ounce sirloins and get no more fat than you would get in one 13-ounce rib eye steak? The rib eye is cut from a fattier part of the steer. Remember, getting

three-quarters of your day's harmful fat in an entrée alone doesn't allow you much more in your dinner—or your day.

The Bottom Line: *If you insist on a rib eye instead of a sirloin, skip the fatty fried Onion Strings that come on top of Stuart Anderson's rib eye.*

NEW YORK STRIP STEAK
(570 calories and 34 grams of fat, 18 of them saturated)

This is a fatty cut, and restaurants serve three-quarters of a pound of it, which is three times the government's recommended serving (4 ounces uncooked, or 3 ounces after cooking). You get almost a day's saturated fat here without the sides, smart or otherwise. And that's if the strip steak is trimmed.

The Bottom Line: *Enjoy half, and take the rest home for a steak sandwich the next day.*

T-BONE STEAK
(690 calories and 44 grams of fat, 23 of them saturated)

The 11 ounces of trimmed meat from a 1-pound T-bone contain more than an entire day's saturated fat. Pair it with a Caesar salad and a buttered spud and you'll lard your arteries with two days' worth of bad stuff and wrap 1,400 calories around your middle.

The Bottom Line: *Order a far less fatty filet mignon and enjoy.*

PORTERHOUSE STEAK
(930 calories and 64 grams of fat, 32 of them saturated)

Do you really think that a porterhouse is four times as delicious as a sirloin? Well, don't order one unless you do, because a porterhouse contains four times the saturated fat of a sirloin steak. "But it's a splurge," you may be thinking. True, but so is eating an entire large Domino's Hand Tossed Cheese Pizza, and that has less saturated fat.

The Bottom Line: *When you see "porterhouse" on the menu, think "portliness" and make another choice.*

PRIME RIB
(980 calories and 62 grams of fat, 38 of them saturated)

A prime rib dinner is the iconic steak-house platter. Unfortunately, if you eat that 1-pound serving with all of its fat intact, you'll consume almost 100 grams of fat, over half of it saturated. That's as much as a serving of fettuccine Alfredo, the dish we call a "heart attack on a plate." And you'll walk away with 1,280 calories. Add a Caesar salad and spud to even a trimmed prime rib and you'll leave the restaurant 1,700 calories heavier.

The Bottom Line: *If you eat just half, trimmed of the fat, and add smart sides, you'll get the fat down to "only" 38 grams, about half of it saturated.*

When Your Favorite Is Not on the List

Many of the appetizers and nonsteak entrées on steak-house menus are similar to those served at dinner houses. See chapter 12, Where Everybody Knows Your Name: Dinner Houses, page 223, for the nutrition numbers on Buffalo wings, chicken fingers, stuffed potato skins, fried mozzarella sticks, entrée-size chicken Caesar salads, bacon and cheese grilled chicken sandwiches, BBQ baby back ribs, and hamburgers. See the chapter on seafood restaurants (page 189) for the lowdown on grilled fish and batter-fried shrimp dishes.

Lone Star and other steak houses offer beef kebabs. Although we didn't analyze this dish (see page 181 for our analyses of kebabs offered at Greek restaurants), it looks like a good option, since steak houses often make theirs from leaner meat, the portion of beef is smaller than an entire steak, and they're usually skewered with vegetables. The rice pilaf that customarily accompanies kebabs probably doesn't add much fat, although it would push up the sodium.

Steak Strategy

• **Replace red meat with another choice.** There's no rule that says you *must* order steak at a steak house. Try grilled seafood or grilled or barbecue chicken. Steak houses offer these alternatives because they're tasty and a lot of health-conscious customers request them.

• **Keep it lean.** Hands down, sirloin and filet mignon are the best nutritional bets among all the red-meat entrées we tested.

• **Make it leaner.** Regardless of which type of steak you order, it can always be made more healthful by trimming off all the visible fat from around the edges. For a large, fatty cut like porterhouse, that can spare you 18 grams of fat, or about 20 percent of the total fat.

• **Downsize entrée portions.** For our study we ordered the steak sizes that appeared most often on menus, but many steak houses also offer smaller versions of the same cuts. For example, Bugaboo Creek has a 7-ounce filet mignon. Steak and Ale offers a 6-ounce filet as well as a 6-ounce sirloin and an 8-ounce prime rib.

• **Look for low-fat appetizers.** Skip fanciful creations like a deep-fried whole onion or those mountains of cheese fries, both of which are nutritional disasters. Check the menu for saner options such as shrimp cocktail, grilled shrimp, or a noncreamy soup. Or have a green salad and bread (they're often complimentary) as your first course.

• **Avoid creamy sauces.** Watch out for the fatty sauces served with some dishes. The flavorful *jus* that accompanies prime rib will be far less fatty than a béarnaise sauce.

• **Choose smart sides.** If you pair your steak with a not-so-smart Caesar salad and a baked potato with butter, you'll consume up to four times more fat than if you'd ordered a mixed green side salad with light dressing and a baked potato with a tablespoon of sour cream. Or you could order a side of the vegetable of the day. If these seem too ho-hum, scout the menu for interesting alternatives like the baked sweet potato offered by Lone Star and LongHorn, or the corn on the cob at Tony Roma's.

• **Don't forget a doggie bag.** Eat only half of your steak and fill up on salad, a baked potato with a tablespoon of sour cream, and plenty of vegetables. Take the other half of the steak home for a meal the next day.

The Steak Name Game

••••••••••••••••••

Popular cuts of the same steak may be known by various names in different parts of the country or even from one steakhouse chain to another. For example, Lone Star sells an 11-ounce rib eye that it calls Delmonico steak. And some places call a New York strip steak a shell or sirloin club steak. If your favorite isn't on our list, ask the server if it's known by a different name.

Within each category, dishes are ranked from best to worst—that is, from the least to most saturated fat in the appetizer or entrée (not the full platter). Steaks and chops are ranked on their trimmed numbers; all weights, except prime rib, are for raw meat. Entrées and platters marked with a ✔

Reminder

Recommended limits for a 2,000-calorie diet:

Total fat: 65 grams
Saturated fat: 20 grams
Cholesterol: 300 milligrams
Sodium: 2,400 milligrams

are Best Bites. Best Bites are relatively low in saturated fat, but they may contain more saturated fat than many Best Bites elsewhere in this book.

STEAK-HOUSE FOODS

Menu Item	Calories	Total Fat (g)	Saturated Fat (g)	Cholesterol (mg)	Sodium (mg)
APPETIZERS					
Fried whole onion (3 cups—21 oz.)	1,690	116	*44*	40	3,040
plus dipping sauce (5 Tb.)	2,130	163	*57*	55	3,840
Cheese fries (4 cups—27 oz.)	2,380	151	*79*	190	4,020
plus ranch dressing (8 Tb.)	3,010	217	*91*	220	4,890
ENTRÉES AND PLATTERS					
✔ Barbecue chicken breast (10 oz.)	280	5	*2*	125	860
✔ plus house salad with fat-free dressing (2 Tb.) and baked potato with sour cream (1 Tb.)	730	11	*4*	125	1,610
✔ plus house salad with fat-free dressing (2 Tb.) and vegetable	550	14	*5*	130	1,580
plus Caesar salad and baked potato with butter (1½ Tb.)	990	47	*18*	180	1,720

STEAK-HOUSE FOODS (continued) Menu Item	Calories	Total Fat (g)	Saturated Fat (g)	Cholesterol (mg)	Sodium (mg)
✔ Sirloin steak, untrimmed (12 oz.)	410	18	9	170	470
✔ Sirloin steak, trimmed	390	15	8	165	470
✔ plus house salad with fat-free dressing (2 Tb.) and baked potato with sour cream (1 Tb.)	840	21	10	170	1,220
plus Caesar salad and baked potato with butter (1½ Tb.)	1,100	58	24	225	1,330
✔ Filet mignon, untrimmed (9 oz.)	360	19	10	125	330
✔ Filet mignon, trimmed	350	18	9	125	330
✔ plus house salad with fat-free dressing (2 Tb.) and baked potato with sour cream (1 Tb.)	800	24	11	130	1,080
plus Caesar salad and baked potato with butter (1½ Tb.)	1,060	60	25	180	1,190
Pork chops, untrimmed (13 oz.)	600	37	15	180	1,030
Pork chops, trimmed	480	26	11	165	1,020
plus house salad with fat-free dressing (2 Tb.) and baked potato with sour cream (1 Tb.)	930	32	12	170	1,770
plus Caesar salad and baked potato with butter (1½ Tb.)	1,200	68	27	225	1,890
Rib eye steak, untrimmed (13 oz.)	610	36	18	180	320
Rib eye steak, trimmed	550	30	16	175	320
plus house salad with fat-free dressing (2 Tb.) and baked potato with sour cream (1 Tb.)	1,000	36	17	175	1,070
plus Caesar salad and baked potato with butter (1½ Tb.)	1,260	73	31	230	1,180

STEAK-HOUSE FOODS (continued)

Menu Item	Calories	Total Fat (g)	Saturated Fat (g)	Cholesterol (mg)	Sodium (mg)
New York strip steak, untrimmed (12 oz.)	630	40	21	185	240
New York strip steak, trimmed	570	34	18	175	230
plus house salad with fat-free dressing (2 Tb.) and baked potato with sour cream (1 Tb.)	1,020	40	19	180	080
plus Caesar salad and baked potato with butter (1½ Tb.)	1,280	76	33	230	1,100
T-bone steak, untrimmed (16 oz.)	800	56	28	165	520
T-bone steak, trimmed	690	44	23	145	510
plus house salad with fat-free dressing (2 Tb.) and baked potato with sour cream (1 Tb.)	1,140	50	24	150	1,260
plus Caesar salad and baked potato with butter (1½ Tb.)	1,400	86	38	205	1,380
Porterhouse steak, untrimmed (20 oz.)	1,100	82	40	260	520
Porterhouse steak, trimmed	930	64	32	235	510
plus house salad with fat-free dressing (2 Tb.) and baked potato with sour cream (1 Tb.)	1,380	71	34	240	1,260
plus Caesar salad and baked potato with butter (1½ Tb.)	1,640	107	48	295	1,370
Prime rib, untrimmed (16 oz.)	1,280	94	52	195	620
Prime rib, trimmed	980	62	38	150	600
plus house salad with fat-free dressing (2 Tb.) and baked potato with sour cream (1 Tb.)	1,430	68	39	155	1,350
plus Caesar salad and baked potato with butter (1½ Tb.)	1,690	104	53	210	1,470

STEAK-HOUSE FOODS *(continued)*

Menu Item	Calories	Total Fat (g)	Saturated Fat (g)	Cholesterol (mg)	Sodium (mg)
SIDE DISHES					
House salad with fat-free dressing (2 Tb.)	170	4	0	0	560
House salad with light dressing (2 Tb.)	200	9	1	1	51
Baked potato with sour cream (1 Tb.)	280	3	*2*	5	200
Vegetable of the day (1 cup)	90	6	*3*	5	160
Baked potato with sour cream (3 Tb.)	330	9	*5*	15	210
Caesar salad (2 cups)	310	26	*7*	45	620
Baked potato with butter (1½ Tb.)	400	17	*8*	15	240
French fries (2 cups)	590	31	*12*	5	460
Loaded baked potato (with bacon, butter, cheese, and sour cream)	620	31	19	70	570

Note: Numbers for house salad and salad dressing are from USDA Nutrient Database for Standard Reference and manufacturers. Saturated fat numbers in *italics* include artery-clogging *trans* fat.

Chapter 12

Where Everybody Knows Your Name: Dinner Houses

In the late 1960s, when a young, unmarried businessman living on New York City's Upper East Side wanted to meet his unmarried female neighbors, he discovered that there was no suitable casual place to share a glass of wine or an inexpensive meal. He bought an abandoned beer joint, transformed it with hanging plants and Tiffany-style lamps, and started an American institution by creating a neighborhood pub called T.G.I.F. It was an enormous success and eventually became T.G.I. Friday's, a chain of lively, casual restaurants that cater to patrons seeking a big meal in a bright and informal atmosphere.

The restaurant industry calls such places "dinner houses," but most of us know T.G.I. Friday's and its imitators—Applebee's, Chili's, Hard Rock Cafe—as affable establishments that follow a basic party formula of food and fun. Surrounded by a jungle of hanging ferns (or rock memorabilia), crowds of boisterous diners flock to these restaurants to socialize with friends and family. They are lively, high-entertainment venues, with snazzier food than fast-food joints and lower prices than more sedate, white-tablecloth places.

The food choices at dinner houses are designed to eliminate what the restaurant industry calls "the veto factor." This means that while you're tucking into a dish of pasta, Uncle Joe can enjoy a burger, and your friend can have tacos. Since the menu has something for everybody, everybody wins. But do they really win?

Dinner houses may offer lots of options, but don't kid yourself. That doesn't necessarily mean you're getting a healthy meal. In fact, when we analyzed the most popular dinner-house dishes, we found that, nutritionally speaking, *they make fast food look good.* It may be hard to believe, but chances are you won't get out of a dinner house without having consumed at least 1,000 calories, as well as your whole day's limit of fat and saturated fat—and that's *without* an appetizer and a dessert.

The good news is that it *is* possible to eat a healthful meal at a dinner house. Many, like Bennigan's and Chili's, have healthy or

---

Dinner-House Makeover
··

With a little effort, dinner houses (and other restaurants, for that matter) could overhaul their regular menus without anyone even noticing. They could start using leaner ground beef, stop using hydrogenated shortenings, leave hamburger and sandwich buns unbuttered, cut down on breading, bake the french fries, add less salt, and serve salad dressings and other high-calorie toppings on the side. It's worth noting that, although many dinner houses offer light dressings for side salads, most of the entrée salads we surveyed, including Caesar or Oriental chicken salads, come with "special" (high-calorie) dressings that should also be served on the side.

Dinner houses always seem primed to jump on the latest food trend, whether it's batter-fried jalapeño peppers or Cajun-style chicken. Let the manager of your local franchise know that healthful foods are a bona fide food trend, and that you and your wallet just might walk if things don't change. Are you listening Hard Rock Café, Houlihan's, Red Robin, and friends?

light dishes on their menus. And there are also some common-sense strategies that will help lessen the load that comes with a typical dinner-house meal.

The Dishes and the Data

We bought take-out portions of 20 popular appetizers, entrées, and side dishes at 39 dinner houses in Chicago, Denver, Los Angeles, and Washington, D.C. (For more on our methodology, see pages 12–14.) We analyzed dishes from some of the largest chains: Applebee's, Bennigan's, Chart House, Chili's, T.G.I. Friday's, Grady's American Grill, Hard Rock Cafe, Houlihan's, Houston's, Marie Callender's, Planet Hollywood, Red Robin, and Ruby Tuesday. Countless other restaurants, chain or independent, offer similar food.

Within each category, we've ranked the dishes from best to worst—that is, from least to most saturated fat.

Appetizers

CHILI
(350 calories and 16 grams of fat, 8 of them saturated)
A 1½ cup serving of spicy beef and beans eats up a quarter of your day's quota of fat and almost half of your allowance of satu-rated fat. Too bad none of the restaurants we surveyed offered a vegetarian chili. This worthy substitute is low in saturated fat and a great source of fiber.

The Bottom Line: Your best bet is to turn this into a meal rather than an appetizer by pairing it with bread and a salad with light dressing. If the chili comes topped with cheese, ask that it be omitted or served on the side so you can use just a sprinkling.

BUFFALO WINGS
without blue cheese dressing (700 calories and 48 grams of fat, 16 of them saturated), **with blue cheese dressing** (1,010 calories and 80 grams of fat, 22 of them saturated)

People joke that eating chicken wings is nothing but gnawing on bones, but we found "chewing the fat" to be a better description. If you eat an average 12-wing order, you'll use up three-quarters of your daily quota for total fat, saturated fat, and sodium, plus nearly a day's cholesterol. And that doesn't include any blue cheese dressing. Dip until there's none left—a typical portion is ¼ cup and contains 32 fat grams—and you'll eat more than 1,000 calories and more saturated fat than you'd get in an *entire* rotisserie chicken, skin and all.

The Bottom Line: *You can't resist temptation. Order something else.*

FRIED MOZZARELLA STICKS
(830 calories and 51 grams of fat, 28 of them saturated)

Our numbers here don't include the marinara dipping sauce, but the low-calorie sauce is hardly the problem. Each modest-size stick contains about 100 calories and as much fat as you'd find in two strips of bacon. There are typically nine sticks in an order. You might as well sit down and eat a half-stick of butter.

The Bottom Line: *Just say no.*

STUFFED POTATO SKINS
without sour cream (1,120 calories and 79 grams of fat, 40 of them saturated), **with sour cream** (1,260 calories and 95 grams of fat, 48 of them saturated)

The scooped-out skins are topped with cheese, bacon, and scallions or chives. An eight-skin order has 1,120 calories and 79 grams—18 teaspoons!—of fat, not including the sour cream that is served on the side. To your heart, that will feel like 2½ pounds of Tater Tots. Or visualize the appetizer this way: a whole order is the equivalent of gorging on eight strips of bacon, eight pats of butter, *and* eight tablespoons of sour cream. Still want to dig in? Bear in mind that even half an order uses up a day's saturated fat and more than 500 calories.

The Bottom Line: *These skins are anything but skinny!*

Entrées and Platters

GRILLED CHICKEN
(270 calories and 8 grams of fat, 3 of them saturated)

It's time for some good news. This chicken breast is one of the lowest-fat restaurant foods we've ever analyzed. Although many restaurants marinate the chicken, that doesn't seem to add fat. The average serving size was just over 6 ounces, cooked. Accompanied by a baked potato with a tablespoon of sour cream and a vegetable of the day, the entire meal clocks in at

Chicken... Again!?

Although grilled chicken topped our honor roll as the best dinner-house entrée, we'll certainly understand if you think you'll sprout feathers at the mention of another skinless, boneless... you know what. Relax. Many of the most healthful entrées from other cuisines we've looked at are also on dinner-house menus. Look for blackened seafood, grilled shrimp or veggie pasta, and veggie fajitas.

640 calories and 14 grams of fat. Be aware: Order your chicken with a loaded baked potato or fries and you triple the fat. Some restaurants pair grilled chicken with rice pilaf, which probably won't add much fat, but it will add quite a bit of sodium.

The Bottom Line: *Order this dish and enjoy it.*

SIRLOIN STEAK
(410 calories and 20 grams of fat, 10 of them saturated)

Despite its bad reputation, steak is a good choice compared to the other options we analyzed. Because sirloin is one of the leanest cuts of beef (only round steak has less fat), you'll use up "only" half a day's saturated fat allowance. The 7 ounces of cooked steak at dinner houses is smaller than what's served at a steak house. (The sizes served at dinner houses ranged from 5½ to 10½ ounces, after cooking.) Sirloin is the only entrée we tested that had fewer than 400 milligrams of sodium.

The Bottom Line: *Choose a baked potato with one tablespoon of sour cream and the vegetable of the day as side dishes, and you'll have yourself a decent meal.*

CHICKEN CAESAR SALAD WITH DRESSING
(660 calories and 46 grams of fat, 11 of them saturated)

The classic salad of romaine leaves, croutons, Parmesan cheese, and garlicky dressing is topped with skinless chicken breast. Although the cheese and croutons don't help, it's the full-fat dressing that causes the calories to climb to 660. Unfortunately, not one of the restaurants whose salads we tested offered a lower-fat Caesar dressing.

The Bottom Line: *Ask for the dressing on the side and drizzle a tablespoon or two onto the salad.*

BACON AND CHEESE GRILLED CHICKEN SANDWICH
(650 calories and 30 grams of fat, 12 of them saturated)

Bacon, cheese, and mayonnaise turn a healthy grilled chicken sandwich from trim to grim. The fat in one sandwich is equal to that in four Wendy's Grilled Chicken Sandwiches. If you add french fries, the fat and sodium shoot up to nearly a day's worth and the calories to a belt-busting 1,230. Low-fat mayo, reduced-fat cheese, and turkey bacon would cut the fat in half, but they're not an option at most places.

The Bottom Line: *Skip the mayo, bacon, and cheese, and pile on the lettuce, tomato, onion, and mustard.*

STEAK FAJITAS WITH TORTILLAS
(860 calories and 31 grams of fat, 12 of them saturated)

After we tested Mexican restaurant foods, chicken fajitas was one of the few dishes we could recommend and then only without accompaniments like the fatty beans, sour cream, and guacamole. Steak fajitas at dinner houses aren't in the same class. They've got a third more fat than those made with chicken, and over twice as much saturated fat. The sour cream, guacamole, and cheese boost the fat and salt to a day's worth and the saturated fat to one and a half day's worth.

The Bottom Line: *Get chicken, shrimp, or veggie fajitas instead. Top each one with a teaspoon of sour cream and as much salsa or pico de gallo as you want.*

ORIENTAL CHICKEN SALAD WITH DRESSING
(750 calories and 49 grams of fat, 12 of them saturated)

Steer clear of this salad entrée if you're watching your weight. Eat it as it comes and you'll get 750 calories—nearly as much as you would get in 15 McDonald's Chicken McNuggets. How does a quarter pound of skinless chicken breast on a bed of romaine lettuce, red cabbage, carrots, and other praiseworthy salad fixings cost you 750 calories and more than half a day's fat? Well, some restaurants top it with nuts and fried noodles (one restaurant added 1⅓ cup of noodles!), but it's primarily the dressing that's the downfall in this otherwise terrific meal. Be sure to find out what kind of chicken is used. Although most places use roasted chicken breast, Applebee's uses breaded and fried chicken fingers.

The Bottom Line: *Ask for dressing on the side, and use a couple of tablespoons. Have the kitchen hold the fried noodles or nuts, and make sure they don't use fried ("crunchy") chicken!*

CHICKEN FINGERS
(620 calories and 34 grams of fat, 13 of them saturated)

A typical five-finger order will have the same effect on your arteries as a Burger King Whopper. If you add fries, coleslaw, and honey mustard dipping sauce, your spree will cost one and a half days' quota of fat, more than a whole day's sodium, and more than 1,600 calories.

The Bottom Line: *Forget the fingers and stick with grilled chicken.*

HAMBURGER
(660 calories and 36 grams of fat, 17 of them saturated)

You'd expect a Super Double Bacon Deluxe Wham-o Cheeseburger to be Fat City. But a plain hamburger on a bun topped with mustard, lettuce, tomato, and onion? Alas, the dinner-house burgers we tested had almost twice the fat of a McDonald's Quarter Pounder and nearly a full day's allotment of saturated fat. Why? They're just much bigger than their fast-food cousins. Many dinner-house chains start with a 6-ounce (uncooked) patty. A Quarter Pounder hits the griddle at 4 ounces. With an order of fries, the calories of the dinner-house version reach 1,240 and the saturated fat hits 1½ days' worth. Succumb to onion rings instead of fries and you've made it a two-day fix.

The Bottom Line: *Order a veggie burger, if there's one on the menu. They are deli-*

Fancy Burgers
••••••••••••••••••••

Burgers come in all kinds of designer dress at dinner houses. You can order them with bacon and cheese, barbecue sauce, or Mexican-style with guacamole. Red Robin even serves one topped with a fried egg! We don't have numbers for each of those variations, but start with the numbers for the plain hamburger or the mushroom cheeseburger and estimate. Veggie burgers are sprouting up on more and more menus. Just be careful that they're not smothered with cheese or mayonnaise and served with a side of fries.

cious, and are usually much lower in saturated fat than hamburgers.

BBQ BABY BACK RIBS
(770 calories and 54 grams of fat, 21 of them saturated)

We all know that a pound of pork ribs isn't a low-fat or low-calorie choice. But did you know that you could eat an entire turkey dinner with the works (stuffing, mashed potatoes with gravy, a vegetable, and cranberry sauce), then eat half of that again—and end up with the same amount of saturated fat as in one lone order of ribs? The usual sidekicks of french fries and coleslaw raise the ante to 36 grams of saturated fat and more than 1,500 calories. That's nearly two days' worth of saturated fat, or what you'd get in three turkey dinners.

The Bottom Line: *If you are in the mood for red meat, order a sirloin steak instead.*

MUSHROOM CHEESEBURGER
(900 calories and 57 grams of fat, 28 of them saturated)

A plain burger is spa food compared to a mushroom cheeseburger. The latter is a cheeseburger gussied up with sautéed mushrooms and sometimes sautéed onions, depending on where you're ordering it. Some restaurants add to the calorie count by slathering the patty with mayo. Even with nothing on the side, a mushroom cheeseburger dumps 1½ days' worth of saturated fat into your blood vessels. Get it with onion rings and you'll double the dose. Or, to put it another, more graphic way, your meal's 1,800 calories will contain the combined fat of five strips of bacon, four Hostess Twinkies, three slices of a large Domino's Hand Tossed Pepperoni Pizza, two Dairy Queen Banana Splits and a McDonald's Big Mac. Honest.

The Bottom Line: *Forget about this one!*

Side Dishes and Desserts

VEGETABLE OF THE DAY
(60 calories and 3 grams of fat, 1 of them saturated)

Now you're talkin'—a cup of some combination of vitamin-packed carrots, broccoli, zucchini, and yellow squash. All dinner houses offer vegetables, and the more times people order them, the more likely it is the restaurants will expand their offerings. Even the bit of butter or oil added to enhance the flavor won't use up too big a bite from the day's fat quota.

The Bottom Line: You can't eat too many veggies!

COLESLAW
(170 calories and 14 grams of fat, 2 of them saturated)

A cup of cabbage and carrots is loaded with nutrients and low in calories. The 170 calories in this side dish come from the two tablespoons of mayonnaise-based dressing. If you are watching your weight, a green salad with a couple of tablespoons of light dressing would have half the calories.

The Bottom Line: If you're concerned about calories, order a vegetable or a side salad with light dressing.

FRENCH FRIES
(590 calories and 31 grams of fat, 12 of them saturated)

Ahhhh ... fries. Who doesn't love them? If only they loved us back! A typical side order contains over half a day's quota of saturated fat. The problem is that many restaurants are still frying in hydrogenated shortening, which contains cholesterol-raising *trans* fat. At least fast-food joints give you a choice of size. On average, our dinner houses dished out a two-cup serving—and three restaurants served up three cups (900 calories worth)! Once they're on your plate, it's tough not to eat them.

The Bottom Line: Feeling weak? Just remember the "french fry factor": adding an order of fries to your dinner is the equivalent of eating a bacon-and-cheese grilled chicken sandwich along with your meal.

LOADED BAKED POTATO
(620 calories and 31 grams of fat, 19 of them saturated)

When this potato leaves the kitchen, it's already stuffed with butter, sour cream, bacon bits, and cheese—*and* a full day's allotment of saturated fat and more than 600 calories. All this from a baked potato, for heaven's sake!

The Bottom Line: *It's the culinary equivalent of a loaded pistol! Order a plain baked potato and use a tablespoon of sour cream.*

ONION RINGS
(900 calories and 64 grams of fat, 23 of them saturated)

A side dish? One order, about 11 rings, has more fat than a sirloin steak dinner or an order of BBQ baby back ribs. The rings provide 900 calories and more saturated fat than any of the entrées we tested at dinner houses except the infamous mushroom cheeseburger.

The Bottom Line: *You do the math.*

FUDGE BROWNIE SUNDAE
(1,130 calories and 57 grams of fat, 30 of them saturated)

No one expects this kind of dessert to be low-cal or fat-free, but this astonishing creation packs more than 1,000 calories and as much saturated fat as two Pizza Hut Personal Pan Cheese Pizzas *plus* one Dairy Queen Banana Split. Enough said.

The Bottom Line: *If enough people ask for healthier desserts, dinner houses will eventually provide them. In the meantime, a few chains already offer lower-fat desserts. Applebee's features a Low-Fat & Fabulous Brownie Sundae and Bennigan's has a Health Club Cheesecake by Eli's.*

When Your Favorite Is Not on the List

We discuss many of the other dishes dinner houses serve in other chapters in this book. For example, we cover fettuccine Alfredo, a dinner-house favorite, and fried calamari in chapter 6, Use Your Noodle: Italian Restaurants, pages 127 and 121. For enchiladas, chicken fajitas, and cheese nachos, see chapter 8, Drop the Chalupa: Mexican Restaurants, pages 164–168. Chapter 11, Here's the Beef: Steak Houses, covers barbecue chicken breast, New York strip steak, filet mignon, pork chops, and that omnipresent appetizer, a fried whole onion (pages 207–220). Chapter 13, Home away from Home: Family-Style Restaurants lists our analyses of pot roast, country-fried steak, and Philly cheese steak sandwiches (pages 240 and 242); and you'll get the scoop on broiled salmon and fried shrimp in chapter 10, Catch of the Day: Seafood Restaurants, pages 197 and 198. Read about cheesecake in chapter 15, Sweet Nothings: Pastry and Desserts, (page 263).

Dinner-House Strategy

Nobody is making you order foods like buffalo wings, fried mozzarella sticks, and stuffed potato skins, so why not use the almost unlimited dinner-house menus to your advantage and find substitutes? Grilled chicken or fish, shrimp or vegetable fajitas, chicken or veggie stir-fries, or pasta with marinara sauce are all delicious, reasonably healthy dishes that can be substituted for less healthful ones.

• **Look for special menus.** If the dinner house has "light" or "healthy" selections, choose from those.

• **Beware of special-flavored dressings.** If you're partial to some of the entrée salads that dinner houses offer, like Chili's Grilled Caribbean Salad, Applebee's Santa Fe Chicken Salad, or Houlihan's Caribbean Salad with Chicken, keep in mind our findings and advice about chicken Caesar and Oriental chicken salads. It's safe to assume that a special-flavored dressing is high in calories unless the menu states otherwise. And don't forget the added calories that toppings like cheese, tortilla strips, or fried noodles will add. They can mean the difference between nutritional boom or bust.

• **Ask about substitutions.** Don't be shy about this. Although upscale restaurants with inventive or temperamental chefs might not be willing to alter a creation just for you, dinner houses are far more flexible. Even if the menu says that platters come with coleslaw and fries, many places will be happy to serve you a baked potato, vegetable of the day, or salad instead. You can also ask that steak fajitas be heavy on the veggies and pico de gallo and light on the meat. And always ask for reduced-fat sour cream. Every time you ask, you're sending a message.

• **Find out the preparation method.** Restaurant menus are sometimes unspecific about how a dish is made. Ask the server in advance how a dish is prepared. You may think you're getting grilled skinless chicken on an entrée salad, only to be surprised and dismayed to find fried chicken nuggets garnishing the greens.

• **Choose a sensible spud.** Boiled, roasted, and baked potatoes are all healthful. Top off your spud with a tablespoon of sour cream, or even light salad dressing or salsa.

• **Assume nothing.** Veggie burgers are always better than hamburgers, but don't automatically assume they are low-fat. Many are topped with melted cheese and accompanied by a side of fries. If that's the case, ask to have the cheese and fries left in the kitchen.

• **Look for burger alternatives.** If you're craving red meat, sirloin steak, which is one of the leanest cuts of beef, is a far better choice than a burger.

• **Hold the cheese.** It seems to show up on everything—burgers, baked potatoes, pasta, chicken sandwiches, salads. Skip it and save yourself the calories and saturated fat.

• **Don't forget the doggie bag.** Considering the calories (at least 1,000) in most dinner-house meals, you may well feel full after eating only half of your meal, so don't hesitate to take the rest home. Eat half today and half tomorrow.

Within each category, items are ranked from best to worst—that is, from least to most saturated fat in the entrée (not the full platter). Entrées and platters marked with a ✔ are Best Bites. Best Bites are relatively low in saturated fat.

Reminder

Recommended limits for a 2,000-calorie diet:

Total fat: 65 grams
Saturated fat: 20 grams
Cholesterol: 300 milligrams
Sodium: 2,400 milligrams

DINNER HOUSE DISHES

Menu Item	Calories	Total Fat (g)	Saturated Fat (g)	Cholesterol (mg)	Sodium (mg)
APPETIZERS					
Chili (1½ cups)	350	16	8	75	1,230
Buffalo wings (12 wings—13 oz.)	700	48	16	240	1,750
plus blue cheese (4 Tb.) and celery (5 sticks)	1,010	80	22	250	2,460
Fried mozzarella sticks (9 sticks—8 oz.)	830	51	28	75	1,890
Stuffed potato skins (8 skins—12 oz.)	1,120	79	40	80	1,270
plus sour cream (5 Tb.)	1,260	95	48	105	1,300
ENTRÉES AND PLATTERS					
✔ Grilled chicken (6 oz.)	270	8	3	145	650
✔ plus baked potato with sour cream (1 Tb.) and vegetable (1 cup)	640	14	5	150	820
plus loaded baked potato and vegetable (1 cup)	950	42	23	220	1,370
✔ Sirloin steak (7 oz.)	410	20	10	170	390
✔ plus baked potato with sour cream (1 Tb.) and vegetable (1 cup)	780	26	13	175	560
plus french fries (2 cups) and vegetable (1 cup)	1,060	54	23	175	1,000
plus loaded baked potato and vegetable (1 cup)	1,090	54	31	245	1,110
Chicken Caesar salad with dressing (4 cups)	660	46	11	130	1,490
Bacon and cheese grilled chicken sandwich	650	30	12	145	1,650
plus french fries (2 cups)	1,230	61	24	145	2,110
plus onion rings (11)	1,550	94	36	150	2,700
Steak fajitas with tortillas (4)	860	31	12	135	1,660
plus guacamole, sour cream, and cheese	1,190	63	28	190	2,810

DINNER HOUSE DISHES (continued) Menu Item	Calories	Total Fat (g)	Saturated Fat (g)	Cholesterol (mg)	Sodium (mg)
Oriental chicken salad with dressing (5 cups)	750	49	*12*	110	1,140
Chicken fingers (5 pieces—9 oz.)	620	34	*13*	110	1,450
plus french fries (2 cups), coleslaw (1 cup),	1,640	106	*30*	130	2,640
Hamburger	660	36	*17*	130	810
plus french fries (2 cups)	1,240	67	*29*	135	1,270
plus onion rings (11)	1,550	101	*40*	135	1,860
BBQ baby back ribs (14 ribs—16 oz.)	770	54	*21*	195	770
plus french fries (2 cups) and coleslaw (1 cup)	1,530	99	*36*	215	1,610
Mushroom cheeseburger	900	57	*28*	150	1,070
plus french fries (2 cups)	1,490	88	*40*	155	1,540
plus onion rings (11)	1,800	122	*52*	160	2,130
SIDE DISHES AND DESSERTS					
Vegetable of the day (1 cup)	60	3	*1*	3	150
Baked potato with sour cream (1 Tb.)	310	3	*2*	5	30
Coleslaw (1 cup)	170	14	*2*	15	380
French fries (2 cups)	590	31	*12*	5	460
Loaded baked potato (bacon, butter, cheese, etc.)	620	31	*19*	70	570
Onion rings (11)	900	64	*23*	5	1,050
Fudge brownie sundae (10 oz.)	1,130	57	*30*	115	400

Note: For celery, baked potato, sour cream, and blue cheese dressing, we used numbers from USDA Nutrient Database for Standard Reference. For guacamole and pico de gallo, we used numbers from food service suppliers. Saturated fat numbers in *italics* include artery-clogging *trans* fat.

Chapter 13

Home away from Home: Family-Style Restaurants

Perhaps it's because we have become such avid consumers of fast-food and take-out meals that Americans have developed a romanticized notion of "home cooking." The meals many of us grew up on—or wished we had grown up on—featured plates laden with gravy-smothered meat and mashed potatoes served with love. It's this sturdy, basic fare that we call comfort food today.

Americans flock to family-style restaurants, drawn by the promise of a real meal like Mom used to make. We're seeking some culinary coddling, and pot roast is the answer. To many Americans, a plate of meat loaf or roast turkey or a golden-topped chicken potpie seems more nutritious than McSandwiches. This homey food is wholesome, right? Not exactly. In the results of our tests of food from 14 family-style restaurant chains, you'll see that what comforts your soul can also break your heart. Although the food may be no worse, nutritionally speaking, than many dishes served at more upscale dinner houses, that's cold comfort indeed. Don't forget that this kind of 1950s down-home chow helped make the 1960s—when heart attack death rates peaked in the United States—the heart attack decade of the twentieth century.

Of course, these places do offer some healthier options. Most family restaurant menus include grilled fish or chicken and heart-friendly accompaniments like a side salad with light dressing and a baked potato with sour cream on the side. Some, like Big Boy and Denny's, even have "healthy" or "light" selections on their menus.

The Dishes and the Data

Here's the lowdown on the 13 popular main dishes and side dishes we analyzed. We went to 26 family-style restaurants in Chicago, Denver, Green Bay, Los Angeles, San Antonio, and Washington, D.C. We analyzed food from some of the largest family-style restaurant chains: Bakers Square, Big Boy, Bob Evans, Carrows, Coco's, Country Kitchen, Cracker Barrel, Denny's, Friendly's, IHOP, Marie Callender's, Perkins, Shoney's, and Village Inn. Many other restaurants serve similar food. (For more on our methodology, see pages 12–14.)

Within each category we've ranked the dishes from best to worst—that is, from least to most saturated fat.

Entrées and Platters

POT ROAST
(370 calories and 16 grams of fat, 7 of them saturated)
The relatively small, 6-ounce portion of lean beef contains a third of a day's saturated fat, an amount that's comparable to a trimmed 12-ounce sirloin steak. Pot roast often comes with a half-cup of carrots, celery, and onion in the gravy, plus mashed potatoes and another side of veggies. With the 1½ cups of vegetables, you've already got three of the five to nine servings of vegetables and fruits you need each day. Unfortunately, the sides also boost the sodium from an admirably low 570 milligrams to 1,310 milligrams.

The Bottom Line: *A relatively low-fat comfort food, and one of your best choices at a family-style restaurant.*

CHICKEN STIR-FRY
(700 calories and 23 grams of fat, 7 of them saturated)
Think of this dish as a skinless chicken breast, a cup of vegetables, 1½ cups of rice, a tablespoon or two of oil—and a whole teaspoon of salt. The scarcity of vegetables in most restaurant meals makes

this one look great. Unfortunately, the stir-fry comes with more than 2,300 milligrams of sodium, a day's worth and about what you'd get from a similar dish in a Chinese restaurant. Ask the chef to go easy on the salt or soy sauce. And ask the waiter to serve the rice separately, so you can use a fork to lift the chicken and vegetables out of the salty sauce and onto your plate of rice.

The Bottom Line: *Overall, a decent choice. The side salad that accompanies this dish at some restaurants is a nutritional bonus, assuming you ask for a light dressing.*

TURKEY WITH STUFFING
(500 calories and 19 grams of fat, 9 of them saturated)

Turkey is the lowest-fat poultry you can buy, but this dish is a classic example of how accompaniments can sabotage even the wisest choices. In this case, it's not the gravy but the stuffing that is the major contributor to the half a day's worth of saturated fat. Adding the fixings—mashed potatoes and gravy, a vegetable, and cranberry sauce—sends the sodium soaring past a day's allowance.

The Bottom Line: *You could substitute a salad or a side of vegetables for of the stuffing, but then, of course, it wouldn't be turkey with stuffing.*

HAMBURGER
(510 calories and 27 grams of fat, 14 of them saturated)

Even with nothing but lettuce, tomato, and onion on it, a family-restaurant burger is still a fattier choice than a McDonald's Quarter Pounder. Although it's not as bad as the bigger burgers from dinner houses like Chili's or Applebee's (those are 40 percent larger), this main dish still uses up three-quarters of a day's saturated fat. With an order of fries, the calories climb to 1,100 and the saturated fat tops a day's worth.

The Bottom Line: *If the restaurant offers Gardenburgers or other tasty veggie burgers, as do Carrows, Marie Callender's,* *and some Denny's restaurants, order one of those instead. They're likely to have less fat and saturated fat than beef burgers. But avoid fatty cheese toppings, and substitute a salad or vegetable of the day for the fries.*

PHILLY CHEESE STEAK SANDWICH
(680 calories and 35 grams of fat, 17 of them saturated)

When you eat a version of this famous Philadelphia favorite (steak smothered with fried onions and melted American or mozzarella cheese, served on a long roll), you're taking in almost a day's quota of saturated fat. Three six-inch Subway Steak & Cheese subs have less saturated fat than one six-inch Philly Cheese Steak. If you have fries along with it, you'll hit 1,270 calories, a day's fat, and 1½ day's saturated fat.

The Bottom Line: Meat, cheese, fried onions—you can't make it healthy. If you crave meat, order a roast beef sandwich with light mayo, mustard, or barbecue sauce instead.

CHICKEN POTPIE
(680 calories and 37 grams of fat, 17 of them saturated)

When you think of comfort food, chicken potpie probably comes to mind. But the things that make it special—that cream sauce and pastry crust—contain so much saturated fat (almost an entire day's worth in one pie) that they outweigh the benefits of the veggies and poultry. The typical family-style restaurant serves a potpie twice the size, with about twice the calories, of a frozen Swanson or Banquet version. You can't take comfort in the fact that, to your arteries, it's the equivalent of eating a 13-ounce rib eye steak.

The Bottom Line: Order a grilled chicken dinner instead.

COUNTRY-FRIED STEAK
(650 calories and 42 grams of fat, 18 of them saturated)

Country-fried steak, also called chicken-fried steak in some parts of the country, is a southern specialty better relegated to your memory than to your plate. The beef is breaded and fried before being smothered in gravy. With twice as much breading and gravy as beef, it's equal in fat to two McDonald's Quarter Pounders. And that's without any sides.

The Bottom Line: *Satisfy your craving for red meat with pot roast or a sirloin steak instead.*

CHEF SALAD
(930 calories and 71 grams fat, 18 of them saturated)

How does a mountain of iceberg lettuce, 4 ounces of turkey and ham, and 1½ ounces of cheese end up having 930 calories and a day's fat? Most of the fat is in the full-fat Thousand Island dressing that restaurants often serve with this. All but one of the restaurants swamped the salad with half to a full cup of dressing; we used a half cup in calculating our numbers. Had we used less, the salad's score would have improved considerably. The rest of the fat comes from the cheese, which is why a chef salad has more saturated fat than a chicken Caesar or an Oriental chicken salad with dressing from a more upscale dinner house like Applebee's.

The Bottom Line: *This is easy to improve. Order light dressing on the side and use only a couple of tablespoons. Ask the kitchen for extra turkey in place of the ham and for only half of the cheese.*

MEAT LOAF
(570 calories and 38 grams of fat, 19 of them saturated)

A typical order of meat loaf is just over half a pound. That will lard your arteries with more fat than a pound of baby back ribs. And that's a day's supply of dangerous saturated fat before you've eaten a crumb of anything else.

The Bottom Line: *There's no comfort in this comfort food's fat numbers. If you're in the mood for meat, order pot roast.*

PATTY MELT
(770 calories and 50 grams of fat, 25 of them saturated)

"Fatty melt" might be a more accurate name for this sandwich. It's a cheeseburger with fried onions served on two slices of rye bread that have been spread with butter or margarine and grilled. It has more than a day's allowance of saturated fat, which is more than you'd get from two McDonald's Big Macs. If you add a side order of fries, you'll consume 81 grams (18 teaspoons) of fat, including a two-day allotment of saturated fat. This meal would cost you 1,350 calories.

The Bottom Line: *You can't make this good enough to eat.*

Side Dishes and Desserts

MASHED POTATOES WITH GRAVY
(190 calories and 8 grams of fat, 3 of them saturated)

Like the mashed potatoes at KFC and other fast-food outlets, this ¾-cup serving may not be as fatty as you thought. Too bad it's got 600 milligrams of sodium, thanks in part to the gravy.

The Bottom Line: *To cut the fat in half, order a plain baked potato with a tablespoon of sour cream instead.*

APPLE PIE
(540 calories and 28 grams of fat, 13 of them saturated)

A typical slice at a family-style restaurant has more than twice the fat of McDonald's Baked Apple Pie because it is more than twice the size. An apple pie with a single crust is likely to be less fatty than one with a lattice crust; which, in turn, is less fatty than one with a double crust. Don't even ask about the numbers for a slice à la mode.

The Bottom Line: *If splitting a slice of pie in half isn't for you, order fresh fruit instead, or opt for frozen yogurt or sherbet.*

VANILLA MILK SHAKE

(620 calories and 30 grams of fat, 21 of them saturated)

When restaurants tout their shakes as "old-fashioned," they might be referring to the whole milk and full-fat ice cream used to make them. They pump half a day's worth of fat and a full day's saturated fat into a 620-calorie, 13-ounce drink. Ounce for ounce, the family-style restaurant version is about three times as fatty as a shake from Burger King, McDonald's, or Wendy's.

The Bottom Line: *Skip it. Instead, head to Friendly's and ask for a Reduced Fat Milk Shake or a Sherbet Cooler.*

When Your Favorite Is Not on the List

You'll find many other family-style menu standbys in other chapters:

- grilled cheese, tuna salad, and bacon, lettuce, and tomato sandwiches (Sandwiches, pages 89–91)
- lasagna and spaghetti with marinara or meat sauce (Italian, pages 126, 122, and 124)
- pork chops, sirloin, and T-bone steaks (Steak Houses, pages 212–214)
- fried shrimp, fried seafood combos, and grilled fish (Seafood, pages 195–199)
- taco salads, nachos, and cheese quesadillas (Mexican, pages 170 and 164)
- buffalo wings, fried mozzarella sticks, chicken Caesar and Oriental chicken salads, grilled chicken, mushroom cheeseburgers, onion rings, and brownie sundaes (Dinner Houses, pages 226–233)

If you're a breakfast-anytime fan, check out chapter 3, Rise and Dine: Breakfast (page 67) for nutrition information on those round-the-clock breakfast platters, omelettes, and pancakes.

Family-Style Strategy

One of the hallmarks of those laminated family-restaurant menus is their length. You should have no trouble finding an alternative to meat loaf, country-fried steak, Philly cheese steak sandwiches, patty melts, and other entrées that can't be salvaged.

• **Look for special menus.** If the restaurant has "light" or "healthy" selections, choose from those.

• **Build a vegetable plate.** Another characteristic of family restaurants is the wide variety of vegetable side dishes they offer. This means you can put together your own vegetable plate. Bob Evans offers a vegetable stir-fry dinner as well as numerous vegetable sides like glazed baby carrots and grilled garden vegetables. Cracker Barrel has a vegetable-heavy entrée called a Country Vegetable Plate and also offers sides like vitamin-rich turnip greens. Other restaurants may let you order three or four veggies from a list that might include green beans, corn, carrots, cooked greens, pinto or baked beans, baked potatoes, applesauce, or a garden salad. Just steer clear of higher-fat dishes like home fries, french fries, and hash browns. Also, see if you can substitute a dinner roll for the biscuit that sometimes accompanies these plates.

• **Take advantage of the soup-and-salad bar.** You should be able to compose a healthy and delicious meal by making judicious choices at the soup-and-salad bar. Just be sure to avoid creamed soups, mayo-based salads, full-fat salad dressings, fried noodles, grated cheeses, and other fixings you know are high in fat and calories.

• **Don't hesitate to ask for substitutions.** The menu may say that the pot roast comes with a biscuit, but you might be able to get a dinner roll instead, or a baked potato and green salad rather than french fries and coleslaw.

- **Making the best beef choice.** If you want red meat, pot roast and sirloin steak are far better for you than burgers, meat loaf, and country-fried steak.

- **Salad sense.** Many family restaurants offer entrée salads that include chicken. Be sure to order the chicken grilled, not fried. Hold the cheese that often comes with these salads, and if they contain nuts, ask for them on the side. Always inquire about the dressings, and choose a light one served on the side.

- **Portion control.** Many family restaurants court senior citizens by offering them smaller portions at lower prices. Let the restaurant know you'd like one, whether or not you're a senior. The worst they can do is say no. If that's their answer, eat half your portion and take home a doggie bag for the next day.

Battle of the Burgers

Here's the proof that all burgers are not created equal. And here's also why you can't rely on calorie-counting guides that don't make the distinction among burgers served at fast-food establishments, family restaurants, and dinner houses.

Burger	McDonald's Quarter Pounder	Family-Style Restaurant	Dinner-House Restaurant
Calories	430	510	660
Total fat	21	27	36
Saturated Fat	8	*14*	*17*

Note: Saturated fat numbers *in italics* include artery-clogging *trans* fat.

Within each category, the dishes that we analyzed are ranked from best to worst—that is, from least to most saturated fat in the entrée (not the full platter). Entrées and platters marked with a ✔ are Best Bites. Best Bites are relatively low in saturated fat and rich in vegetables.

Reminder

Recommended limits for a 2,000-calorie diet:

Total fat: 65 grams
Saturated fat: 20 grams
Cholesterol: 300 milligrams
Sodium: 2,400 milligrams

FAMILY-STYLE FOODS

Menu Item	Calories	Total Fat (g)	Saturated Fat (g)	Cholesterol (mg)	Sodium (mg)
ENTRÉES AND PLATTERS					
✔ Pot roast (10 oz.)	370	16	7	115	570
✔ plus vegetable (1 cup) and mashed potatoes with gravy (¾ cup)	620	26	11	125	1,310
✔ Chicken stir-fry with rice (3½ cups)	700	23	7	15	2,330
Turkey (6 oz.) with stuffing (1 cup) and gravy	500	19	9	140	2,190
plus mashed potatoes with gravy (¾ cup), vegetable (1 cup), and cranberry sauce (⅛ cup)	880	30	13	155	2,960
Hamburger (7 oz.)	510	27	14	105	570
plus french fries (2 cups)	1,100	58	25	105	1,040
Philly cheese steak sandwich (6-inch)	680	35	17	100	1,330
plus french fries (2 cups)	1,270	66	29	100	1,790
Chicken potpie (13 oz.)	680	37	17	70	1,590
Country-fried steak (9 oz.)	650	42	18	70	1,250
plus vegetable (1 cup) and mashed potatoes with gravy (¾ cup)	900	52	21	85	1,990

FAMILY-STYLE FOODS *(continued)* Menu Item	Calories	Total Fat (g)	Saturated Fat (g)	Cholesterol (mg)	Sodium (mg)
Chef salad (5 cups) with dressing (½ cup)	930	71	*18*	285	2,510
Meat loaf (9 oz.)	570	38	*19*	180	1,510
plus vegetable (1 cup) and mashed potatoes with gravy (¾ cup)	820	49	*23*	195	2,260
Patty melt (9 oz.)	770	50	*25*	125	1,130
plus french fries (2 cups)	1,350	81	*37*	130	1,600
SIDE DISHES AND DESSERTS					
Vegetable of the day (1 cup)	60	3	*1*	3	150
Baked potato with sour cream (1 Tb.)	310	3	*2*	5	30
Mashed potatoes with gravy (¾ cup)	190	8	*3*	10	600
French fries (2 cups)	590	31	*12*	5	460
Apple pie (8 oz.)	540	28	*13*	5	440
Milk shake, vanilla (13 oz.)	620	30	*21*	110	230

Note: For baked potato, sour cream, and cranberry sauce, we used numbers from the USDA Nutrient Database for Standard Reference. Saturated fat numbers in *italics* include artery-clogging *trans* fat.

Chapter 14

In the Drink: Beverages

n the 1950s, a "family-size" bottle of Coca-Cola was 26 ounces, presumably enough to last Mom, Dad, Sis, and Junior from one weekly grocery run to the next. Over the years, however, serving sizes have steadily crept up, and we're now awash in sugary sodas. The plain truth is that serving sizes for beverages are ballooning—right along with Americans' waistlines.

Current soft drink sizes at McDonald's range from a 12-ounce kids' size (1½ cups) to a 42-ounce super size (more than 5 cups). A "Double Gulp" at 7-Eleven convenience stores holds a ridiculous 64 ounces. That's eight cups—a huge serving even if you order it with extra ice. And the soft drinks at movie theaters like Loew's and some AMCs (which can hit 44 ounces) often come with free refills. Sit-down restaurant chains like Applebee's, Chili's, Denny's, The Olive Garden, Outback Steakhouse, and T.G.I. Friday's start you off with 14 to 22 ounces of soda, then also offer free refills. Mom's old admonition not to "fill up on soda" has gone the way of the advice to chew each bite of food a hundred times—it's largely forgotten.

Soft drinks aren't the only beverage giants. A venti Starbucks Caffè Latte is 20 ounces, and at McDonald's a large shake weighs in at 32 ounces. Even cocktails are burgeoning in size. T.G.I. Friday's sells 18-ounce cocktails like the Ultimate Daiquiri, Hawaiian Volcano, Long Island Iced Tea, Margarita, and Mudslide. Order a beer on tap at restaurants like Applebee's, T.G.I Friday's, or The Olive Garden and you'll be offered a choice between a

16-ounce draft or a 22-ounce one. (A can or bottle of beer is generally around 12 ounces.)

With obesity the norm in the United States, it's important to stop and think before you order a beverage. It takes only a few seconds to consider how many calories you'll be sucking up through that straw. Twenty ounces of most beverages—even juice or fat-free milk—means 200 to 450 calories.

"Beverages are a huge contributor to obesity," says Richard Mattes of Purdue University in West Lafayette, Indiana. "They're major players that often get overlooked." And the problem isn't just that beverages are bigger. According to a growing body of evidence, it's very possible that your body may not register the calories you *drink* as well as it does the calories you *eat*. So when you down that latte before lunch or drink a soda or other liquid calories with a meal, you may not eat less food later in the day to compensate. "We found that people compensate for about two-thirds of the calories in solid foods, one-third of the calories in semisolid foods, but none of the calories in liquids," says Mattes. "Liquid calories don't trip our satiety mechanisms."

In one three-week study, women who were given 40 ounces a day of regular cola to drink gained more weight, whereas those who were given diet soda gained none. "It doesn't matter if you drink them with a meal or before a meal," according to Barbara Rolls of the Pennsylvania State University, author of *Volumetrics: Feel Full on Fewer Calories*. "The calories from most drinks add on to—rather than displace—food calories."

Beverage Strategy

Before you wet your whistle with a beverage, remember to check out the chart on page 254 and take to heart the following strategies for ordering drinks. Follow them, and you'll save yourself a bellyful of calories.

• **Order "kiddie" or "small" sizes.** At McDonald's and many other restaurants, a child's serving is 12 ounces. Most fast-food places offer a "small" 16-ounce drink (two cups).

• **Ask for extra ice.** The more ice in the cup, the less you drink and the fewer calories you'll consume.

• **Share with a friend.** If no small-size beverage is available, order a large one, but ask for an empty glass and split it with a friend.

• **Forget about refills.** If the server brings around the refill pitcher, ask for water instead. Most restaurants will happily bring you ice water with a slice of lemon, orange, or lime. A squeeze, a stir, *et voilà,* a no-cal drink that's also free!

• **Be inventive.** To cut calories, ask for a mix of orange juice, cranberry juice, or pineapple juice and club soda. You may even find that it's more refreshing than a heavily sugared soft drink.

• **Don't forget fat-free or 1 percent low-fat milk.** The calcium, protein, and other nutrients in a glass of milk make it well worth the 100-or-so calories.

• **Diet soft drinks are better than regular soda.** Diet soda has a leg up on regular soda because it is calorie- and sugar-free. However, questions have been raised about the safety of aspartame (NutraSweet), the most widely used artificial sweetener. Some people believe that it causes dizziness, hallucinations, or headaches, but controlled studies have not confirmed those problems. In addition, aspartame needs to be tested better to confirm that it does not cause cancer.

• **Avoid excess caffeine.** If you guzzle caffeinated soda, coffee, or tea all day, it may leave you jittery and unable to sleep. Many coffee drinkers experience headaches, irritability, sleepiness, and other withdrawal symptoms when they go cold turkey. Because caffeine may increase the risk of miscarriages (and possibly birth defects) and inhibits fetal growth, women who are pregnant or considering becoming pregnant should avoid it. Caffeine may also make it harder to get pregnant.

Here's a rundown of popular drinks, ranked from least to most number of calories. We didn't choose Best Bites because beverages are rarely interchangeable. For example, you wouldn't order milk with Chinese food or a glass of orange juice instead of a beer. Some of the serving sizes may surprise you—but we swear we didn't make them up!

DRINKS BY THE NUMBERS

Beverage (serving size)	Calories
Water or seltzer	0
Diet soda (20 oz.)	5
Coffee, with one liquid creamer (8 oz.)	30
Tea, with two packets of sugar (8 oz.)	50
Milk, fat-free (8 oz.)	90
Beer, light (12 oz.)	100
Milk, 1% low-fat (8 oz.)	100
Apple or orange juice (8 oz.)	110
Au Bon Pain Iced Cappuccino, small (9 oz.)	110
Starbucks Cappuccino made with skim milk, grande (16 oz.)	110
Irish coffee, without whipped cream (8 oz.)	120
Cranberry juice (8 oz.)	140
Au Bon Pain Iced Cappuccino, medium (12 oz.)	150
Beer, regular (12 oz.)	150
Grape juice (8 oz.)	150
Mimosa (8 oz.)	150

Beverage (serving size)	Calories
Martini (2½ oz.)	160
Starbucks Caffè Latte made with skim milk, grande (16 oz.)	160
Wine, white (8 oz.)	160
Gin & tonic, on the rocks (7½ oz.)	170
Wine, red (8 oz.)	170
Milk, whole (8 oz.)	180
Starbucks Cappuccino made with whole milk, grande (16 oz.)	180
Ginger ale (20 oz.)	200
Smoothie King Slim & Trim Orange-Vanilla, small (20 oz.)	200
Dairy Queen Misty, small (16 oz.)	220
7-Up, Coca-Cola, or root beer (20 oz.)	250
Starbucks Caramel Macchiato, made with whole milk, grande (16 oz.)	250
Au Bon Pain Iced Cappuccino, large (20½ oz.)	270
Starbucks Caffè Latte made with whole milk, grande (16 oz.)	270
Au Bon Pain Strawberry Banana Split Blast (16 oz.)	280
Beer, regular, draft (22 oz.)	280
Margarita (from mix), on the rocks (8 oz.)	290
Orange soda (20 oz.)	300
Starbucks Coffee Frappuccino, venti (24 oz., with ice)	300
McDonald's Coca-Cola classic, large (32 oz.)	310
McDonald's Chocolate Shake, small (14 oz.)	360
McDonald's Coca-Cola classic, super size (42 oz.)	410
Burger King Vanilla Shake, medium (14 oz.)	430
Dairy Queen Misty, large (32 oz.)	440
Au Bon Pain Malt Shoppe Blast (16 oz.)	460
McDonald's Hi-C Orange Drink, super size (42 oz.)	460
Au Bon Pain Original Frozen Mocha Blast, large (24 oz.)	480
Jamba Juice, Razzmatazz, power size (32 oz.)	590

Beverage (serving size)	Calories
Starbucks White Chocolate Mocha made with whole milk and whipped cream, venti (20 oz.)	600
Dunkin' Donuts Coolatta made with cream, large (32 oz.)	820
McDonald's Chocolate Shake, large (32 oz.)	1,030
Baskin-Robbins Chocolate Milkshake, large (24 oz.)	1,130
Smoothie King Strawberry Hulk, king size (40 oz.)	1,910

Note: The numbers were provided by the manufacturers and the USDA Nutrient Database for Standard Reference.

Chapter 15

Sweet Nothings: Pastry and Desserts

hile touring Europe in 1878, a homesick Mark Twain fantasized about the American foods he was eagerly looking forward to tasting again at home. The list encompassed dozens of dishes, which Twain later enumerated in *A Tramp Abroad* (1880). Among the delicacies he craved were fried and stewed oysters, porterhouse steak, trout, hot biscuits, soft-shell crabs, buttered corn, mashed potatoes, and maple syrup. And at the end of the list, Twain mused about his favorite desserts: apple dumplings and apple fritters, peach cobbler, pumpkin pie and squash pie, plus "all sorts of American pastry." Like most Americans, Twain had a prodigious appetite for sweets.

Indeed, a sweet tooth seems to be an integral part of the American character, despite the fact that many of us have known for some time that we indulge in these temptations at no small price. As one of Twain's contemporaries, popular cookbook author Sarah Tyson Rorer, cautioned her nineteenth-century readers, "desserts are both unhealthy and unnecessary as articles of food. . . . All of these things look so good but they are so deadly." It's so true.

Although twentieth-century research has revealed the nutritional pitfalls of the butter, eggs, cream, chocolate, and sugar in so many of our favorite sweets, this knowledge is sometimes easy to ignore. The spicy aroma of baking pastry and the promise of icing are an almost irresistible combination to anyone within sniffing distance of Cinnabon, whose warm, hyper-size cinnamon rolls are widely sold in malls and airports. "O-o-o-h-h-h-h. I knew they were bad, but I didn't know they were *that* bad," moaned a Cinnabon devotee after she read our initial report on sweets in *Nutrition Action Healthletter.* That was also our reaction when we sized up 14 popular sweets from some of the most popular mall outlets and storefronts around the country. We weren't expecting to find nutritional powerhouses; we just hoped to find some favorites that weren't outrageous. What we found instead was that many pastries and sweets contain not only a dinner's worth of calories, but also a day's worth of saturated fat.

Of course, eating a sticky bun once in a while is not going to kill you. But for too many people, a sticky bun is not an unusual extravagance. Instead, it is part of a daily diet that might include a McDonald's Sausage Biscuit for breakfast, a ham-and-cheese sandwich for lunch, and kung pao chicken takeout for dinner. Few people (except maybe marathon runners) are able to afford the calories in sky-high layer cakes and softball-sized muffins.

It's clear from their popularity that the Double Fudge Brownies from Mrs. Fields, the chocolate croissants from Vie de France, and countless other readily available sweets are not just an occasional splurge for many people. Cinnabon has sold countless millions of rolls in the last 16 years, the majority from its 500-plus bakeshops in 17 countries. Mrs. Fields had sales of $158 million in 2000, according to *Restaurants and Institutions*, an industry trade publication. And along with the advent of Starbucks and other specialty beverage spots have come thousands of new opportunities to buy high-calorie pastries more often than as an accompaniment to that morning brew. No wonder more than half of all adult Americans are overweight or obese. In addition to the super-size, overstuffed, high-calorie restaurant meals, sweet pastries and desserts are now consumed from breakfast to bedtime.

Being prudent need not mean being deprived. After a closer look at the facts, the wiser alternatives to some of the richest offerings may become appealing. Let the following numbers be your guide the next time you're drawn to those sweet aromas drifting from a storefront. This information will help you decide when you can—and can't—afford to satisfy your sweet tooth. At least now when you splurge, you'll know the cost.

The Dishes and the Data

We analyzed 14 of the most popular sweets from 70 outlets, including Au Bon Pain, The Cheesecake Factory, Cinnabon, Mrs. Fields, Starbucks, and Vie de France, in Atlanta, Boston, Chicago, Denver, Houston, Los Angeles, and Washington, D.C. (For more on our methodology, see pages 12–14.)

Before we give you the hard numbers, we can sum up in a nutshell the trouble with the items we analyzed: They are sweets on steroids. It's that simple. On average, the pastries are at least twice the size of similar items made by Entenmann's, Little Debbie, Pepperidge Farm, Sara Lee, and lesser-known brands of packaged sweet treats. Here's the rundown on sweets, ranked from best to worst—that is, from least to most saturated fat.

AU BON PAIN TRIPLE BERRY LOW FAT MUFFIN
(260 calories and 4 grams of fat, 1 of them saturated)

Au Bon Pain makes the lowest-fat item we analyzed. It weighs 4 ounces—twice the size of a typical supermarket muffin. Its 4 grams of fat are about what you get in a McDonald's Lowfat Apple Bran Muffin (also 4 ounces; see page 292). Not bad. The 260 calories are about what you'd get in some low-fat frozen entrées or a low-fat fruit-flavored yogurt. That's not negligible, but it's far fewer calories than you'll find in most pastries. Incidentally, Au Bon Pain says that the Triple Berry Low Fat Muffins and the Chocolate Cake Low Fat Muffin (which has about the same amount of fat and calories) sell well.

AU BON PAIN BLUEBERRY MUFFIN
(430 calories and 18 grams of fat, 4 of them saturated)

Here's an example of why it's so important to get in the habit of ordering only low-fat muffins. Thanks to its margarine and butter, this 4½-ounce muffin harbors more than four times the fat of the Triple Berry Low Fat version. The 430 calories are as many as you'd get in a McDonald's Quarter Pounder. And don't be fooled by that healthy-sounding Carrot Walnut Muffin on Au Bon Pain's menu (page 322). The company reports that the Carrot Walnut contains 580 calories and 30 grams of fat. That's fattier than the Corn and the Chocolate Chip Muffins, which are fattier than the Blueberry.

MRS. FIELDS DEBRA'S SPECIAL (OATMEAL RAISIN WALNUT) COOKIE
(240 calories and 12 grams of fat, 6 of them saturated)

There's no good nutritional news about cookies. Usually made with flour, butter, sugar, and eggs, and frequently flavored with chocolate, molasses, raisins and nuts, they're irresistible. But they're sweet suicide for cookie lovers. With more than 500 bakeries, Mrs. Fields sells more fresh-baked cookies than anyone else. Her oatmeal cookies are about twice as large as most packaged cookies. But even ounce for ounce, the Fields's recipe squeezes in three times as much saturated fat. We wish the emphasis were on the whole-grain goodness, but there's more white flour, butter, sugar, and eggs than oatmeal. The best you can say about these cookies is that they have fewer calories than some other snacks . . . if you stop at one.

MRS. FIELDS MILK CHOCOLATE CHIP COOKIE
(250 calories and 13 grams of fat, 8 of them saturated)

At 2 ounces, this cookie is nearly twice as big as the oversize Pepperidge Farm Nantucket Double Chocolate Chunk Cookie and five times the size of a regular Chips Ahoy! Its 5 teaspoons of sugar, plus butter, eggs, and more chocolate chips than flour explain the numbers. Eating just one gives you as much saturated fat as a 12-ounce sirloin steak.

MRS. FIELDS WHITE CHUNK MACADAMIA COOKIE
(270 calories and 16 grams of fat, 9 of them saturated)

Of course they taste good. But if you eat just one, you'll blow half a day's saturated fat quota. One of Pepperidge Farm's smaller Tahoe White Chocolate Macadamia Cookies, which is equally yummy, would give you only one-third the saturated fat.

VIE DE FRANCE BUTTER CROISSANT, LARGE
(350 calories and 18 grams of fat, 12 of them saturated)

Think of a butter croissant as a dinner roll spread with almost five pats of butter. Blowing half a day's saturated fat on one food is a recipe for coronary overload. Even a medium-size one has enough saturated fat—8 grams—to lard your arteries. Save its 250 calories and 13 grams of fat for something better. If you're in the habit of ordering sandwiches made with a croissant instead of bread or a roll, you'll be half a day's worth of saturated fat in the hole before the filling is even added.

CINNABON
(670 calories and 34 grams of fat, 14 of them saturated)

Jerilyn Brusseau, the baker/restaurateur who developed the Cinnabon recipe, described the product in an interview with the *Seattle Times* as "wonderful, rich everyday food." We won't quibble with the first two, but "everyday"!? We don't know who can afford to use up three-quarters of a day's saturated fat and nearly 700 calories on one serving of junk food. At some locations you can watch the cooks slather margarine on the raw dough and cream cheese frosting on the fresh-baked rolls. If you simply can't resist this confection, at least opt for the smaller Minibon instead. That way you will consume "only" 300 calories and 11 grams of fat, 5 of them saturated. (Too bad that Cinnabon dropped its lower-fat Minibon Delight, which had just 7 grams of fat.) When the server offers extra frosting, just say "NO!"

VIE DE FRANCE CHOCOLATE CROISSANT
(430 calories and 23 grams of fat, 15 of them saturated)

The yen for an occasional chocolate croissant is easy to understand but hard on your heart. Just keep in mind that neither an overstuffed corned beef sandwich nor a 12-inch Subway Classic Steak & Cheese sub contains this much saturated fat.

MRS. FIELDS DOUBLE FUDGE BROWNIE
(420 calories and 25 grams of fat, 16 of them saturated)

Betty Crocker, Duncan Hines, and Little Debbie don't even come close to these sweets. Their brownies have no more than 3 grams of saturated fat in smaller, far more sensible servings. Mrs. Fields's 2-inch-by-3-inch brownie may look modest, but her double-fudge wonder has the saturated fat of three slices of a large Domino's Hand Tossed Pepperoni Pizza. Some snack!

STARBUCKS CINNAMON SCONE
(530 calories and 26 grams of fat,16 of them saturated)

According to industry analysts, the average Starbucks customer stops in 15 to 20 times a month. If that customer is picking up one of these scones with every stop, he or she is in trouble. Starbucks's scone may not look like two pork chops with mashed potatoes and gravy, but that's how your arteries will see it. The 500-plus calories are a quarter of a day's worth. Plus, the 16 grams of saturated fat gobble up three-quarters of your daily maximum.

AU BON PAIN ALMOND CROISSANT
(630 calories and 42 grams of fat, 18 of them saturated)
Before you treat yourself to one of these with your tea, keep in mind that a Swanson's Hungry-Man Salisbury Steak dinner has fewer calories and less saturated fat. And that's for the *average* Au Bon Pain Almond Croissant. Au Bon Pain's Almond Croissants tend to be inconsistent in size. Of the 12 we sampled, the largest supplied 23 grams of saturated fat, 7 teaspoons of sugar, and 820 calories.

AU BON PAIN PECAN ROLL
(800 calories and 45 grams of fat, 20 of them saturated)
Denny's Original Grand Slam breakfast platter has two slices of bacon, two sausage links, two eggs, and two hotcakes, and it uses up three-quarters of a day's allowance of saturated fat. That's less than one Au Bon Pain Pecan Roll delivers! Like the Grand Slam, nearly all of this roll's key ingredients are fatty: pecans, shortening, margarine, and palm kernel oil. Can you handle 11 teaspoons of sugar and an extra 800 calories?

AU BON PAIN SWEET CHEESE DANISH
(520 calories and 31 grams of fat, 23 of them saturated)
The fat and saturated fat in one of these are equal to what's in a pint of Breyers All Natural Ice Cream. The fats, and the facts, speak for themselves.

THE CHEESECAKE FACTORY ORIGINAL CHEESECAKE
(710 calories and 49 grams of fat, 31 of them saturated)
It's not easy to find a food that uses up all of today's—and half of tomorrow's—quota of saturated fat. Two slices of Pizza Hut's The

Sweet Statistics

••••••••••••••••••••••••••

Ask if there is nutrition information available. Some shops and restaurants may have information about their baked goods but not display it or even advertise that it's available. (If they do have it, it's usually kept in notebooks behind the counter.) Au Bon Pain, Cinnabon, Starbucks, and Vie de France, for example, claim that every outlet has nutrition information for most menu items.

Big New Yorker Pepperoni Pizza plus two Dairy Queen Banana Splits would do it, and so would one slice of this *plain* cheesecake. (You can also choose from varieties like Triple Chocolate Chip and White Chocolate Chunk Macadamia Nut.) But the worst dessert on the menu (according to the company's numbers) at The Cheesecake Factory isn't the cheesecake—it's the Carrot Cake. One slice has 1,560 calories and 84 grams of fat (23 of them—a day's worth—are saturated). The Factory's Black Out, Linda's Fudge, and Fabulous Chocolate Mousse are in the same ballpark. A slice of each has about 1,400 calories. (In case you've forgotten, most people need only 2,000 calories in an entire day.) These desserts make the Original Cheesecake look like a bargain at "only" 710 calories.

When Your Favorite Is Not on the List

We discuss many other desserts in other chapters of this book. For example, we cover doughnuts offered at Dunkin' Donuts in chapter 17, Shop Till You Drop: Mall Food, page 303. We also discuss a number of other sweets sold at Au Bon Pain in the same chapter. For apple pie, see chapter 13, Home away from Home: Family-Style Restaurants, page 239. You'll get the scoop on a fudge brownie sundae in chapter 12, Where Everybody Knows Your Name: Dinner Houses, page 223. Read about desserts offered at fast-food restaurants in chapter 16, On the Run: Fast-Food Restaurants, page 271.

Sweets Strategy

• **Check out the competition.** Outlets like Mrs. Fields and Cinnabon are usually in malls, airports, and other high-traffic locations where they are surrounded by lots of other food vendors. Take a look at what else is offered before succumbing to a high-calorie treat. You may find there's a place selling bagels, baguettes, fruit, or low-fat frozen yogurt right around the corner. See the mall food chapter (page 303) and the fast-food chapter (page 271) for more information.

• **Look for low-fat treats.** If a shop or restaurant offers low-fat options, choose one of them. But keep in mind that these products may not be low in calories.

The Secret Life of Sweets

Cheesecake *sounds* nutritious if you've never baked one at home and have no idea what goes into one. Why is it so fatty? Well, most cookbook recipes list the principal ingredients as cream cheese (which is more cream than cheese), eggs, and sugar. Recipes may also include other fatty ingredients like whipping cream and chocolate.

Scones sound as dainty and demure as a tea party, but they're actually big, brawny biscuits made from white flour, eggs, cream or milk, butter, baking powder, and sugar. Starbucks Cinnamon Scone is as bad for your arteries as two McDonald's Quarter Pounders.

Croissants are quite simply super-saturated with butter. That tender, flaky interior is created by layering rolled-out yeast dough with slabs of butter, then repeatedly folding it over on itself until all of the butter is incorporated.

• **Buy a bagel.** Places like Au Bon Pain and Vie de France sell bagels and French rolls. Instead of a croissant or a Danish, have a bagel or roll with preserves.

• **Size does matter.** Smaller is always better when it comes to sweets. A Minibon, for example, has roughly 50 percent less saturated fat and calories than a full-size Cinnabon. But don't confuse "less" with "low." Even a Minibon has 300 calories. And a modest-size Double Fudge Brownie from Mrs. Fields has as much saturated fat as two corned beef sandwiches.

• **"Cholesterol-free" is no guarantee of healthfulness.** A product touted as "cholesterol-free" is not necessarily low in fat or calories.

• **Avoid super-size sweets.** Monster-size pastries contain monstrous amounts of calories. And remember, even one ordinary-size take-out cookie may contain as much saturated fat as a full breakfast.

The Bagel Option

•••••••••••••••••••••••••••••••••••••••

Who says a quick stop in a bakeshop has to send your cholesterol soaring? Au Bon Pain and Starbucks, two of the chains whose products we studied, offer bagels at some of their outlets (and, of course, bagels are available at many other venues across the country). In fact, at Au Bon Pain, bagels are the best-selling breakfast item.

According to numbers provided by Au Bon Pain, a Plain, Cinnamon Raisin, Honey 9 Grain, or Wild Blueberry bagel will set you back 350 to 390 calories but have no more than 2 grams of fat, almost none of it saturated. The Cranberry Walnut bagel has the most calories and total fat among the sweet flavors—460 calories and 4 grams of fat, only 1 gram of which is saturated.

Of course, you could up the numbers by ordering your bagel with full-fat cream cheese. Just 1 tablespoon has 50 calories and 5 grams of fat, 3 of them saturated. Many shops trowel the cheese onto their bagels like mortar, using as much as 4 tablespoons! That brings your bagel to about 600 calories and more than half a day's saturated fat. Look for light cream cheese, which many chains offer. It's just as tasty and frequently comes mixed with fruit or crunchy chopped raw veggies. Whether it's light or regular, spread only a thin layer on your bagel. A little cream cheese goes a long way.

See chapter 17, Shop Till You Drop: Mall Food (page 303) for additional information.

he "Sugars" number includes both refined sugars and (generally) much smaller amounts of naturally occurring sugars from fruit and milk. The U.S. Department of Agriculture's recommended limit for refined sugars is 40 grams per day, or 10 teaspoons. (That's the amount in a typical 12-ounce soft drink.) We've ranked sweets from best to worst—that is, from least to most saturated fat. Items marked with a ✔ are Best Bites. Best Bites are relatively low in saturated fat.

Reminder
Recommended limits for a 2,000-calorie diet:
Total fat: 65 grams
Saturated fat: 20 grams
Cholesterol: 300 milligrams
Sodium: 2,400 milligrams
Refined sugars: 40 grams

SWEETS

Menu Item	Calories	Total Fat (g)	Saturated Fat (g)	Cholesterol (mg)	Sugars (g)
✔ Au Bon Pain Triple Berry Low Fat Muffin (4 oz.)	260	4	*1*	15	30
Au Bon Pain Blueberry Muffin (4½ oz.)	430	18	*4*	80	36
Mrs. Fields Debra's Special (Oatmeal Raisin Walnut) Cookie (2 oz.)	240	12	*6*	25	19
Mrs. Fields Milk Chocolate Chip Cookie (2 oz.)	250	13	*8*	25	23
Mrs. Fields White Chunk Macadamia Cookie (2 oz.)	270	16	*9*	20	19
Vie de France Butter Croissant, large (3 oz.)	350	18	*12*	45	7
Cinnabon (7½ oz.)	670	34	*14*	65	49
Vie de France Chocolate Croissant (3½ oz.)	430	23	*15*	40	18
The Cheesecake Factory Linda's Fudge Cake (1 slice, 14 oz.)	1,400	52	15	95	168
Mrs. Fields Double Fudge Brownie (3 oz.)	420	25	*16*	70	47
Starbucks Cinnamon Scone (5 oz.)	530	26	*16*	125	15
Au Bon Pain Almond Croissant (5 oz.)	630	42	*18*	90	23

SWEETS *(continued)*

Menu Item	Calories	Total Fat (g)	Saturated Fat (g)	Cholesterol (mg)	Sugars (g)
Au Bon Pain Pecan Roll (6½ oz)	800	45	*20*	45	42
Au Bon Pain Sweet Cheese Danish (4½ oz)	520	31	*23*	80	23
The Cheesecake Factory Carrot Cake (1 slice, 14 oz.)*	1,560	84	23	190	143
The Cheesecake Factory Black Out Cake (1 slice, 14 oz.)*	1,490	72	29	140	150
The Cheesecake Factory Original Cheesecake (1 slice, 7 oz.)	710	49	*31*	215	49
The Cheesecake Factory Fabulous Chocolate Mousse Cake (1 slice, 12 oz.)*	1,250	71	35	280	111

*Numbers were provided by the company.

Note: Saturated fat numbers in *italics* include artery-clogging *trans* fat.

Chapter 16

On the Run: Fast-Food Restaurants

mericans eat at fast-food places far more than at any other type of restaurant, according to a survey by *Restaurants and Institutions*, an industry trade magazine. Nearly half (44 percent) of those surveyed stop in at least once a week. The same survey also found that the three most popular offerings at these restaurants are the familiar fast-food triumvirate of hamburgers, french fries, and soft drinks.

So what's new in the ever-evolving world of fast food? Chains are tripping over one another to build bigger burgers, and in the process they've devised a range of sizes in which "small" is rarely an option. Orders of fries have exploded into "super" and "king" sizes that have as many calories as a McDonald's Big Mac. Sugar-laden sodas now come in bucket-sized cups. And although chicken nuggets, fish, and potatoes are no longer fried in beef fat, the hydrogenated vegetable shortening that replaced it is just about as artery-clogging.

Ironically, as consumers have become more health conscious, the fast-food restaurants have abandoned some of the improvements they made in the early 1990s. McDonald's has ditched its McLean Deluxe burger. The company's grilled chicken sandwich (although still better than a fried chicken sandwich) has gained 150 extra calories because of a thick layer of mayo, and its shakes and ice cream cones are no longer low-fat. Taco Bell's Border Lights lower-fat menu is just a memory, as is KFC's Tender Roast rotisserie chicken.

Yet if you look carefully, you can find some fast foods worth crossing the street for. A handful of salads, baked potatoes, grilled chicken sandwiches, wraps, and McDonald's Fruit 'n Yogurt Parfait make up a short list of fast food that's decent.

Because we're looking at menu offerings chain by chain, we've divided the dishes into "Picks" and "Pans." "Picks" are usually lower in saturated fat and may provide a serving of vegetables. "Pans" usually contain at least half a day's limit of saturated fat. Our discussion focuses on core menu items, but you'll find nutrition numbers for other products in the accompanying chart. Note that all nutrition information was provided by the companies, except for a few fried items that we analyzed for artery-clogging *trans* fat.

Burger King

If a Burger King outlet is your only fast-food option at lunch, you might want to consider brown-bagging it. The nation's No. 2 burger giant (8,310 restaurants in the United States) has the fewest healthy-eating options of any of the chains we examined.

In early 2002, Burger King announced that it would revamp its menu with 14 new items, including new burgers and desserts. Most, like the King Supreme hamburger and 1/4 Lb. Burger, will likely be in keeping with Burger King's fatty, calorie-laden menu. The new Old Fashioned Vanilla Milkshake has 700 calories and 41 grams of fat, 26 of them saturated. That's essentially a Whopper's worth of fat and calories for a *medium*. Burger King declined to reveal numbers for a large.

The only bright spot: Burger King may be the first nationwide burger chain to offer a vegetarian burger. McDonald's has sold them at a few selected locations for years, but never anywhere else. Finally, Burger King is taking the plunge. Its Veggie Burger has 330 calories, and that includes light mayonnaise. Congratulations, Burger King. What took you so long?

Picks: Your best bet is the BK Broiler Chicken Sandwich; order it without the mayo to slash the fat by two-thirds and save 160 calories. In place of the mayo, use mustard, ketchup, or the Barbecue Dipping Sauce that comes with the Chicken Tenders. None of Burger King's burgers qualified for "Picks," but if you can't live without one, go for the regular Hamburger. But be aware that it's larger than a McDonald's Hamburger and has about twice the saturated fat.

Pans: Flame-broiled or not, Burger King's specialties are some of the most artery-damaging burgers you can eat at a fast-food restaurant. The Double Whopper and Double Whopper with Cheese will not only cost you 900 to 1,000 calories, but at least a day's allowance of saturated fat as well. A Bacon Double Cheeseburger, a Double Cheeseburger, and a Whopper with Cheese all have nearly double the Big Mac's saturated fat—about a day's worth. Burger King's signature sandwich, the Whopper, has 50 percent more saturated fat than a McDonald's Quarter Pounder. Burger King's Chicken Sandwich and BK Big Fish Sandwich may sound better than a burger, but they're both deep-fried in *trans* fat–laden shortening, which makes them about as bad for your heart as a Whopper.

Fries accompany about 80 percent of all burger orders at fast-food restaurants. That hair-raising statistic spells trouble for frequent customers because Burger King serves some of the most artery-clogging fries you can find. (Like other major fast-food chains, Burger King and McDonald's cook their fries in hydrogenated shortening.) A king-size order of Burger King's fries contains 600 calories and 30 grams of fat (16 of them saturated, which is three-fourths of a day's worth). Not only is that side of fries worse for your arteries than a Whopper, but the 6-ounce serving also has one and a half times as much saturated fat as a 7-ounce serving of McDonald's super-size fries. And that's not all—along with all that fat, BK's king-size french fries harbor a whopping 1,140 milligrams of sodium, compared to 390 milligrams in a McDonald's super size.

Breakfast at Burger King is as unkind to your health and waistline as lunch. The BK Croissan'wich and Biscuit sandwiches topped with sausage all have as much saturated fat as a Whopper. And the Biscuit with Sausage, Cini-minis (cinnamon rolls with icing), French Toast Sticks, or a small order of Hash Brown Rounds are each as bad for your arteries as a BK Cheeseburger.

A Word About Meals: Burger King's Value Meals are some of the least healthful among fast-food chains. They typically include a burger or chicken or fish sandwich plus medium fries and medium drink. One of the lowest-calorie Value Meals, the Whopper Jr., medium fries, and a medium Coca-Cola Classic, has 1,000 calories and nearly a day's allowance of saturated fat (18 grams). If you order your Value Meal with large or king-size fries and drink, the numbers are far worse. For example, a Whopper, large fries, and a large Coca-Cola Classic hits 1,500 calories and more than a day's quota of saturated fat (26 grams). A Double Whopper with Cheese, king-size fries, and a king-size Coca-Cola Classic soars to 2,050 calories and two days' worth of saturated fat (43 grams). Our advice: Skip the Value Meals and order a BK Broiler Chicken Sandwich without the mayo and an orange juice. The meal will cost you 530 calories. That's about the best you can do at Burger King.

KFC

KFC, the world's largest fried chicken chain, proves you can thrive in the fast-food biz with nary a burger on the menu. Indeed, Colonel Sanders was decades ahead of today's home-meal-replacement industry when he promoted his buckets of chicken and side dishes as "Sunday Dinner, Seven Days a Week." But a lack of beef on the menu doesn't automatically mean there are healthful meals. Unfortunately, with a couple of exceptions, most of KFC's offerings still have a date with the deep fryer.

Picks: Your best bet for a light lunch is the Tender Roast Chicken Sandwich, with or without sauce. Sauceless, the sandwich provides only 5 grams of fat, 2 of them saturated. That's as healthful a sandwich as you can get anywhere. You can also make a meal out of side dishes. The best is the Corn on the Cob, which is low in both fat and sodium. Another notable accompaniment, the BBQ Baked Beans, pack a quarter of a day's fiber. However, like most canned bean dishes, it comes at a price—760 milligrams of sodium. As for potatoes, your best bet would be Mashed Potatoes with Gravy. You could eat two orders of Mashed Potatoes with Gravy and still get less fat and fewer calories than you would get by eating one order of Potato Wedges. Coleslaw and potato salad are your next-best choices.

You can turn any fried chicken into a pick by not eating the skin. It doesn't matter whether you order Original Recipe, Hot & Spicy, or Extra Crispy chicken—as long as you remove the skin and breading, you end up with the same amount of fat. Skinning chicken cuts the fat by about half. Although ounce for ounce a skinned breast is leaner than a skinned drumstick, a drumstick actually has less fat because it's a smaller piece. The thigh and wing are the fattiest pieces (and it's virtually impossible to pull the skin off the wing).

Pans: The worst item on KFC's menu is baked, not fried. KFC's Chunky Chicken Pot Pie contains 770 calories and two-thirds of a day's saturated fat (13 grams).

Also stay away from the breaded and fried Crispy Strips, Hot Wings, and Popcorn Chicken. Our numbers don't tell the whole story because they omit the *trans* fat in KFC's vegetable shortening. Based on other chains, it's a good bet that the "saturated fat" numbers in our KFC chart should be twice as high. And finally, avoid KFC's Biscuits—just one will supply a third of a day's saturated fat.

A Word About Meals: KFC's Combo Meals typically include two or three pieces of chicken plus a biscuit and choice of a side dish. A typical three-piece meal—Extra Crispy Drumstick, two Extra Crispy Thighs, plus Potato Wedges and a Biscuit—hits 1,420 calories and 89 grams of fat (28 of them saturated). That's more than a day's quota of fat and saturated fat. Choosing Mashed Potatoes with Gravy or Corn on the Cob instead of fried Potato Wedges saves around 150 calories. Substituting Original Recipe for Extra Crispy chicken shaves off another 300 calories. You'd be better off constructing you own combo meal. For example, the Tender Roast Sandwich with sauce paired with Corn on the Cob has just 500 calories and 3 grams of saturated fat.

McDonald's

The biggest restaurant chain on the planet, McDonald's operates close to 13,000 restaurants in the United States and another 16,000 abroad. Every day the company serves a mind-boggling 45 million people worldwide. Given the tons of ground beef, cheese, hydrogenated vegetable shortening, and sugar that this chain shovels into the nation's gullets on a daily basis, it's hard to praise its menu. And the fast-food colossus has a habit of introducing new items that make its older selections look good. The small 280-calorie Hamburger—still a fixture in kids' Happy Meals—has been pushed aside by the 430-calorie Quarter Pounder, the 590-calorie Big Mac, and the 540-calorie Big N' Tasty.

Likewise, orders of french fries keep expanding. In the 1950s and 1960s, McDonald's had only one size of french fries. Like today's "small," it had 200 calories. In the early 1970s, the chain introduced a 320-calorie "large." But in the 1980s, the 1970s' "large" became a "medium," and the new "large" swelled to 400 calories. By the mid 1990s, the "large" had grown to 450 calories, and customers could order a "super size" with 540 calories. By 2000, the "large" had became a "medium," the "super size" had become "large," and the new 7-ounce "super size" provided 610 calories. As go McDonald's fries, so goes the nation.

On the other hand, McDonald's has introduced some of the healthiest items you can buy at a fast-food restaurant. You can't buy a Fruit 'n Yogurt Parfait—or anything like it—at any other chain. The McSalad Shaker makes it easier to take your veggies and run. And the Lowfat Apple Bran Muffin, 1-percent low-fat milk, and orange juice make for a good breakfast.

Picks: Thank heaven there's more to this burger giant than the burgers. McDonald's has figured out how to make salads something you can eat on the run. McSalad Shaker Salads are lettuce and fixings in a tall, clear plastic container with a snazzy dome lid. Add some dressing, give it a shake, and dig in. Try a Garden Salad, Grilled Chicken Caesar, or Chef Salad with a packet of Fat Free Herb Vinaigrette (just 40 calories) or Red French Reduced Calorie Dressing (130 calories). The full-fat Ranch dressing, however, will add 170 calories.

You can order the Chicken McGrill sandwich without the mayo and save 110 calories. Try topping it with a packet of Light Mayonnaise, Barbeque Sauce, or Honey Mustard Sauce. Each adds about 50 calories to your sandwich.

None of the regular-size burgers at *any* of the fast-food restaurants we looked at was low enough in saturated fat to qualify as a "Pick." But if you've got to have a burger, your best bet is the smallest one. At McDonald's, it's the regular hamburger, which is also used in children's Happy Meals. The meat isn't lean, but you get no more than 1½ ounces of it, which makes this burger among the lowest-fat sandwiches at any burger chain.

McDonald's leads the fast-food pack in respectable breakfast choices. For something quick, try a plain English muffin or bagel that you can top with preserves and wash down with an orange juice or 1-percent low-fat milk. Or try a Lowfat Apple Bran Muffin, which has one-sixth the fat of the Cinnamon Roll that's offered at some outlets. The Hotcakes are also a reasonable option, but to keep them that way you'll need to skip the margarine and go easy on the syrup. The restaurant gives you nearly enough condiments to double the fat and boost the calories to 600.

McDonald's now offers a refreshing and healthful low-fat Fruit 'n Yogurt Parfait at most outlets. The parfait layers rich-tasting, but low-fat, vanilla yogurt with fabulous, frozen blueberries and sliced strawberries. A sprinkle of low-fat granola on top adds a nice crunchy counterpoint. Although the yogurt does contain added sugar, the Fruit 'n Yogurt Parfait provides just a few grams of fat and a good chunk of your daily calcium and vitamin C, plus fiber (especially if you add the granola). Bravo!

Pans: Unless you stick with our "Picks," it's tough to walk out of McDonald's without eating at least half a day's quota of saturated fat. A Big Mac will do it. So will a Quarter Pounder with Cheese; a Big N' Tasty (with or without cheese); a large or super-size French Fries; a Bacon, Egg & Cheese Biscuit; a Sausage Biscuit with Egg; a Sausage McMuffin with Egg; a Spanish Omelet; a Steak, Egg & Cheese Bagel; or a Hot Fudge Sundae.

You could make your meal even worse by topping it off with a soft-serve McFlurry, in which bits of candies or cookies are mixed with reduced-fat vanilla ice cream. The result is a line of desserts ranging from 570 calories (the Oreo McFlurry) to 630 calories (the M&M, the Nestlé Crunch, and the Butterfinger). The McFlurries are also fat city. All four flavors contain at least two-thirds of your day's saturated-fat allotment.

But the large shakes make even the McFlurries look good. McDonald's Shakes used to be admirably low in fat, but the company switched from skim to whole milk, sending the fat content soaring to 29 grams (19 of them saturated!) in a large (32-ounce) shake. We don't know anyone who can afford to drink 1,000 calories with a meal!

A Word About Meals: McDonald's Value Meals are kind to your wallet but not to your waistline. Value Meals usually feature a burger, a chicken or fish sandwich, or McNuggets plus medium fries, and a medium Coca-Cola Classic. They hover around 1,200 calories and use up about three-quarters of a day's saturated fat. Super-sizing a Value Meal for another 40 cents tacks on another 400 or so calories. For example, a Quarter Pounder with Cheese plus super-size Fries and a super-size Coca-Cola Classic has 1,550 calories, not to mention a day's saturated fat (23 grams). To keep the calories around 600, skip the Value Meals altogether, and order a Chicken McGrill sandwich and a Garden McSalad Shaker with Fat Free Herb Vinaigrette dressing, or try a Grilled Chicken Caesar McSalad Shaker with Fat Free Herb Vinaigrette and a Fruit 'n Yogurt Parfait. Yum.

Taco Bell

Its zany talking-Chihuahua commercials may have been a hit, but many of the menu items offered at the nation's largest Mexican-style fast-food chain are a miss. The guts of most of their dishes—ground beef, cheese or cheese sauce, and sour cream—aren't exactly what the doctor ordered.

Picks: Want to get half (12 grams) your day's requirement of fiber in a quick, convenient lunch? Order a Bean Burrito. The sodium is on the high side, but its 1,080 milligrams is lower than all but three of Taco Bell's other burritos. Picks also include the Beef, Chicken, or Steak Gordita Nacho Cheese; the Chicken Gordita Santa Fe; the Chicken or Steak Gordita Baja; the Chicken or Steak Soft Taco; and the Chicken or Steak Fiesta Burrito.

Pans: It probably would not surprise you to learn that a Beef Double Burrito Supreme, Beef Enchirito, Cheesy Gordita Crunch, or Nachos BellGrande will use up about half a day's allowance of saturated fat. So will the Chicken Quesadilla, whose saturated fat comes from cheddar cheese, as well as the Cheese Quesadilla.

Lest you think a salad must be better than a double burrito, numbers for the Taco Salad dwarf almost everything else on Taco Bell's menu. The fried tortilla shell that holds the salad sends the fat soaring from 22 to 52 grams and the calories from 400 to 850. But even without the shell, the salad has more saturated fat and calories than a Double Decker Taco. By far the worst item on Taco Bell's menu is the Mucho Grande Nachos. With 1,320 calories and 82 grams of fat, 25 of which are saturated (more than a day's quota), it makes even the biggest burger look petite.

A Word About Meals: Many of Taco Bell's Combo Meals manage to stay just under 1,000 calories (not including a beverage), but they also supply at least half a day's limit of saturated fat. For example, a Burrito Supreme Combo Meal, which includes a Beef Burrito Supreme and a Double Decker Taco, has 810 calories and half of a day's quota of saturated fat (12 grams). However, if you order a Bean Burrito and a Chicken Soft Taco instead, you could cut the saturated fat in half and save 250 calories.

Wendy's

Wendy's, the nation's fifth-largest restaurant chain, provides several options for nutrition-conscious customers. Mixed in with the usual burgers, fries, fried chicken nuggets, and shakes you can find a handful of healthier items—like baked potatoes and chili—that other chains don't offer. You can also find salads that go beyond iceberg lettuce, and grilled chicken sandwiches that aren't smothered with mayo. At some locations, you can still find a Fresh Stuffed Pita sandwich. It's a pocket bread filled with fresh vegetables, dressing, and in some varieties, chicken. Unfortunately, it's no longer a standard on the menu, so you can't depend on it.

Picks: A couple of Wendy's Garden Sensation salads lead the lineup of good choices. While most chains just tear up some iceberg lettuce and call it a salad, Wendy's usually jazzes up its salads with romaine and red baby lettuce, carrots, cucumbers, red onions, and grape tomatoes. Pair the Mandarin Chicken Salad with a warm Soft Breadstick to make the salad more of a meal. Just think twice before you drench it in full-fat Oriental Sesame dressing. To cut calories, try the Fat Free French Style Low Fat Honey Mustard or Reduced Fat Creamy Ranch dressing instead.

The Grilled Chicken Sandwich is another fine choice. Because the chicken breast is dressed with a reduced-calorie honey mustard sauce, Wendy's sandwich has less than half the fat of McDonald's Chicken McGrill.

Wendy's also offers baked potatoes as a delicious alternative to shortening-laden fries. The Broccoli & Cheese, Bacon & Cheese, and Sour Cream & Chives varieties are all fairly low in saturated fat. But with so much sodium (820 milligrams) in the Bacon & Cheese, your best bet is the Sour Cream & Chives (80 milligrams) or the Broccoli & Cheese (470 milligrams). If a 400-or-so calorie potato isn't enough to fill you up, order a Side Salad to go with it.

Wendy's Chili has half the fat of the chili you'd get at dinnerhouse chains like Applebee's or Chili's. As for burgers, only one— the Jr. Hamburger with 3 grams of saturated fat—is a reasonable choice. You could eat two Jr. Hamburgers (not that you *should*, of course) and still get less fat and fewer calories than you'd get in one Big Bacon Classic.

Pans: Of course, you'll want to avoid some Wendy's offerings. If you don't want to blow more than half a day's quota of saturated fat on a single item, skip the Big Bacon Classic. A Taco Supreme Salad with Sour Cream and Taco Chips uses up three-quarters of a day's saturated fat. A Classic Double with Everything hits a day's allowance of saturated fat, and a Classic Triple with Everything climbs to one and a half day's worth of saturated fat and tops 1,000 calories.

Don't reward yourself for having a salad by eating a medium Frosty Dairy Dessert. It has about the same calories—440—as a Classic Single with Everything.

A Word About Meals: Wendy's Combo Meals usually include a burger or chicken sandwich plus medium fries and a medium drink. One of their best combo meals includes a Grilled Chicken Sandwich, medium fries, and a medium cola. But with 850 calories (and nearly half a day's saturated fat), it's hardly a diet plate. If you design your own combo meal by ordering the Grilled Chicken Sandwich and a Side Salad with Fat Free French Style dressing and an unsweetened iced tea, you can cut the calories in half and the saturated fat by three-quarters. A large Chili and a Side Salad with Low Fat Honey Mustard Dressing is another good choice and clocks in at just 470 calories. Unfortunately, many combo meals are beyond fixing. A Classic Triple with Everything made with three slices of cheese, Biggie Fries, and Biggie cola hits 1,700 calories and socks you with nearly 2 days' saturated fat (36 grams). Opting for medium fries and a medium cola instead of the biggie size would save you only 130 calories.

When Your Favorite Is Not on the List

We looked at the most common menu items offered at five of the largest fast-food chains. However, new products are always being tested, old products are sometimes dropped, and some sandwiches appear only as limited-time specials or regional offerings. If noontime finds you hankering for sandwiches and subs instead of burgers and fries, check out chapter 4, Hold the Mayo: Sandwich Shops (page 85) and chapter 17, Shop Till You Drop: Mall Food (pages 311, 334–341) for the best nutrition deals at delis and sub chains like Subway, Blimpie, and Schlotzsky's Deli. Pizza, another lunchtime favorite, is covered in chapter 7, Any Way You Slice It: Pizzerias (page 135) as well as in chapter 17, Shop Till You Drop: Mall Food (pages 316, 350).

Fast-Food Strategy

• **Think salads.** The best bet at fast-food restaurants are salads— *if* you can get them. (Burger King doesn't sell salads.) Grilled chicken or garden salad beats a fatty taco salad. Remember to use light or reduced-calorie dressings.

• **Choose chicken over beef.** Grilled chicken is generally the best fast-food sandwich choice, but watch out for the (usually) high-calorie mayo-based dressing. Substitute light mayo if you can, or use mustard, ketchup, or barbecue sauce.

• **Order the smallest burger.** If nothing but a burger will do, choose the smallest size on the menu. You can usually get a beef patty that's no larger than 2 ounces. And have it your way: Ask for extra lettuce, tomatoes, and onions.

• **Remove the breading.** Remove all or at least some of the fatty skin and breading on fried chicken. Removing all of it can cut the fat by about half.

• **Stick to small portions.** Whatever you're ordering, if the server asks, "Can I super size that for you?" just say *no*.

• **Make yourself heard.** Reward fast-food chains that offer nutritionally sound choices by giving them your business. Don't hesitate to tell the manager what items you'd like to see added to the menu, such as veggie burgers; chicken nuggets and french fries that are baked instead of fried; and more fruit-filled, low-fat treats like McDonald's Fruit 'n Yogurt Parfait.

Other than Burger King, which supplies *trans*-fat numbers for most of its items, and a few items we had analyzed (McDonald's Hashbrowns and Sausage Biscuit with Egg), the saturated fat numbers in the charts do not include (artery-clogging) *trans* fat. If they did, the saturated fat numbers would be even higher. Exception: The saturated fat numbers for McDonald's French Fries and Chicken McNuggets and Wendy's French Fries include our estimates for *trans* fat (neither chain supplies *trans* numbers). All other numbers in the charts were provided by the companies. Within each restaurant chain, the items are ranked from best to worst—that is, from least to most saturated fat. Entrées and meals marked with a ✔ are Best Bites. Best Bites are relatively low in saturated fat.

Reminder

Recommended limits for a 2,000-calorie diet:

Total fat: 65 grams
Saturated fat: 20 grams
Cholesterol: 300 milligrams
Sodium: 2,400 milligrams

FAST FOODS

Menu Item

	Calories	Total Fat (g)	Saturated Fat (g)	Cholesterol (mg)	Sodium (mg)
BURGER KING					
Burgers and Sandwiches					
✔ BK Broiler Chicken Sandwich without mayo (8½ oz.)	390	8	2	90	1,010
✔ BK Broiler Chicken Sandwich (9 oz.)	550	25	5	105	1,110
Hamburger (4½ oz.)	320	14	7	45	530
Whopper Jr. (6 oz.)	410	23	8	50	520
Cheeseburger (5 oz.)	370	18	10	55	750
Whopper Jr. with Cheese (6½ oz.)	460	27	11	60	740
Chicken Sandwich (8 oz.)	660	39	11	70	1,330
Chicken Club Sandwich (9 oz.)	740	44	12	85	1,530

FAST FOODS *(Burger King continued)* Menu Item	Calories	Total Fat (g)	Saturated Fat (g)	Cholesterol (mg)	Sodium (mg)
Whopper (10 oz.)	680	39	*13*	80	940
BK Big Fish Sandwich (9½ oz.)	710	38	*16*	50	1,200
Double Cheeseburger (7 oz.)	570	34	*19*	110	1,020
Whopper with Cheese (10½ oz.)	780	47	*19*	105	1,390
Bacon Double Cheeseburger (7 oz.)	610	37	*20*	120	1,170
Double Whopper (12½ oz.)	920	57	*22*	150	1,020
Double Whopper With Cheese (13½ oz.)	1,020	65	*27*	170	1,460
Fries, Tenders, etc.					
French Fries, small (2½ oz.)	230	11	*6*	0	630
Chicken Tenders, 5 pieces (2½ oz.)	220	12	*6*	30	530
Onion Rings, medium (3½ oz.)	320	16	*8*	0	460
Chicken Tenders, 8 pieces (4½ oz.)	340	19	*9*	50	840
French Fries, medium (4 oz.)	360	18	*10*	0	690
French Fries, large (5½ oz.)	500	25	*13*	0	940
Onion Rings, king (5¼ oz.)	550	27	*13*	0	800
French Fries, king (6 oz.)	600	30	*16*	0	1,140
Sauces (1 package)					
Ketchup	20	0	0	0	180
Marinara Dipping Sauce	20	0	0	0	280
Sweet and Sour Dipping Sauce	40	0	0	0	70
Barbecue Dipping Sauce	40	0	0	0	400
Honey Flavored Dipping Sauce	90	0	0	0	0
Honey Mustard Dipping Sauce	90	6	1	10	150

FAST FOODS (Burger King continued)

Menu Item	Calories	Total Fat (g)	Saturated Fat (g)	Cholesterol (mg)	Sodium (mg)
Ranch Dipping Sauce	120	13	2	5	90
Tartar Sauce	70	8	4	5	100
Breakfasts					
Biscuit (3 oz.)	300	15	4	0	830
Biscuit with Egg (4½ oz.)	390	22	5	150	1,020
Hash Brown Rounds, small (2½ oz.)	240	15	9	0	450
French Toast Sticks (5 sticks, 4 oz.) with syrup	470	20	9	0	460
Cini-minis with icing (4 rolls, 5 oz.)	550	26	10	25	750
Biscuit with Sausage (4½ oz.)	510	35	10	30	1,190
Croissan'wich with Sausage & Cheese (4 oz.)	410	29	13	40	830
Biscuit with Sausage, Egg & Cheese (6½ oz.)	650	46	14	190	1,600
Hash Brown Rounds, large (4½ oz.)	550	25	15	0	760
Croissan'wich with Sausage, Egg & Cheese (5½ oz.)	500	36	15	190	1,020
Drinks and Desserts					
Tropicana Pure Orange Juice (10 oz.)	140	0	0	0	0
Coca-Cola Classic, small (16 oz.)	160	0	0	0	N/A
Coca-Cola Classic, medium (22 oz.)	230	0	0	0	N/A
Coca-Cola Classic, large (32 oz.)	330	0	0	0	N/A
Coca-Cola Classic, king (42 oz.)	430	0	0	0	N/A
1% Reduced Fat Milk (8 oz.)	110	3	2	10	120
Shake, medium (14 oz.)[1]	460	8	5	30	320
Dutch Apple Pie (4 oz.)	340	14	6	0	470
Hershey's Sundae Pie (3 oz.)	310	18	15	10	140

FAST FOODS *(Burger King continued)*

Menu Item	Calories	Total Fat (g)	Saturated Fat (g)	Cholesterol (mg)	Sodium (mg)
Our Burger King Best Bite Meal					
✔ BK Broiler Chicken Sandwich and Tropicana Pure Orange Juice	690	25	5	105	1,110
Burger King Value Meals					
Whopper Jr., medium Fries, and medium Coca-Cola Classic	1,000	41	*18*	50	1,210
Chicken Sandwich, medium Fries, and medium Coca-Cola Classic	1,250	57	*21*	70	2,020
Whopper, medium Fries, and medium Coca-Cola Classic	1,270	57	*23*	80	1,630
Whopper, large Fries, and large Coca-Cola Classic	1,510	64	*26*	80	1,880
Bacon Double Cheeseburger, medium Fries, and medium Coca-Cola Classic	1,200	55	*30*	120	1,860
Bacon Double Cheeseburger, large Fries, and large Coca-Cola Classic	1,440	62	*33*	120	2,110
Whopper with Cheese, king Fries, and king Coca-Cola Classic	1,810	77	*35*	105	2,530
Double Whopper with Cheese, large Fries, and large Coca-Cola Classic	1,850	90	*40*	170	2,400
Double Whopper with Cheese, king Fries, and king Coca-Cola Classic	2,050	95	*43*	170	2,600

KFC

Menu Item	Calories	Total Fat (g)	Saturated Fat (g)	Cholesterol (mg)	Sodium (mg)
Chicken					
✔ Tender Roast Sandwich without sauce (6 oz.)	270	5	2	65	690
Original Recipe Drumstick (2 oz.)	140	9	2	75	420
Original Recipe Whole Wing (1½ oz.)	140	10	3	55	410
Hot & Spicy Drumstick (2½ oz.)	180	10	3	75	360

FAST FOODS (KFC continued)

Menu Item	Calories	Total Fat (g)	Saturated Fat (g)	Cholesterol (mg)	Sodium (mg)
Extra Crispy Drumstick (2½ oz.)	200	12	3	75	380
✔ Tender Roast Sandwich with sauce (7½ oz.)	350	15	3	75	880
Extra Crispy Whole Wing (2 oz.)	220	15	4	55	420
Colonel's Crispy Strips (3 pieces, 4 oz.)	300	16	4	55	1,170
Hot & Spicy Whole Wing (2 oz.)	210	25	4	55	350
Triple Crunch Sandwich without sauce (6½ oz.)	390	15	5	50	650
Triple Crunch Zinger Sandwich without sauce (6 oz.)	390	15	5	50	650
Original Recipe Thigh (3 oz.)	250	18	5	95	750
Honey BBQ Crunch Melt (8 oz.)	560	26	5	60	1,010
Popcorn Chicken, small (3½ oz.)	360	23	6	45	610
Original Recipe Breast (5½ oz.)	400	24	6	135	1,120
Triple Crunch Sandwich with sauce (6½ oz.)	490	29	6	70	710
Hot & Spicy Thigh (4 oz.)	360	26	7	125	630
Extra Crispy Thigh (4 oz.)	380	27	7	120	630
Triple Crunch Zinger Sandwich with sauce (7½ oz.)	550	32	7	85	830
Twister (8½ oz.)	600	34	7	50	1,430
Extra Crispy Breast (6 oz.)	470	28	8	160	870
Hot & Spicy Breast (6½ oz.)	510	29	8	160	1,170
Hot Wings (6 pieces, 5 oz.)	470	33	8	150	1,230
Honey BBQ Pieces (6 pieces, 7 oz.)	610	38	10	190	1,150
Popcorn Chicken, large (6 oz.)	620	40	10	75	1,050
Chunky Chicken Pot Pie (13 oz.)	770	42	13	70	2,160

FAST FOODS *(KFC continued)*

Menu Item	Calories	Total Fat (g)	Saturated Fat (g)	Cholesterol (mg)	Sodium (mg)
Side Items					
Corn on the Cob (5½ oz.)	150	2	0	0	20
BBQ Baked Beans (5½ oz.)	190	3	1	5	760
Mashed Potatoes with Gravy (5 oz.)	120	6	1	0	440
Cole Slaw (5 oz.)	230	14	2	10	280
Potato Salad (5½ oz.)	230	14	2	15	540
Macaroni & Cheese (5½ oz.)	180	8	3	10	860
Potato Wedges (5 oz.)	280	13	4	5	750
Biscuit (2 oz.)	180	10	7	0	560
Desserts					
Apple Pie slice (4 oz.)	310	14	3	0	280
Little Bucket Parfait, Fudge Brownie (3½ oz.)	280	10	4	145	190
Double Chocolate Chip Cake (2½ oz.)	320	16	4	55	230
Pecan Pie slice (4 oz.)	490	23	5	65	510
Little Bucket Parfait, Strawberry Shortcake (3½ oz.)	200	7	6	10	220
Little Bucket Parfait, Lemon Creme (4½ oz.)	410	14	8	20	290
Strawberry Creme Pie slice (2½ oz.)	280	15	8	15	130
Little Bucket Parfait, Chocolate Cream (4 oz.)	290	15	11	15	330
Our KFC Best Bite Meals (drink not included)					
✔ Tender Roast Sandwich with sauce and Corn on the Cob	500	17	3	75	900
✔ Cole Slaw, Corn on the Cob, and BBQ Baked Beans	570	18	3	15	1,060

FAST FOODS *(KFC continued)*

Menu Item	Calories	Total Fat (g)	Saturated Fat (g)	Cholesterol (mg)	Sodium (mg)
KFC Combo Meals (drink not included)					
Original Recipe Chicken (Drumstick and Thigh), Cole Slaw, and Biscuit[2]	800	51	16	180	2,010
Original Recipe Chicken (Breast and Whole Wing), Mashed Potatoes with Gravy, and Biscuit[2]	840	50	17	190	2,530
Extra Crispy Chicken (Breast and Whole Wing), Mashed Potatoes with Gravy, and Biscuit[2]	990	59	20	215	2,290
Hot and Spicy Chicken (Breast and Whole Wing), Mashed Potatoes with Gravy, and Biscuit[2]	1,020	70	20	215	2,520
Extra Crispy Chicken (Drumstick and Thigh), Potato Wedges, and Biscuit[2]	1,040	62	21	200	2,310
Original Recipe Chicken (Drumstick and 2 Thighs), Potato Wedges, and Biscuit[2]	1,100	68	22	270	3,300
Extra Crispy Chicken (Drumstick and 2 Thighs), Potato Wedges, and Biscuit[2]	1,420	89	28	320	3,230

McDONALD'S

Burgers and Sandwiches					
✔ Chicken McGrill without mayo (7½ oz.)	340	7	2	50	890
✔ Chicken McGrill (8 oz.)	450	18	3	60	970
✔ Hamburger (4 oz.)	280	10	4	30	590
Filet-O-Fish (5½ oz.)	470	26	5	50	890
Crispy Chicken (8½ oz.)	550	27	5	50	1,180
Cheeseburger (4½ oz.)	330	14	6	50	830
Quarter Pounder (6 oz.)	430	21	8	70	840
Big N' Tasty (9 oz.)	540	32	10	80	970
Big Mac (7½ oz.)	590	34	11	85	1,090

FAST FOODS *(McDonald's continued)*

Menu Item	Calories	Total Fat (g)	Saturated Fat (g)	Cholesterol (mg)	Sodium (mg)
Big N' Tasty with Cheese (9½ oz.)	590	37	12	95	1,210
Quarter Pounder with Cheese (7 oz.)	530	30	13	95	1,310
Fries and Nuggets					
French Fries, small (2½ oz.)[3]	210	10	*3*	0	140
Chicken McNuggets (6 piece, 4 oz.)[3]	290	17	*5*	55	540
French Fries, medium (5 oz.)[3]	450	22	*8*	0	290
Chicken McNuggets (9 piece, 5½ oz.)[3]	430	25	*8*	80	810
French Fries, large (6 oz.)[3]	540	26	*9*	0	350
French Fries, super size (7 oz.)[3]	610	29	*10*	0	390
Sauces (1 package)					
Honey	50	0	0	0	0
Sweet 'N Sour	50	0	0	0	140
Barbeque	50	0	0	0	250
Hot Mustard	60	4	0	5	240
Honey Mustard	50	5	1	10	90
Light Mayonnaise	50	5	1	10	100
McSalad Shaker Salads (weight without dressing)					
✔ Grilled Chicken Caesar Salad (5½ oz.)	100	3	2	40	240
✔ Garden Salad (5½ oz.)	100	6	3	75	120
✔ Chef Salad (7½ oz.)	150	8	4	95	740
Salad Dressings (1 package—3 Tb.)					
Fat Free Herb Vinaigrette	40	0	0	0	260
Red French Reduced Calorie	130	6	1	0	360

FAST FOODS (McDonald's continued)

Menu Item	Calories	Total Fat (g)	Saturated Fat (g)	Cholesterol (mg)	Sodium (mg)
Thousand Island	130	9	2	15	350
Honey Mustard	160	11	2	15	260
Caesar	150	13	3	10	400
Ranch	170	18	3	15	460
Drinks and Desserts					
Orange Juice (6 oz.)	80	0	0	0	20
Coca-Cola Classic, small (16 oz.)	150	0	0	0	20
Coca-Cola Classic, medium (21 oz.)	210	0	0	0	20
Coca-Cola Classic, large (32 oz.)	310	0	0	0	30
Coca-Cola Classic, super size (42 oz.)	410	0	0	0	40
1% Lowfat Milk (8 oz.)	100	3	2	10	120
✔ Fruit 'n Yogurt Parfait without granola (11 oz.)	280	4	2	15	120
✔ Fruit 'n Yogurt Parfait with granola (11½ oz.)	380	5	2	15	240
Vanilla Reduced Fat Ice Cream Cone (3 oz.)	150	5	3	20	80
Baked Apple Pie (2½ oz.)	260	13	4	0	200
Shake, small (14 oz.)[1]	360	9	6	40	230
Hot Fudge Sundae without nuts (6½ oz.)	340	12	9	30	170
Hot Fudge Sundae with nuts (6.½ oz.)	380	16	9	30	230
McFlurry (12½ oz.)[1]	610	22	14	75	250
Shake, large (32 oz.)[1]	1,010	29	19	115	530
Breakfasts					
✔ Bagel (3½ oz.) with Strawberry Preserves	280	1	0	0	390
✔ English Muffin (2½ oz.) with Strawberry Preserves	180	2	0	0	210

FAST FOODS (McDonald's continued) Menu Item	Calories	Total Fat (g)	Saturated Fat (g)	Cholesterol (mg)	Sodium (mg)
✔ Lowfat Apple Bran Muffin (4 oz.)	300	3	1	0	380
✔ Hotcakes, plain (5½ oz.)	340	8	2	20	630
Hotcakes with margarine and syrup (8 oz.)	600	17	3	20	770
Hash Browns (2 oz.)	130	8	4	0	330
Egg McMuffin (5 oz.)	290	12	5	235	790
Cinnamon Roll (3½ oz.)	390	18	5	65	310
Breakfast Burrito (4 oz.)	290	16	6	170	680
Sausage McMuffin (4 oz.)	360	23	8	45	740
Ham, Egg & Cheese Bagel (7½ oz.)	550	23	8	255	1,490
Sausage Biscuit (4½ oz.)	410	28	8	35	930
Sausage McMuffin with Egg (5½ oz.)	440	28	10	255	890
Bacon, Egg & Cheese Biscuit (6 oz.)	480	31	10	250	1,410
Steak, Egg & Cheese Bagel (8½ oz.)	700	35	13	290	1,290
Spanish Omelet Bagel (9 oz.)	690	38	14	280	1,570
Sausage Biscuit with Egg (6½ oz.)	490	33	16	245	1,110
Our McDonald's Best Bite Meals					
✔ Grilled Chicken Caesar McSalad Shaker with Fat Free Herb Vinaigrette, Fruit 'n Yogurt Parfait with granola, and Iced Tea (unsweetened)	520	8	4	55	740
✔ Chicken McGrill, Garden McSalad Shaker with Fat Free Herb Vinaigrette, and 1% Lowfat Milk	690	27	8	145	1,470
McDonald's Value Meals					
Chicken McNuggets (6 pieces), medium Fries, and medium Coca-Cola Classic[4]	950	39	13	55	850
Crispy Chicken sandwich, medium Fries, and medium Coca-Cola Classic[4]	1,210	49	13	50	1,490

FAST FOODS (McDonald's continued)

Menu Item	Calories	Total Fat (g)	Saturated Fat (g)	Cholesterol (mg)	Sodium (mg)
Crispy Chicken sandwich, super-size Fries, and super-size Coca-Cola Classic[4]	1,570	56	15	50	1,610
Big N' Tasty, medium Fries, and medium Coca-Cola Classic[4]	1,200	54	18	80	1,280
Big Mac, medium Fries, and medium Coca-Cola Classic[4]	1,250	56	19	85	1,400
Big Mac, super-size Fries, and super-size Coca-Cola Classic[4]	1,610	63	21	85	1,520
Quarter Pounder with cheese, medium Fries, and medium (21 oz.) Coca-Cola Classic[4]	1,190	52	21	95	1,620
Quarter Pounder with cheese, super-size Fries, and super-size (42 oz.) Coca-Cola Classic[4]	1,550	59	23	95	1,740

TACO BELL

Burritos

Menu Item	Calories	Total Fat (g)	Saturated Fat (g)	Cholesterol (mg)	Sodium (mg)
✔ Chicken Fiesta Burrito (6½ oz.)	370	12	4	35	1,000
✔ Steak Fiesta Burrito (6½ oz.)	370	12	4	25	1,020
✔ Bean Burrito (7 oz.)	370	12	4	10	1,080
Chili Cheese Burrito (5 oz.)	330	13	5	25	900
Beef Fiesta Burrito (6½ oz.)	380	15	5	30	1,100
Chicken Burrito Supreme (4 oz.)	410	16	6	45	1,120
Steak Burrito Supreme (9 oz.)	420	16	6	35	1,140
Chicken Double Burrito Supreme (9 oz.)	460	17	6	70	1,200
Beef Burrito Supreme (9 oz.)	430	18	7	40	1,210
Steak Double Burrito Supreme (9 oz.)	470	18	7	55	1,230
7-Layer Burrito (10 oz.)	520	22	7	25	1,270
Grilled Stuft Chicken Burrito (10½ oz.)	690	29	8	70	1,900

FAST FOODS *(Taco Bell continued)*

Menu Item	Calories	Total Fat (g)	Saturated Fat (g)	Cholesterol (mg)	Sodium (mg)
Grilled Stuft Steak Burrito (10½ oz.)	690	30	8	60	1,970
Beef Double Burrito Supreme (10½ oz.)	510	23	9	60	1,500
Grilled Stuft Beef Burrito (10½ oz.)	730	35	11	65	2,090
Chalupas					
Chicken Chalupa Nacho Cheese (5½ oz.)	350	19	5	25	640
Steak Chalupa Nacho Cheese (5½ oz.)	350	19	5	20	660
Chicken Chalupa Baja (5½ oz.)	400	24	5	40	660
Beef Chalupa Nacho Cheese (5½ oz.)	370	22	6	25	740
Steak Chalupa Baja (5½ oz.)	400	24	6	30	680
Chicken Chalupa SantaFe (5½ oz.)	420	26	6	40	560
Steak Chalupa SantaFe (5½ oz.)	430	27	6	35	580
Chicken Chalupa Supreme (5½ oz.)	360	20	7	45	490
Steak Chalupa Supreme (5½ oz.)	360	20	7	35	500
Beef Chalupa Baja (5½ oz.)	420	27	7	35	760
Beef Chalupa SantaFe (5½ oz.)	440	29	7	35	660
Beef Chalupa Supreme (5½ oz.)	380	23	8	40	580
Gorditas					
✔ Chicken Gordita Nacho Cheese (5½ oz.)	290	13	3	25	690
✔ Steak Gordita Nacho Cheese (5½ oz.)	290	13	3	20	700
Beef Gordita Nacho Cheese (5½ oz.)	310	15	4	25	780
✔ Chicken Gordita Baja (5½ oz.)	340	18	4	40	710
✔ Steak Gordita Baja (5½ oz.)	340	18	4	35	760
✔ Chicken Gordita Santa Fe (5½ oz.)	370	20	4	40	610

FAST FOODS *(Taco Bell continued)*

Menu Item	Calories	Total Fat (g)	Saturated Fat (g)	Cholesterol (mg)	Sodium (mg)
Chicken Gordita Supreme (5½ oz.)	300	13	5	45	530
Beef Gordita Supreme (5½ oz.)	300	14	5	35	550
Steak Gordita Supreme (5½ oz.)	300	14	5	35	550
Steak Gordita Santa Fe (5½ oz.)	370	20	5	35	620
Beef Gordita Baja (5½ oz.)	360	21	5	35	810
Beef Gordita Santa Fe (5½ oz.)	380	23	5	35	700
Cheesy Gordita Crunch (6½ oz.)	560	33	11	60	980
Cheesy Gordita Crunch Supreme (8 oz.)	610	37	13	70	990
Tacos					
✔ Chicken Soft Taco (3½ oz.)	190	7	3	35	480
Beef Soft Taco (3½ oz.)	210	10	4	30	570
✔ Steak Soft Taco (3½ oz.)	280	17	4	35	630
Taco (3 oz.)	210	12	4	30	330
Double Decker Taco (6 oz.)	380	17	5	30	740
Taco Supreme (4 oz.)	260	16	6	40	350
Double Decker Taco Supreme (7 oz.)	420	21	8	40	760
Miscellaneous					
Pintos 'n Cheese (4½ oz.)	180	8	4	15	640
Mexican Rice (5 oz.)	190	9	4	15	750
Nachos (3½ oz.)	320	18	4	5	560
Tostada (6½ oz.)	250	12	5	15	640
MexiMelt (5 oz.)	290	15	7	45	830
Nachos Supreme (7 oz.)	440	24	7	35	800

FAST FOODS *(Taco Bell continued)*

Menu Item	Calories	Total Fat (g)	Saturated Fat (g)	Cholesterol (mg)	Sodium (mg)
Chicken Enchirito (7½ oz.)	350	16	8	55	1,210
Steak Enchirito (7½ oz.)	350	16	8	45	1,220
Mexican Pizza (7 oz.)	390	25	8	45	930
Beef Enchirito (7½ oz.)	370	19	9	50	1,300
Taco Salad with Salsa, without shell (16½ oz.)	400	22	10	70	1,510
Cheese Quesadilla (5 oz.)	490	28	11	55	1,080
Nachos BellGrande (11 oz.)	760	39	11	35	1,300
Chicken Quesadilla (6½ oz.)	540	30	12	80	1,270
Taco Salad with Salsa, with shell (19 oz.)	850	52	14	70	2,250
Mucho Grande Nachos (18 oz.)	1,320	82	25	75	2,670
Our Taco Bell Best Bite Meal (drink not included)					
✔ Bean Burrito with Chicken Soft Taco	560	19	6	45	1,560
Taco Bell Combo Meals (drink not included)					
Burrito Supreme Combo (1 Beef Burrito Supreme with 1 Double Decker Taco)	810	35	12	70	1,950
Mexican Pizza Combo (1 Mexican Pizza with 1 Taco)	600	37	12	75	1,260
Beef Gordita Combo (2 Baja Beef Gorditas with 1 Taco)	930	54	14	100	1,950
Nachos BellGrande Combo (1 Nachos BellGrande with 1 Taco)	970	51	15	65	1,630
Taco Supreme Combo (3 Taco Supremes)	780	48	18	120	1,050

WENDY'S

Burgers and Sandwiches					
✔ Grilled Chicken Sandwich (6½ oz.)	300	7	2	55	740
✔ Jr. Hamburger (4 oz.)	270	9	3	30	620

FAST FOODS (Wendy's continued)

Menu Item	Calories	Total Fat (g)	Saturated Fat (g)	Cholesterol (mg)	Sodium (mg)
Spicy Chicken Sandwich (7½ oz.)	410	14	3	65	1,280
Chicken Breast Fillet Sandwich (7½ oz.)	430	16	3	55	750
Chicken Club Sandwich (7¾ oz.)	470	20	5	65	940
Jr. Cheeseburger (4½ oz.)	310	12	6	45	800
Jr. Cheeseburger Deluxe (6½ oz.)	350	16	6	50	860
Jr. Bacon Cheeseburger (6 oz.)	380	19	7	55	870
Classic Single with Everything (7½ oz.)	410	19	7	70	920
Big Bacon Classic (10 oz.)	580	30	12	100	1,460
Classic Double with Everything made with 2 slices of cheese (11 oz.)	760	45	19	175	1,730
Classic Triple with Everything made with 3 slices of cheese (14¼ oz.)	1,030	65	29	245	2,280
Fries and Nuggets					
Chicken Nuggets (5 pieces, 2½ oz.)	230	16	3	30	470
French Fries, small (3 oz.)[3]	270	13	4	0	90
French Fries, medium (5 oz.)[3]	420	20	6	0	130
French Fries, Biggie (5½ oz.)[3]	470	23	7	0	150
French Fries, Great Biggie (6½ oz.)[3]	570	27	8	0	180
Sauces (1 package)					
Ketchup	10	0	0	0	80
Sweet and Sour Sauce	50	0	0	0	120
Barbeque Sauce	50	0	0	0	160
Mayonnaise	30	3	0	5	60
Honey Mustard Sauce	130	12	2	10	220

FAST FOODS *(Wendy's continued)*

Menu Item	Calories	Total Fat (g)	Saturated Fat (g)	Cholesterol (mg)	Sodium (mg)
Baked Potatoes and Chili					
✔ Plain Baked Potato (10 oz.)	310	0	0	0	30
✔ Chili, small (8 oz.)	210	7	3	30	800
✔ Broccoli & Cheese Baked Potato (14½ oz.)	470	14	3	5	470
✔ Sour Cream & Chives Baked Potato (11 oz.)	370	5	4	15	80
✔ Chili, large (12 oz.)	310	10	4	45	1,190
✔ Bacon & Cheese Baked Potato (13½ oz.)	530	17	4	25	820
Breadstick and Side Salads					
Soft Breadstick (1½ oz.)	130	3	1	5	250
Caesar Side Salad (3½ oz.)	70	4	2	15	240
homestyle garlic croutons (1 pkt.)	70	3	0	0	120
Entrées Salads					
✔ Mandarin Chicken Salad (12 oz.)	160	2	0	10	650
crispy rice noodles (1 pkt.)	60	2	1	0	180
roasted almonds (1 pkt.)	130	12	1	0	70
Spring Mix Salad (11 oz.)	180	11	6	30	240
honey roasted pecans (1 pkt.)	130	13	1	0	65
Chicken BLT Salad (13 oz.)	310	16	8	60	1,140
homestyle garlic croutons (1 pkt.)	70	3	0	0	120
Taco Supremo Salad (17½ oz.)	360	17	9	65	1,090
salsa (1 pkt.)	30	0	0	0	440
taco chips (1 pkt.)	220	11	2	0	150
sour cream (1 pkt.)	60	6	4	15	20

FAST FOODS (Wendy's continued)

Menu Item	Calories	Total Fat (g)	Saturated Fat (g)	Cholesterol (mg)	Sodium (mg)
Salad Dressings (1 pkt.—5 Tbs.—unless otherwise noted)					
Fat Free French Style	90	0	0	0	240
Low Fat Honey Mustard	120	4	0	0	370
Reduced Fat Creamy Ranch	110	9	2	15	60
Caesar (1 pkt.—2 Tbs.)	150	16	3	20	240
House Vinaigrette	220	20	3	0	830
Oriental Sesame	280	21	3	0	620
Creamy Ranch	250	25	5	15	640
Honey Mustard	310	29	5	25	410
Blue Cheese	290	30	6	45	870
Drinks and Desserts					
Cola, small (16 oz.)	100	0	0	0	10
Cola, medium (20 oz.)	130	0	0	0	10
Cola, biggie (32 oz.)	210	0	0	0	20
Frosty, junior (6 oz.)[1]	170	4	3	20	100
Frosty, small (12 oz.)[1]	330	8	5	35	200
Frosty, medium (16 oz.)[1]	440	11	7	50	260
Our Wendy's Best Bite Meals					
✔ Grilled Chicken Sandwich, Side Salad with Fat Free French Style dressing, and Iced Tea (unsweetened)	430	10	2	55	1,200
✔ Large Chili, Side Salad with Low Fat Honey Mustard Dressing, and Iced Tea (unsweetened)	470	14	4	45	1,580
✔ Broccoli & Cheese Baked Potato, Side Salad with Fat Free French Style dressing, and Iced Tea (unsweetened)	600	17	4	5	930

FAST FOODS *(Wendy's continued)*

Menu Item	Calories	Total Fat (g)	Saturated Fat (g)	Cholesterol (mg)	Sodium (mg)
Wendy's Combo Meals					
Grilled Chicken Sandwich, medium Fries, and medium Cola[4]	850	27	8	55	880
Chicken Breast Fillet Sandwich, medium Fries, and medium Cola[4]	980	36	9	55	890
Classic Single with Everything, medium Fries, and medium Cola[4]	960	39	13	70	1,060
Big Bacon Classic, medium Fries, and medium Cola[4]	1,130	50	18	100	1,600
Big Bacon Classic, Biggie Fries, and Biggie Cola[4]	1,260	53	19	100	1,630
Classic Double with Everything, medium Fries, and medium Cola[4]	1,310	65	25	175	1,870
Classic Double with Everything, Biggie Fries, and Biggie Cola[4]	1,440	68	26	175	1,900
Classic Triple with Everything, medium Fries, and medium Cola[4]	1,580	85	35	245	2,420
Classic Triple with Everything, Biggie Fries, and Biggie Cola[4]	1,710	88	36	245	2,450

Note: Saturated fat numbers in *italics* include artery-clogging *trans* fat. N/A=not available

[1]Line average.

[2]Saturated fat numbers include artery-clogging *trans* fat from the biscuit.

[3]CSPI *trans* fat estimate.

[4]Saturated-fat numbers include our estimate of artery-clogging *trans* fat from the french fries and/or chicken nuggets.

Chapter 17

Shop Till You Drop: Mall Food

In the days of downtown shopping, before the advent of the mall, hungry lunchers had only a handful of choices. If they didn't indulge in a leisurely ladylike lunch at an elegant department store restaurant, the alternative was to pop into a cafeteria or grab a fast bite at a drugstore or dimestore lunch counter. These days the shopping action is in malls, where the entire environment is geared toward consumption. So it's not surprising that, hungry or not, many mall-goers nosh while they shop. The possibilities are numerous, varied, and almost irresistible. Shoppers can drop into a coffee bar, hesitate at a pretzel stand, or line up at the gourmet ice cream shop, the cookie store, or the fruit smoothie vendor. Or the weary shopper can relax in the food court, where the choices range from Chinese and Italian to deli food, burgers, and more. Even folks who haven't set foot inside a mall in years (all ten of them) can't escape recreational eateries. Food courts are ubiquitous at airports, train stations, sports arenas, and service areas on the interstate. What's cooking? You might be surprised.

Because mall food does not come with Nutrition Facts labels, it's hard to know how many calories are in a cinnamon sugar pretzel or how much fat is in a caffè mocha. But it is possible for consumers to find out. Many food-court chains have nutrition numbers for at least part of their menus. They're just not about to advertise them. But we are. We don't have information on every chain in your local mall, but most Chinese, Italian, steak-and-potato, pretzel, and deli eateries are probably fairly similar to one another. Still, the numbers from the chains may not be accurate, for several reasons:

Mall chains are more likely to estimate nutrients based on their recipes rather than to commission lab analyses. That leaves lots of room for error. At one chain, we bought several foods and sent them to an independent lab because we suspected that the chain's numbers were wrong. As it turned out, some were accurate, but others were not. In addition, restaurants rarely know how much *trans* fat their foods contain. Without *trans*, which comes from hydrogenated vegetable oils, margarine, and shortening, the saturated-fat numbers in our charts underestimate the risk that many mall foods pose to your arteries.

Finally, many chains don't insist that their employees use precise measures when they cook or serve. It's not just about how much pepperoni goes on the pizza or how much mayo goes into the tuna. One of the biggest unknowns is how much food you're being served. We found that one Sbarro outlet, for example, might serve a portion of lasagna that weighed twice as much as another one. As a result, you may end up with more or less on your plate than the serving sizes listed in our charts.

Nevertheless, some information is better than none at all. Here's what several major mall and food-court chains say they serve. Within each category, we've ranked the dishes from best to worst—that is, from least to most saturated fat.

Bakeries—Au Bon Pain

Boston-based Au Bon Pain has more than 240 bakery cafés in the United States and several other countries and offers upscale pastries, breads, sandwiches, and salads that range from terrific to terrible.

Bagels—like Americans—have grown larger over the years. A 4-ounce bagel from bakeries like Au Bon Pain has about 350 calories, with nothing on it. If you add regular cream cheese, you'll hit half a day's saturated fat. With about 550 calories, it's what you'd wind up with if you ordered Au Bon Pain's Egg on a Bagel Sandwich with Bacon or Cheese.

We're pleased that Au Bon Pain offers a selection of "lite" cream cheeses with one-third less saturated fat and calories than the regular version. You'll also find two low-fat muffins—Triple Berry and Chocolate Cake. At around 280 calories, each has about half the calories that you'd get in some of the company's popular monster muffins.

If you've got a sweet tooth, think of each Danish, cookie bar, brownie, scone, or shortbread cookie you eat as 400 to 550 calories to schlep around the mall. As for the Pecan Roll, how does 800 calories sound?

If you're not stuck on pastries, there are several terrific options at Au Bon Pain. The fresh fruit cup (only 90 calories) or yogurt with berries or granola (around 200 calories and only 4 grams of fat) is a great way to start the day. The scrumptious Thai Chicken Sandwich and the Honey Smoked Turkey Wrap are also low in saturated fat, as are the Oriental Chicken Salad and Pesto Chicken Salad. Just watch the dressing if you're watching your weight. A 6-tablespoon portion of dressing ranges from 70 calories for the Fat Free Tomato Basil to the mid-200s for the Lite Italian or Lite Honey Mustard. The calorie count for full-fat dressings runs as high as 300 to 400. If a salad isn't enough, add a Rosemary-Garlic Breadstick.

Bakeries—Dunkin' Donuts

Dunkin' Donuts (and many other doughnut shops) sell two types of doughnuts: "Yeast" doughnuts are raised by yeast, so they have more air; the denser "cake" doughnuts are made with baking powder. Both types of doughnuts have a big Achilles heel. Though the companies' ingredient information rarely mentions it, they're all fried in vegetable shortening that contains *trans* fat. When we analyzed five of Dunkin' Donuts most popular doughnuts (marked with an * in our chart), we found that they typically had about as much *trans* fat as saturated fat. For example, a Glazed Donut has 220 calories, and 3 grams of saturated fat. But our analysis found another 3 grams of *trans* fat—yielding a total of nearly a third of a day's worth of heart-damaging fat. And doughtnut lovers seldom stop at one.

Regardless of which type of doughnut you choose, remember that a chocolate or coconut coating adds insult to injury because the fats in both of these coatings are both more saturated than lard. For example, our analysis found that the Dunkin' Donuts Chocolate Glazed Cake Donut has 340 calories of sugar, and 22 grams of fat, 12 of them saturated or *trans*. That's more than half a day's worth of artery-clogging fat.

Dunkin' makes it tough for consumers to be virtuous, what with its frequent promotions like "Buy six, get six free." And don't let your eyes wander over to those crullers, fritters, or coffee rolls while you're waiting in line. Think of each as 250 to 300 calories of deep-fried sugar-coated flour.

Dunkin' also sells muffins. Unlike the petite 2-ouncers sold in grocery stores, the ones from Dunkin' Donuts hit the 5-ounce mark. And that means calories in the 500 to 600 range, 15 to 24 grams of fat, and 8 to 13 teaspoons of total sugars (including the sugar from berries or other fruit).

Because the muffins are so large, they are not much of a threat to your arteries than the fat in doughnuts, Danish, and croissants. Four to 6 grams per muffin are saturated (exception: Dunkin' Donuts Chocolate Chip Muffin hits 10).

The Honey Bran Raisin muffin does have 5 grams of fiber, so you will get some of the bran's phytochemicals and nutrients. But realistically, you're still talking mostly white flour, fat, and sugar for breakfast or a snack.

Your best bet at Dunkin' Donuts is a bagel . . . as long as you eat it unadorned (not so hard if it's cinnamon raisin, blueberry, or some other interesting flavor) or if you use just a thin layer of light cream cheese. A plain bagel with regular cream cheese has 540 calories and 22 grams of fat, 14 of them saturated, which is three-quarters of a day's worth. And don't think you're getting much protein from the cream cheese. It's more cream than cheese. Also steer clear of the bagel or croissant sandwiches. Most will run you 500 to 600 calories and half a day's fat, saturated fat, and sodium. That's like eating a McDonald's Big Mac for breakfast. And forget about the salt bagel: It has more than a day's worth of sodium.

Bakery Strategy

• **Buy a bagel.** Instead of a fatty croissant or a doughnut, have a bagel with preserves.

• **Look for low-fat treats.** If a shop offers low-fat options, choose one of them. An Au Bon Pain low-fat muffin has about half the calories you'd get in some of the company's regular muffins.

Chinese — Panda Express

If you're at a food court, one of your choices is bound to be Chinese. That's a good thing. Chinese is one of the few cuisines that serves vegetables beyond iceberg lettuce and a slice of pale tomato. Plus there's no cheese to boost the saturated fat. On the other hand, you can't let the server pile on a bargain "combo" meal of two or three entrées plus fried rice or lo mein. Chinese mall food stays reasonable only if you choose steamed rice plus one entrée or possibly two, if the second is mixed vegetables.

Take Panda Express, the largest Chinese food-court chain. If you order just one entrée as part of your typical "combo" meal, it will cost you only 200 to 300 calories and about 10 grams of fat, 2 of them saturated. There are exceptions: spicy chicken with peanuts and sweet and sour pork with sauce hit 400 to 500 calories and 20 to 30 grams of fat, 5 to 7 of them saturated. But if you dodge nuts, sweet sauces, and deep-fried dishes, you should stay under 300 calories. Of course, all combo meals come with a choice of steamed rice (220 calories), lo mein (270 calories), vegetable chow mein (300 calories), or vegetable fried rice (410 calories). So now your 200 to 300 calorie entrée has reached the 400 to 500 range. The problem is that at Panda Express and similar places it costs only another dollar or so apiece to add a second or third entrée to your combo. This temptation can raise the stakes to 600 to 800 calories for two entrées plus steamed rice, or 800 to 1,100 calories for three entrées plus rice. And it means at least 1,000 to 2,000 milligrams of sodium. The only saving grace: Even for larger Chinese meals, saturated fat is still rock-bottom compared to any other cuisine.

Chinese Strategy

• **Stick with steamed rice.** An order of steamed rice has half the calories of an order of fried rice.

• **Choose one entrée only.** A single entrée with steamed rice has a reasonable 400 to 500 calories. Two entrées plus rice hits 600 to 800 calories, and three entrées plus rice climbs to 800 to 1,100 calories.

Coffee—Starbucks

"Cream and sugar?" used to be the only question a coffee drinker had to answer. But with the rise of coffee emporiums like Starbucks, the questions are now endless. Choosing the drink can sometimes be a bewildering Italian lesson for the uninitiated, with names like Cappuccino, Frappuccino, Caffè Latte, Caffè Mocha, and Caramel Macchiato vying for attention. Then there's the size (tall, grande, or venti). And you'll need to advise your server about the type of milk (skim, whole, half-and-half, or soy); beverage temperature (hot or iced); and caffeine level (full-caf, half-caf, or decaf). As if that weren't enough, you can add syrups, whipped cream, and extra espresso to almost any coffee. Making a few simple decisions at the counter is a small price to pay for the civilized treat of enjoying a conversation over a coffeehouse concoction. Just take care not to unwittingly turn that simple cup of coffee into a 600-calorie coffee-flavored milk shake. That's a Starbucks venti-size White Chocolate Mocha made with whole milk and whipped cream. It has more calories and saturated fat than a McDonald's Quarter Pounder with Cheese!

Coffee addicts should be mindful of caffeine. Regardless of Starbuck's ambience and coffee's flavor, caffeine is a mildly addictive stimulant drug. Consuming too much can cause insomnia and anxiety. And there is evidence that, for women who are or may become pregnant, caffeine could increase the risk of miscarriage or reduce fertility. Those women should avoid caffeine. Decaf coffee, of course, is one solution and herbal tea another.

Coffee Strategy

• **Make it skim.** Substituting skim for whole milk keeps the calories down around 100 (Cappuccino) or 150 (Caffè Latte) for a 16-ounce "grande." Whole milk puts these drinks in the 200- to 300-calorie range and dispenses anywhere from a quarter of a day's saturated fat allowance (Cappuccino) to half a day's worth (Latte). Add about 50 more calories for a "venti" (20 ounces). With half-and-half? Don't ask.

• **Don't get whipped.** The cloud of cream that automatically comes atop your Caffè Mocha and some other drinks adds 100 calories and a quarter of a day's saturated fat. Cancel that creamy cloud— your brew will be rich and luscious without it.

• **Skip the syrup.** At least a Latte's calories come from milk. A Mocha's calories come from milk *and* syrup. Frappuccinos also have enough added sugar to freight a venti Coffee Frappuccino with 300 calories.

Cookies, Buns, etc.—Cinnabon and Mrs. Fields

You've been on your feet for hours, or so it seems. So what's wrong with one little cookie for some get-up-and-go? If it's one little Mrs. Fields cookie, you're really getting the equivalent of two or three cookies baked into one. It's roughly 300 empty calories, about 40 percent of a day's saturated fat, and 4 to 6 teaspoons of sugar.

Brownies are more caloric, with around 400 calories apiece. That's about as many calories as you'll find in a small Light & Flavorful sandwich at Schlotzsky's Deli. The important difference is that a Dijon Chicken, Albacore Tuna, or Smoked Turkey Breast sandwich contains protein, vitamins, and minerals. Lumberjacks might have room for 400 useless calories, but most shoppers don't.

Then there's the Cookie Cup, a frosted cookie in a cupcake shape with 400-plus calories. And who can spare nearly 700 calories for a Peanut Butter Dreambar? It's not just what's there—a day's saturated fat and sugar; it's what's missing—fruits, vegetables, and whole grains.

If you can't resist the magnetic pull of Mrs. Fields, at least think small. Go for the smallest bag of Nibblers (six half-ounce cookies) and share it with friends, or save some for tomorrow. Some outlets will let you buy just one or two Nibblers.

Use the same strategy at Cinnabon. Skip the 670-calorie Cinnabon or 890-calorie Caramel Pecanbon, each of which weighs half a pound and contains more than half a day's fat quota. If you must indulge, choose the 300-calorie Minibon (if you can find it). Better yet, skip Cinnabon.

Cookies, Buns, etc. Strategy

• **Get the smallest size possible.** Smaller is always better when it comes to sweets. A Minibon, for example, has roughly half the calories of a full-size Cinnabon. But don't confuse "less" with "low." Even a Minibon has 300 calories.

• **Share with a friend.** If no small-sized sweet is available, get the regular size and split it—along with the calories and fat—with a friend.

Delicatessen—Schlotzsky's Deli

Scholtzsky's Deli is one of the nation's largest deli chains. It sells some terrific salads and an entire line of Light & Flavorful sandwiches.

Your best bet is a small Light & Flavorful sandwich. The Chicken Breast, Smoked Turkey Breast, Albacore Tuna, Dijon Chicken, and Pesto Chicken are delish and provide about 350 calories and just a couple of grams of saturated fat. The Santa Fe Chicken and the Vegetarian, which contain about a quarter of a day's worth (5 grams) of saturated fat, just missed qualifying for a Best Bite.

Trouble begins when you order the regular and large sandwiches. The regular Light & Flavorful sandwiches hit 500 calories, which is not unreasonable for a hefty lunch. But the large sandwiches in the Light & Flavorful line pack 1,000 calories.

Schlotzsky's other sandwich lines are much worse. The Large Original sandwich layers three processed meats (lean ham, Genoa salami, and cotto salami) with three cheeses (mozzarella, cheddar, and Parmesan) and garnishes like lettuce, tomato, olives, and pickles on a toasted sourdough bun. That sandwich contains 1,300 calories, 50 grams of fat (25 of them saturated), and 4,400 milligrams of sodium, according to our analysis. That's two-thirds of a day's calories, one day's allowance of saturated fat, and two days' worth of sodium. That's the equivalent of *three* McDonald's Quarter Pounders. Avoid all Original sandwiches, even the Turkey Original, which is no more healthful—thanks to all that cheese and Genoa salami—than the red-meat version. Even the best of the bunch, a small Ham & Cheese Original, has half a day's quota of saturated fat.

And be careful of the Specialty Deli sandwiches, which start at 400 calories for a small and hit 1,100 to 1,800 for a large. The only ones that earned a Best Bite are the small Corned Beef, Roast Beef, and Turkey Guacamole. (Our chart lists mostly regular sandwiches, but you can also order small and large ones. The small is plenty for most people.)

Salads range from 60 calories (Garden) to 150 (Chinese Chicken or Caesar) to 250 (Chicken Caesar, Smoked Turkey Chef, or Ham & Turkey Chef) *without dressing*. Light dressing will add another 100 or so calories, and regular about 250. Having a salad with light dressing along with a small Light & Flavorful sandwich would be a reasonably healthy lunch. That adds up to 500 to 600 calories and fewer than 10 grams of fat. The only problem is the 2,400 milligrams of sodium—a day's quota in one meal.

Delicatessen Strategy

• **Think small.** When a category of sandwiches is available in a variety of sizes, choose the smallest. It will usually be enough to satisfy most appetites.

• **Think light.** Choose from the Light & Flavorful menu, except for the Santa Fe Chicken and the Vegetarian.

Fruit Smoothies—Jamba Juice and Smoothie King

A fruit smoothie can be a wonderful thing: a cup of refreshingly cold, sweet velvet packed with bananas, berries, mango, papaya, peaches, or other succulent treasures. The upside is that you get some fruit and, usually, not much fat. The downside is that at Jamba Juice, Smoothie King, and other similar outlets it's hard to know just how much *fruit* they're actually blenderizing in.

For most of these drinks, fruit is not the only ingredient. They also contain various kinds of sweeteners. At Jamba Juice, it's sherbet and frozen yogurt. At Smoothie King, it's a "carbohydrate mix," honey and turbinado sugar. This means that even the smallest size low-fat shakes, which run between 20 and 24 ounces, generally have 300 to 500 calories. The large ones can run as high as 750 calories at Jamba Juice and more than 1,000 calories at Smoothie King, where the king-size beverages are larger than a quart. The king-size Strawberry Hulk actually contains ice cream and a *weight-gain mix*: If you gulp one down, you'll consume a day's worth of calories (1,910) and fat (58 grams).

Our advice is to take Smoothie King up on its offer, made in the company's nutrition brochure, to leave out the sweeteners. You can also try the Vanilla or Orange-Vanilla Slim & Trim Smoothies, which keep the calories down around 200 for a small beverage.

For a shake that's a meal, look for low-fat versions made with soy milk, yogurt, or some other protein-rich ingredient. (Don't order ones with peanut butter or ice cream, unless you're trying to put on some weight.) Smoothie King's small (20-ounce) Yogurt D-Lite has 13 grams of protein and 340 calories, for example. But beware of the King's "power" shakes. Some have double the usual calories, which your body may store rather than burn.

Smoothie Strategy

• **Check the calories.** The makers of fruit shakes and smoothies often supply a free brochure with calorie counts and other nutrition numbers. Be sure to check it before placing your order.

• **Get the smallest size possible.** At Smoothie King, a small (20-ounce) Angel Food has 330 calories. A King (40-ounce) Angel Food hits 660 calories.

• **Don't believe that herbal "Extras" or "Boosts" added to Smoothies will do anything for you.** Many herbs have little or no benefit. If you want a specific herbal supplement, get it from a pill where you know how much you're getting.

Ice Cream, Frozen Yogurt, etc. — Häagen-Dazs and TCBY

Every food court features places to get a cold and sweet treat to perk you up. Whether you chill out with ice cream, frozen yogurt, or frozen custard, order so it doesn't weigh you down.

Gourmet ice cream establishments like Häagen-Dazs are the riskiest. Just one scoop of most full-fat flavors contains half a day's saturated fat and roughly 300 calories. Thinking about indulging in a double or triple scoop? Do the math.

Luckily, Häagen-Dazs and other shops offer several elegant sorbets that clock in at about 120 fat-free calories. If you're only interested in something creamy, try low-fat ice creams and frozen yogurts (assuming you can find them). They hover around 200 calories and have just a tenth of a day's saturated fat if you stick with just one scoop.

At soft-frozen-yogurt vendors like TCBY, the yogurt is low in fat, so the calories *should* be as low as sorbet. (Fat-free yogurt is also available for those who want to save a couple of grams of saturated fat.) But the serving size may be a problem. A regular cup holds 8 ounces—270 calories' worth—of frozen yogurt. Order a large cup (11 ounces), and you'll wind up with 350 calories.

Remember that cups and cones are not created equal, nor are cones and cones. A regular *cake* cone holds 6 ounces of frozen yogurt, which is as much as a small cup. The cone itself has only 13 calories. But if you choose a regular *waffle* cone, which holds 8 ounces, then you're up to 270 calories, *not including* the 110 calories lurking in the cone itself.

Then, of course, there are the toppings. A scoop of blueberries, peaches, or other fruit adds a negligible 10 calories. But pecans, chocolate chip cookie dough, crumbled fudge brownies, or coconut will tack on 50 to 80 calories. And sprinkles, M&M's, Butterfinger Pieces, hot fudge, walnuts in syrup, or a chocolate topper will add 100 to 160 calories.

Ice Cream and Yogurt Strategy

• **Think small.** Our advice is to order a small cup or regular cone. You might even consider getting a 3-ounce kiddie cup, which has about 100 calories and should easily satisfy a small appetite. After all, ice cream bars are typically about 3 fluid ounces.

• **Choose low-fat or fat-free options.** Low-fat ice cream or frozen yogurt is healthier for your heart than full-fat varieties. But keep in mind that it may not be low in calories.

Italian—Sbarro

Few foods are more American than pizza. And Sbarro serves more pizza—and other Italian dishes—than any other food-court chain. That's Sbad news. (For information about Pizza Hut and other pizza chains, please refer to chapter 7, page 135.)

The nutrition numbers we got from Sbarro were *so* depressing that we sent several dishes to an independent lab for analysis to make sure there had been no mistake. Unfortunately, the company's numbers were usually on target. Just one slice of Sbarro Pepperoni Pizza contains about 500 calories and 21 grams of fat. And 10 of those grams are saturated, which is half a day's worth. The Cheese Pizza is slightly better, whereas the Sausage and Supreme Pizzas are a bit worse. But the real surprise is the Spinach & Broccoli Stuffed Pizza, which had signs of nutritional promise. Unfortunately, one slice reaches 700 calories, and it had as much saturated fat as a slice of Pepperoni Pizza. So much for vegetables. Still worse is a slice of Sausage & Pepperoni Stuffed Pizza, which has nearly 900 calories and 44 grams of fat, including a day's worth of saturated fat and sodium.

Some Sbarro locations sell a Veggie Slice Pizza, which the company says has less fat than the chain's regular Vegetable Pizza because it's made with lower-fat cheese. But Sbarro wouldn't give us numbers for either one, so we can't vouch for what it says.

Stay away from Sbarro's Baked Ziti and Meat Lasagna. They'll fill you with 700 to 800 calories and a day's allowance of saturated fat.

Italian Strategy

• **Select spaghetti with sauce.** Its nutrition numbers are quite reasonable. Sbarro says it has 900 calories, but our analysis revealed the count was closer to 600, and it had hardly any saturated fat.

- **Eat your veggies.** Some Sbarros sell sides of a refreshing cold cucumber salad or hot sautéed garlicky veggies, but the chain has no nutrition numbers for them. Pair either with a side order of spaghetti or a garlic roll for a relatively light lunch.

Pretzels—Auntie Anne's

The soft, warm oversize pretzel—traditionally sold by sidewalk vendors in cities like New York and Philadelphia—has taken on a new life at malls. Enterprises like Auntie Anne's pretzels, which sells 10 flavors of pretzels that you can get with or without butter or eight varieties of dip, are itching to become the Baskin-Robbins of pretzeldom. A Glazin' Raisin Pretzel with butter (510 calories) may taste great with Caramel Dip (140 calories), and it's much lower in fat than, say, a Cinnabon. But those 650 calories make it more like a meal than a snack. The Whole Wheat Pretzel, actually a mixture of whole wheat and refined flour, has a hearty flavor and is the healthiest choice. Unfortunately, many outlets don't carry it. Next best is the Original. And if you just can't resist ordering a dip, try savory rather than sweet ones to cut calories. The fat-free Marinara Sauce (10 calories) and the Sweet Mustard (60 calories) are your best bets. Not surprisingly, pretzels are salty. The Original, Whole Wheat, and Jalapeño hover around 1,000 milligrams. An Original pretzel with butter and Cheese Sauce delivers a whopping 1,400 milligrams of sodium.

Pretzel Strategy

- **Skip the butter.** Our advice is to order your pretzel without butter, although that makes it harder for any topping to stick.

This will keep the calories in the 300- to 350-calorie range. (The exception is Glazin' Raisin, which hits 470 calories, even without butter.)

• **Hold the salt.** Order the Original, Whole Wheat, or Jalapeño pretzel without the salt and do your blood pressure a favor.

Steak and Potatoes—The Great Steak & Potato Company

It's no surprise that a classic steak-and-cheese sandwich is heavy-hitter mall food in every way. At The Great Steak & Potato Company, even if you forgo that main attraction, you'll still be hard-pressed to find much lighter fare. Even the items that sound healthy may not be. For example, thanks to the cheese, the Veggie Delight sandwich has 570 calories and 29 grams of fat, 7 of them saturated. In contrast, the irresistible Chicken Teriyaki knocks the fat down to 17 grams (5 of them saturated), but its sodium approaches 1,500 milligrams.

The Great Salad Experience with Chicken looks good on paper, with only 260 calories and 9 grams of fat, 5 of them saturated. But at some Great Steak locations, the dish itself looks more like The Great Disappointment, with chunks of chicken covered with melted cheese on a bed of iceberg lettuce. Other locations offer a more appealing salad that includes carrots, radishes, romaine lettuce, etc.

If you can't get a Great Steak Sandwich out of your mind, just be aware that even a regular 7-inch steak and cheese sub has 660 calories and 34 grams of fat, 10 of which are saturated—essentially a Big Mac with about 100 extra calories. The large 12-inch version weighs in at a whopping 1,070 calories and 55 grams of fat, 16 of them saturated.

Steak and Potatoes Strategy

• **Think small.** A 7-inch sandwich at The Great Steak & Potato Company has "only" 600 to 700 calories. Jump to a 12-incher (large) and you can expect about 1,000 calories.

• **Hold the cheese and mayo.** As usual, you can cut fat and calories by asking for no cheese. All but the Philadelphia sandwiches taste great without it. You can also have the sandwich maker hold the mayo and add some yourself, if you need it. Inquire if light mayonnaise is available.

• **Share the spuds.** At The Great American Steak & Potato Company, the fries are cooked in lightly hydrogenated peanut oil, so they're a cut above the *trans*-filled fries sold at most fast-food chains, where shortening is used. But we estimate that a small or regular order will hang about 500 calories on your frame, whereas a large will upholster you with 900. As your mom said, share with your friends. (The numbers for fries in our chart are lower than those provided by Great Steak because the company overestimated its serving sizes.)

THE MALL FOOD CHARTS

The numbers in the charts were provided by the restaurant chains, except for the two dozen items that we had analyzed. These are marked with an *. Most numbers do not include artery-clogging *trans* fat; if they did, the saturated-fat numbers—particularly for doughnuts and other sweets made with shortening—would be higher than those indicated. Within each restaurant chain, dishes are ranked from best to worst—that is, from least to most saturated fat—unless otherwise noted. Items marked with a ✔ are Best Bites. Best Bites are relatively low in saturated fat.

BAKERIES

The "Sugars" numbers include both refined sugars and naturally occurring sugars from fruit and milk. Flavored yogurts have both refined (added) sugars and naturally occurring sugars (from milk), whereas all the sugars in fresh fruit are naturally occurring. The U.S. Department of Agriculture's recommended limit for refined sugars is 40 grams, or 10 teaspoons, per day (the amount in a typical 12-ounce soft drink).

Reminder

Recommended limits for a 2,000-calorie diet:

Total fat: 65 grams
Saturated fat: 20 grams
Cholesterol: 300 milligrams
Sodium: 2,400 milligrams
Refined Sugars: 40 grams
(does not include milk or fruit sugar)

MALL FOOD (Au Bon Pain)

Menu Item	Calories	Total Fat (g)	Saturated Fat (g)	Sodium (mg)
Bagels, etc. (weight of each item)				
✔ Plain Bagel (4 oz.)	350	1	0	540
✔ Cinnamon Raisin Bagel (5 oz.)	390	1	0	550
✔ Honey 9 Grain Bagel (4 oz.)	360	2	0	580
✔ Wild Blueberry Bagel (5 oz.)	380	2	0	570
✔ Rosemary-Garlic Breadstick (2 oz.)	180	3	0	550
✔ Everything Bagel (4 oz.)	360	3	0	710
✔ Cranberry Walnut Bagel (5 oz.)	460	4	1	590
Focaccia Bagel (4 oz.)	330	5	1	990
Cheddar & Scallion Bagel (4 oz.)	310	5	3	600
Asiago Cheese Bagel (4 oz.)	380	6	4	690
Jalapeño Double Cheddar Bagel (4 oz.)	390	8	5	710
Cream Cheese (4 Tb.)				
Lite Plain	100	8	5	280

MALL FOOD *(Au Bon Pain continued)* **Menu Item**	Calories	Total Fat (g)	Saturated Fat (g)	Sodium (mg)
Lite Sun-Dried Tomato	120	8	5	320
Lite Raspberry	130	10	7	200
Lite Veggie	130	11	7	230
Lite Honey Walnut	150	11	7	190
Plain	180	18	11	150

Cookies, Scones, etc. (weight of each item)	Calories	Total Fat (g)	Saturated Fat (g)	Sugars (g)
Sour Cream Lemon Scone (4 oz.)	390	8	4	35
Oatmeal Raisin Cookie (2 oz.)	250	10	4	26
Lemon Swirl Danish (4 oz.)	360	11	4	19
7 Layer Bar (4 oz.)	300	10	5	10
Oreo Cookie Bar (5 oz.)	550	29	5	43
Cinnamon Scone (4 oz.)	440	17	7	19
Chocolate Chip Cookie (2 oz.)	280	13	8	26
Orange Scone with Icing (4 oz.)	430	15	8	13
Cinnamon Roll (4 oz.)	340	15	9	13
Mochaccino Bar (4 oz.)	400	24	10	30
Walnut Fudge Brownie (4 oz.)	380	18	11	34
Shortbread Cookie (2 oz.)	390	25	15	13
Chocolate Dipped Shortbread (2 oz.)	410	27	19	17
Pecan Roll (7 oz.)*	800	45	20	42
Sweet Cheese Danish (4 oz.)*	520	31	23	23
Cinnamon Raisin Dessert Croissant (4 oz.)	340	5	3	15
Plain Croissant (2 oz.)	250	6	4	6

MALL FOOD (Au Bon Pain continued)

Menu Item	Calories	Total Fat (g)	Saturated Fat (g)	Sugars (g)
Apple Dessert Croissant (3 oz.)	280	10	6	19
Raspberry Cheese Croissant (4 oz.)	340	11	6	20
Sweet Cheese Croissant (4 oz.)	350	14	8	16
Chocolate Dessert Croissant (3 oz.)	440	23	15	25
Almond Croissant (5 oz.)*	630	42	*18*	23
Fruit and Yogurt (weight of each item)				
✔ Fresh Fruit Cup (8 oz.)	90	1	0	19
✔ Blueberry Yogurt with Fresh Berries (9 oz.)	210	3	1	37
✔ Plain Yogurt with Granola (8 oz.)	230	4	2	33
✔ Strawberry Yogurt with Granola (8 oz.)	230	4	2	37
Muffins (weight of each item)				
✔ Chocolate Cake Low Fat (4 oz.)	290	3	1	43
✔ Triple Berry Low Fat (4 oz.)*	260	4	*1*	30
Blueberry (4 oz.)*	430	18	*4*	36
Pumpkin with Streusel Topping (6 oz.)	570	20	4	40
Corn (5 oz.)	520	23	4	36
Carrot Walnut (5 oz.)	580	30	4	34
Raisin Bran (5 oz.)	450	14	5	33
Cranberry Walnut (5 oz.)	480	26	5	25
Chocolate Chip (4 oz.)	600	26	6	38

Menu Item	Calories	Total Fat (g)	Saturated Fat (g)	Sodium (mg)
Salads (weight of each salad)				
✔ Large Garden Salad, without dressing (11 oz.)	160	2	0	290
✔ Oriental Chicken Salad, without dressing (9 oz.)	270	4	1	700
✔ Thai Chicken Salad, without dressing (10 oz.)	330	8	1	980
✔ Pesto Chicken Salad, without dressing (11 oz.)	230	11	2	250

MALL FOOD *(Au Bon Pain continued)* Menu Item	Calories	Total Fat (g)	Saturated Fat (g)	Sodium (mg)
✔ Chicken Tarragon Salad with Almonds (16 oz.)	470	23	4	500
Tuna Salad (15 oz.)	490	27	5	750
Caesar Salad, without dressing (9 oz.)	270	10	6	800
Chicken Caesar Salad, without dressing (11 oz.)	360	11	6	910
Mozzarella & Roasted Red Pepper Salad, without dressing (14 oz.)	340	18	10	135
Chef Salad, without dressing (12 oz.)	390	26	11	1,460
Field Greens, Gorgonzola & Roasted Walnut Salad, without dressing (6 oz.)	400	34	13	800
Salads & Dressings (6 Tb., unless otherwise noted)				
Fat Free Tomato Basil	70	0	0	650
Thai Peanut (4 Tb.)	130	6	0	1,000
Lite Italian	230	20	2	570
Lemon Basil Vinaigrette	330	32	2	460
Lite Honey Mustard	280	17	3	560
Mandarin Orange	380	33	3	310
Buttermilk Ranch	310	32	4	270
Sesame French	370	30	5	1,010
Caesar	380	39	5	410
Greek	440	50	7	820
Bleu Cheese	410	41	8	910
Sandwiches (weight of each item)				
Egg on a Bagel Sandwich (7 oz.)	500	5	1	880
✔ Thai Chicken Sandwich (8 oz.)	420	6	1	1,320
✔ Honey Smoked Turkey Wrap (15 oz.)	540	7	2	1,520
Egg on a Bagel Sandwich with Bacon (7 oz.)	580	12	4	1,100

MALL FOOD *(Au Bon Pain continued)*

Menu Item	Calories	Total Fat (g)	Saturated Fat (g)	Sodium (mg)
✔ Fields & Feta Wrap (12 oz.)	560	17	4	850
Egg on a Bagel Sandwich with Cheese (7 oz.)	580	12	5	1,010
Egg on a Bagel Sandwich with Bacon & Cheese (8 oz.)	660	19	7	1,240
Chicken Caesar Wrap (10 oz.)	630	31	8	1,140
Soups (12 oz.)				
Garden Vegetable	50	0	0	1,240
Mushroom Orzo	90	3	0	1,300
Vegetarian Chili	210	4	0	1,610
Tomato Florentine	90	2	1	1,550
Chicken Noodle	120	2	1	1,000
Beef Barley	110	3	1	980
Asiago Tomato Lentil	180	3	1	1,310
Maryland Crab & Red Lentil	300	7	1	1,570
Forest Mushroom Bisque with chicken	200	9	5	1,550
Corn & Green Chile Bisque	300	16	9	1,830
Roasted Vegetable Bisque	340	18	10	1,350
Asiago Cheese Bisque	370	25	13	1,050
Cream of Broccoli	330	28	13	1,160
Corn Chowder	390	24	14	1,150
Clam Chowder	400	29	14	1,090

* Numbers from independent lab analyses.
Note: Saturated fat numbers in *italics* include artery-clogging *trans* fat.

MALL FOOD *(Dunkin' Donuts)*

Menu Item	Calories	Total Fat (g)	Saturated Fat (g)	Sugars (g)
Donuts (about 2 oz. unless otherwise noted)				
Sugar Raised Donut	170	8	2	4
Apple N' Spice Donut	200	8	2	7
Black Raspberry Donut	210	8	2	10
Strawberry Donut	210	8	2	11
Lemon Donut	200	9	2	8
Marble Frosted Donut	200	9	2	11
Bavarian Kreme Donut	210	9	2	9
Maple Frosted Donut	210	9	2	12
Strawberry Frosted Donut	210	9	2	12
Vanilla Frosted Donut	210	9	2	12
Apple Crumb Donut	230	10	3	12
Blueberry Crumb Donut	240	10	3	15
Eclair Donut	270	11	3	17
Chocolate Kreme Filled Donut	270	13	3	16
Vanilla Kreme Filled Donut	270	13	3	17
Caramel Apple Krunch Donut	300	14	3	15
Dunkin' Donut	240	15	3	6
Old Fashioned Cake Donut	250	15	3	7
Sugared Cake Donut	250	15	3	9
Cinnamon Cake Donut	270	15	3	12
Powdered Cake Donut	270	15	3	13

MALL FOOD (Dunkin' Donuts continued)

Menu Item	Calories	Total Fat (g)	Saturated Fat (g)	Sugars (g)
Glazed Cake Donut	270	15	3	14
Chocolate Frosted Cake Donut	300	16	3	18
Boston Kreme Donut (3½ oz.)*	300	8	4	21
Bismark, Chocolate Iced Donut	340	15	4	31
Blueberry Cake Donut	290	16	4	16
Bow Tie Donut	300	17	4	10
Double Chocolate Cake Donut	310	17	4	18
Whole Wheat Glazed Cake Donut	310	19	4	14
Butternut Cake Donut Ring	300	16	5	16
Coconut Cake Donut	290	17	5	13
Toasted Coconut Cake Donut	300	17	5	16
Glazed Donut*	220	12	6	7
Chocolate Coconut Cake Donut	300	19	6	12
Chocolate Frosted Donut*	260	13	7	15
Jelly Filled Donut (3 oz.)*	310	13	7	20
Chocolate Glazed Cake Donut (2½ oz.)*	340	22	12	13
Fritters, Crullers, etc. (about 2 oz.)				
Jelly Stick	290	12	3	24
Glazed Fritter	260	14	3	7
Coffee Roll	270	14	3	10
Maple Frosted Coffee Roll	290	14	3	13
Vanilla Frosted Coffee Roll	290	14	3	13
Apple Fritter	300	14	3	12

MALL FOOD *(Dunkin' Donuts continued)* Menu Item	Calories	Total Fat (g)	Saturated Fat (g)	Sugars (g)
Plain Cruller	240	15	3	6
Sugar Cruller	250	15	3	8
Powdered Cruller	270	15	3	11
Glazed Chocolate Cruller	280	15	3	16
Chocolate Frosted Coffee Roll	290	15	3	12
Glazed Cruller	290	15	3	18
Cinnamon Bun	510	15	4	42
Muffins (5½ oz.)				
Honey Bran Raisin	490	16	4	48
Cranberry Orange	470	15	4	41
Corn	500	16	5	34
Blueberry	490	17	6	41
Lemon Poppyseed	580	19	6	53
Apple Cinnamon Pecan	510	21	6	41
Banana Nut	530	23	6	37
Chocolate Chip	590	24	10	50
Bagels (about 4 oz.)				
Salt	340	1	0	3,030
✔ Blueberry	340	3	1	630
✔ Plain	340	3	1	680
✔ Cinnamon Raisin	340	4	1	600
✔ Sesame	380	5	1	720
Cream Cheese (1 packet, about 4 Tb.)				

MALL FOOD (Dunkin' Donuts continued)

Menu Item	Calories	Total Fat (g)	Saturated Fat (g)	Sodium (mg)
Lite Plain	130	11	7	250
Strawberry	180	16	9	170
Garden Vegetable	180	17	11	310
Plain	200	19	13	230
Sandwiches (one sandwich)				
Ham, Egg, and Cheese Omwich on English Muffin	320	12	6	1,340
Pizza Omwich on English Muffin	350	17	6	1,150
Spanish Omwich on English Muffin	370	18	6	1,180
Spanish Omwich on Bagel	570	18	6	1,370
Pizza Omwich on Bagel	560	19	6	1,310
Bacon and Cheddar Omwich on English Muffin	400	21	8	1,440
Bacon and Cheddar Omwich on Bagel	600	21	8	1,630
Egg and Cheese Sandwich on Biscuit	380	22	8	1,250
Spanish Omwich on Biscuit	470	29	9	1,400
Pizza Omwich on Biscuit	500	30	9	1,480
Bacon and Cheddar Omwich on Biscuit	500	32	11	1,660
Pizza Omwich on Croissant	510	34	11	900
Spanish Cheese Omwich on Croissant	530	36	11	930
Bacon and Cheddar Omwich on Croissant	560	38	13	1,190
Sausage, Egg, and Cheese Sandwich on Biscuit	590	42	15	1,620

* Numbers from independent lab analyses.
Note: Saturated fat numbers in *italics* include artery-clogging *trans* fat.

CHINESE

MALL FOOD (Panda Express)

Menu Item	Calories	Total Fat (g)	Saturated Fat (g)	Sodium (mg)
Entrées (5 oz. unless otherwise noted)				
✔ Mixed Vegetables	80	3	0	450
✔ Chicken with Mushrooms	170	9	2	570
✔ Chicken with String Beans	180	9	2	620
✔ Black Pepper Chicken	210	10	2	570
✔ Beef & Broccoli	180	11	3	910
Orange Chicken	310	13	3	420
Spicy Chicken with Peanuts	510	29	5	1,250
Sweet & Sour Pork with sauce (6 oz.)	370	20	7	400
Side Dishes (8 oz.)				
Steamed Rice	220	0	0	10
Vegetable Chow Mein	300	10	2	610
Lo Mein	270	10	2	1,090
Vegetable Fried Rice	410	19	3	440
Other Dishes				
Egg Flower Soup (1½ cups)	80	0	0	640
Hot & Sour Soup (1½ cups)	110	4	1	890
Egg Rolls (2 rolls—3 oz.)	190	6	1	490

COFFEE

The "Sugars" numbers include both refined sugars and naturally occurring sugars from milk. The U.S. Department of Agriculture's recommended limit for refined sugars is 40 grams, or 10 teaspoons, per day. (That's the amount in a typical 12-ounce soft drink.)

MALL FOOD (Starbucks)

Menu Item	Calories	Total Fat (g)	Saturated Fat (g)	Sugars (g)
Coffee Drinks (grande—16 oz.—unless otherwise noted)				
✔ Cappuccino with skim milk	110	0	0	13
✔ Caffè Latte with skim milk	160	1	1	21
Caramel Macchiato with skim milk	190	1	1	32
Caffè Mocha with skim milk	240	3	1	36
Coffee Frappuccino, venti (24 oz.)	300	3	2	52
Cappuccino with whole milk	180	9	6	13
Caramel Macchiato with whole milk	250	9	6	32
White Chocolate Mocha with skim milk	400	11	7	39
Caffè Latte with whole milk	270	14	9	20
White Chocolate Mocha with whole milk and whipped cream, tall (12 oz.)	360	15	9	29
Caffè Mocha with whole milk and whipped cream, tall (12 oz.)	320	17	10	27
White Chocolate Mocha with whole milk and whipped cream	480	20	12	38
Caffè Mocha with whole milk and whipped cream	420	23	13	36

COOKIES, BUNS, ETC.

MALL FOOD (Mrs. Fields) Menu Item	Calories	Total Fat (g)	Saturated Fat (g)	Sugars (g)
Cookies (3 oz. unless otherwise noted)				
Debra's Special Mini Cup (1 oz.)	140	6	3	13
Milk Chocolate Mini Cup (1 oz.)	140	7	4	15
Semi-Sweet Chocolate Mini Cup (1 oz.)	140	7	4	15
Milk Chocolate with Walnuts Mini Cup (1 oz.)	150	8	4	14
Semi-Sweet Chocolate with Walnuts Mini Cup (1 oz.)	150	8	4	14
White Chunk Macadamia Mini Cup (1 oz.)	150	8	4	14
Debra's Special*	240	12	6	25
Debra's Special Nibbler (6 cookies)	300	14	6	24
Milk Chocolate Chip*	250	13	8	23
Semi-Sweet Chocolate Chip	280	14	8	26
Semi-Sweet Chocolate Chip with Walnuts	310	16	8	25
Debra's Special Cookie Cup	410	17	8	41
Milk Chocolate Nibbler (6 cookies)	330	15	9	30
Semi-Sweet Chocolate Nibbler (6 cookies)	330	15	9	30
White Chunk Macadamia*	270	16	9	19
Milk Chocolate Chip with Walnuts	320	17	9	26

MALL FOOD (Mrs. Fields continued)

Menu Item	Calories	Total Fat (g)	Saturated Fat (g)	Sugars (g)
Milk Chocolate with Walnuts Nibbler (6 cookies)	360	18	9	27
White Chunk Macadamia Nibbler (6 cookies)	360	21	11	15
Semi-Sweet Chocolate Chip Cookie Cup	420	20	12	45
Milk Chocolate Cookie Cup	430	20	12	44
Milk Chocolate with Walnuts Cookie Cup	440	23	12	42
Semi-Sweet Chocolate with Walnuts Cookie Cup	440	23	12	45
White Chunk Macadamia Cookie Cup	460	24	12	42
Brownies, etc. (weight of each item)				
Walnut Fudge Brownie (3 oz.)	340	20	9	30
Frosted Fudge Brownie (4 oz.)	440	21	12	41
Double Fudge Brownie (3 oz.)*	420	25	*16*	47
Rocky Mountain Mogul (5 oz.)	610	35	18	60
Peanut Butter Dreambar (5 oz.)	670	42	21	52

* Numbers from independent lab analyses.
Note: Saturated fat numbers in *italics* include artery-clogging *trans* fat.

COOKIES, BUNS, ETC.—CINNABON

The "Sugars" numbers include both refined sugars and (generally) much smaller amounts of naturally occurring sugars from milk. The U.S. Department of Agriculture's recommended limit for refined sugars is 40 grams, or 10 teaspoons, per day. (That's the amount in a typical 12-ounce soft drink.)

MALL FOOD (Cinnabon) Menu Item	Calories	Total Fat (g)	Saturated Fat (g)	Sugars (g)
CINNABON				
Bun (weight of each item)				
Minibon (3 oz.)	300	11	5†	18†
Caramel Pecanbon (8 oz.)*	890	41	*13*	48
Cinnabon (8 oz.)*	670	34	*14*	49

* Numbers from independent lab analyses.
† Our estimate
Note: Saturated fat numbers in *italics* include artery-clogging *trans* fat.

DELICATESSEN

The "Sugars" numbers for desserts include both refined sugars and (generally) much smaller amounts of naturally occurring sugars from fruit and milk. The U.S. Department of Agriculture's recommended limit for refined sugars is 40 grams, or 10 teaspoons, per day. (That's the amount in a typical 12-ounce soft drink.)

MALL FOOD (Schlotzsky's Deli) Menu Item	Calories	Total Fat (g)	Saturated Fat (g)	Sodium (mg)
Sandwiches (weight of each sandwich)				
✔ Dijon Chicken, Light & Flavorful, small (10 oz.)	330	4	1	1,370
✔ Smoked Turkey Breast, Light & Flavorful, small (9 oz.)	340	5	1	1,430
✔ Pesto Chicken, Light & Flavorful, small (9 oz.)	350	6	1	1,300
✔ Dijon Chicken, Light & Flavorful, regular (15 oz.)	500	6	1	2,090
✔ Smoked Turkey Breast, Light & Flavorful, regular (13 oz.)	500	7	1	2,120
✔ Chicken Breast, Light & Flavorful, small (10 oz.)	360	7	2	1,600
✔ Pesto Chicken, Light & Flavorful, regular (14 oz.)	510	9	2	1,930
✔ Corned Beef, Specialty Deli, small (8 oz.)	390	10	2	1,630
Dijon Chicken, Light & Flavorful, large (29 oz.)	970	10	2	3,980
✔ Roast Beef, Specialty Deli, small (9 oz.)	410	11	2	1,160
Smoked Turkey Breast, Light & Flavorful, large (26 oz.)	990	13	2	4,230
✔ Turkey Guacamole, Specialty Deli, small (11 oz.)	450	15	2	1,760
✔ Chicken Breast, Light & Flavorful, regular (15 oz.)	540	10	3	2,370
✔ Albacore Tuna, Light & Flavorful, small (9 oz.)	360	11	3	1,120
Corned Beef, Specialty Deli, regular (12 oz.)	590	15	3	2,490

MALL FOOD *(Schlotzsky's Deli continued)* Menu Item	Calories	Total Fat (g)	Saturated Fat (g)	Sodium (mg)
Pesto Chicken, Light & Flavorful, large (27 oz.)	1,000	15	3	3,800
Roast Beef, Specialty Deli, regular (14 oz.)	620	17	3	1,730
Turkey Guacamole, Specialty Deli, regular (16 oz.)	680	24	3	2,680
Chicken Breast, Light & Flavorful, large (29 oz.)	1,010	15	4	4,520
Albacore Tuna, Light & Flavorful, regular (13 oz.)	530	16	4	1,660
The Vegetarian, Light & Flavorful, small (8 oz.)	350	11	5	890
BLT, Specialty Deli, small (7 oz.)	380	15	5	1,010
Vegetable Club, Specialty Deli, small (8 oz.)	390	16	5	960
Corned Beef, Specialty Deli, large (23 oz.)	1,130	25	5	4,750
Santa Fe Chicken, Light & Flavorful, small (11 oz.)	430	13	6	1,550
Chicken Club, Specialty Deli, small (11 oz.)	460	15	6	1,590
Albacore Tuna, Light & Flavorful, large (25 oz.)	1,000	26	6	3,100
Roast Beef, Specialty Deli, large (27 oz.)	1,190	28	6	3,360
Turkey Guacamole, Specialty Deli, large (32 oz.)	1,320	42	6	5,260
The Vegetarian, Light & Flavorful, regular (12 oz.)	520	17	7	1,330
Corned Beef Reuben, Specialty Deli, small (10 oz.)	530	21	7	2,270
Vegetable Club, Specialty Deli, regular (13 oz.)	580	24	7	1,440
BLT, Specialty Deli, regular (10 oz.)	580	24	7	1,550
Santa Fe Chicken, Light & Flavorful, regular (17 oz.)	640	19	9	2,300
Ham & Cheese Original, small (11 oz.)	540	22	9	2,300
Chicken Club, Specialty Deli, regular (16 oz.)	690	23	9	2,400
The Philly, Specialty Deli, small (11 oz.)	560	22	10	1,470

MALL FOOD (Schlotzsky's Deli continued)

Menu Item	Calories	Total Fat (g)	Saturated Fat (g)	Sodium (mg)
Western Vegetarian, Specialty Deli, small (8 oz.)	450	23	10	790
Roast Beef & Cheese, Specialty Deli, small (11 oz.)	580	24	10	1,670
Pastrami & Swiss, Specialty Deli, small (10 oz.)	570	24	11	2,450
Turkey Reuben, Specialty Deli, small (11 oz.)	580	26	11	2,660
Turkey & Bacon Club, Specialty Deli, small (11 oz.)	600	27	11	2,010
Texas Schlotzsky's, Specialty Deli, small (11 oz.)	560	26	12	2,260
The Vegetarian, Light & Flavorful, large (24 oz.)	970	26	12	2,400
Albacore Tuna Melt, Specialty Deli, small (11 oz.)	560	28	12	1,550
Pastrami Reuben, Specialty Deli, small (11 oz.)	620	29	12	2,680
Ham & Cheese Original, regular (17 oz.)	790	32	12	3,430
Corned Beef Reuben, Specialty Deli, regular (15 oz.)	830	35	13	3,510
Vegetable Club, Specialty Deli, large (25 oz.)	1,110	41	13	2,720
Santa Fe Chicken, Light & Flavorful, large (32 oz.)	1,180	29	14	4,230
The Philly, Specialty Deli, regular (16 oz.)	820	32	14	2,190
Western Vegetarian, Specialty Deli, regular (12 oz.)	650	33	14	1,160
Roast Beef & Cheese, Specialty Deli, regular (17 oz.)	850	34	14	2,450
BLT, Specialty Deli, large (20 oz.)	1,140	46	14	3,070
Turkey & Bacon Club, Specialty Deli, regular (17 oz.)	870	40	15	3,010
Texas Schlotzsky's, Specialty Deli, regular (16 oz.)	820	37	16	3,360
Turkey Reuben, Specialty Deli, regular (16 oz.)	860	39	16	3,890
Albacore Tuna Melt, Specialty Deli, regular (16 oz.)	820	40	16	2,290
Cheese Original, small (10 oz.)	600	31	17	1,430
Pastrami & Swiss, Specialty Deli, regular (15 oz.)	860	37	17	3,720

MALL FOOD *(Schlotzsky's Deli continued)* **Menu Item**	Calories	Total Fat (g)	Saturated Fat (g)	Sodium (mg)
The Original, small (10 oz.)	710	41	17	2,330
Turkey Original, small (12 oz.)	760	41	17	2,790
Chicken Club, Specialty Deli, large (31 oz.)	1,350	45	17	4,680
Pastrami Reuben, Specialty Deli, regular (16 oz.)	920	43	18	3,920
Turkey Original, regular (17 oz.)	1,020	51	20	3,740
The Original (14 oz.)	940	50	22	3,170
Cheese Original, regular (14 oz.)	850	44	23	2,110
Corned Beef Reuben, Specialty Deli, large (31 oz.)	1,590	62	25	6,940
Deluxe Original, small (13 oz.)	1,040	65	26	4,280
Large Original (28 oz.)*	1,300	50	27	4,400
Texas Schlotzsky's, Specialty Deli, large (31 oz.)	1,540	65	27	6,450
Western Vegetarian, Specialty Deli, large (23 oz.)	1,260	61	28	2,240
Ham & Cheese Original, large (33 oz.)	1,630	67	29	6,810
Deluxe Original, regular (19 oz.)	1,300	75	29	5,400
Turkey Reuben, Specialty Deli, large (32 oz.)	1,660	69	31	7,700
The Philly, Specialty Deli, large (33 oz.)	1,710	66	32	4,480
Pastrami & Swiss, Specialty Deli, large (29 oz.)	1,680	69	32	7,210
Roast Beef & Cheese, Specialty Deli, large (33 oz.)	1,750	70	33	4,990
Albacore Tuna Melt, Specialty Deli, large (31 oz.)	1,630	77	34	4,470
Pastrami Reuben, Specialty Deli, large (32 oz.)	1,780	77	34	7,770
Turkey & Bacon Club, Specialty Deli, large (34 oz.)	1,790	80	35	6,090
Turkey Original, large (34 oz.)	2,080	104	45	7,540
Cheese Original, large (29 oz.)	1,860	98	56	4,370

MALL FOOD (Schlotzsky's Deli continued)

Menu Item	Calories	Total Fat (g)	Saturated Fat (g)	Sodium (mg)
Soups (8 oz.)				
Tomato Milano	90	0	0	440
Minestrone	90	1	0	1,050
Beef & Black Bean	150	1	0	1,060
Red Beans and Rice	170	1	0	930
Ravioli Tomato	110	2	0	1,120
Schlotzsky's Vegetable	220	2	0	2,200
Santa Fe Vegetable	120	2	1	680
Chicken Noodle, Old Fashioned	120	2	1	1,100
7 Bean Medley	150	2	1	1,260
Chicken Tortilla	170	3	1	1,030
Vegetable Beef Barley	100	3	1	1,160
Tortellini	120	3	1	1,360
Chicken Gumbo	110	5	1	1,110
Cream of Potato with Bacon	230	13	1	1,210
Boston Clam Chowder	230	15	1	1,060
Vegetable Vegetarian	140	6	2	1,540
Timberline Chili	210	7	3	810
Tuscan Clam Bisque	220	16	3	950
Corn Chowder	280	17	3	1,010
Broccoli Cheese	250	17	4	1,100
Vegetable Cheese	290	19	6	1,340

MALL FOOD *(Schlotzsky's Deli continued)* Menu Item	Calories	Total Fat (g)	Saturated Fat (g)	Sodium (mg)
Wisconsin Cheese	320	25	7	1,100
Chicken with Wild Rice	380	28	12	1,200
Salads (weight of each salad)				
✔ Garden Salad, without dressing (9 oz.)	60	1	0	120
✔ Chinese Chicken, without dressing (9 oz.)	150	3	1	450
Potato Salad, diced with egg (5 oz.)	220	13	2	600
Potato Salad, with mustard and egg (5 oz.)	230	15	2	530
Country Style Cole Slaw (5 oz.)	230	16	3	290
Cole Slaw, shredded (5 oz.)	230	16	3	390
Choice Potato Salad (5 oz.)	250	18	3	530
Caesar Salad, without dressing (7 oz.)	150	8	4	510
Macaroni Salad (5 oz.)	340	23	4	620
Chicken Caesar Salad, without dressing (9 oz.)	250	10	5	940
Smoked Turkey Chef Salad, without dressing (13 oz.)	240	10	5	1,280
Ham & Turkey Chef Salad, without dressing (13 oz.)	250	11	5	1,440
Greek Salad, without dressing (12 oz.)	220	12	8	560
Salad Dressings (3 Tb.)				
Light Italian	90	8	2	690
Light Spicy Ranch	140	11	3	350
Greek Balsamic Vinaigrette	170	17	3	330
Thousand Island	220	21	3	360
Spicy Ranch	230	25	4	310

MALL FOOD (Schlotzsky's Deli continued) Menu Item	Calories	Total Fat (g)	Saturated Fat (g)	Sodium (mg)
Olde World Caesar	260	27	5	250
Traditional Ranch	270	29	5	370
8" Sourdough Crust Pizzas (weight of each pizza)				
Fresh Tomato & Pesto (11 oz.)	540	16	8	1,670
Vegetarian Special (11 oz.)	550	17	8	1,760
Mediterranean (10 oz.)	530	18	8	1,880
Southwestern (13 oz.)	640	19	8	2,020
Smoked Turkey & Jalapeño (13 oz.)	650	19	8	2,590
Chicken & Pesto (13 oz.)	650	19	9	2,190
Thai Chicken (14 oz.)	680	19	9	2,300
Barbeque Chicken (12 oz.)	650	20	9	2,100
New Orleans (13 oz.)	670	20	9	2,490
Double Cheese (10 oz.)	600	21	10	1,770
Bacon, Tomato & Mushroom (11 oz.)	640	24	10	1,890
The Original Combination (12 oz.)	650	25	10	1,990
Double Cheese & Pepperoni (11 oz.)	740	34	16	2,210
Desserts (weight of each item)				
Oatmeal Raisin Cookie (1 oz.)	150	5	1	20
Sugar Cookie (1 oz.)	160	6	1	10
Chocolate Chunk Cookie (1 oz.)	160	7	2	10
Chocolate Pecan Chunk Cookie (1 oz.)	170	8	2	10
Peanut Butter Cookie (1 oz.)	170	8	2	10

MALL FOOD *(Schlotzsky's Deli continued)* Menu Item	Calories	Total Fat (g)	Saturated Fat (g)	Sugars (g)
Chocolate Chip Cookie (1 oz.)	160	7	3	10
Fudge Chocolate Chunk Cookie (1 oz.)	170	8	3	10
Peanut Butter Chocolate Chunk Cookie (1 oz.)	170	8	3	10
White Chocolate Macadamia Nut Cookie (1 oz.)	170	8	3	10
Strawberry Swirl Cheesecake (3 oz.)	300	17	9	20
Cookies & Creme Cheesecake (3 oz.)	330	18	9	30
New York Creamstyle Cheesecake (3 oz.)	310	18	10	20
Fudge Brownie Cake (4 oz.)	410	25	11	30

* Numbers from independent lab analyses.
Note: Saturated fat numbers in *italics* include artery-clogging *trans* fat.

FRUIT SMOOTHIES

We've ranked smoothies from best to worst—that is, from least to most total fat, then calories. We chose Best Bites that are lower in calories because people often drink these beverages with a meal or as a snack.

MALL FOOD *(Jamba Juice)* Menu Item	Calories	Total Fat (g)	Protein (g)	Fiber (g)
Smoothies (regular—24 oz.—unless otherwise noted)				
Kiwi Berry Burner	420	0	3	5
Orange-A-Peel	420	1	8	5
Strawberries Wild	440	1	6	5
Protein Berry Pizazz	470	1	25	6
Orange Berry Blitz	380	2	5	4
Cranberry Craze	390	2	5	4
Caribbean Passion	410	2	2	4
Citrus Squeeze	420	2	4	5
Coldbuster!	430	2	5	6

MALL FOOD (Jamba Juice continued)

Menu Item	Calories	Total Fat (g)	Protein (g)	Fiber (g)
Razzmatazz	440	2	3	4
Orchard Oasis	440	2	2	4
Aloha Pineapple	440	2	7	3
Jamba Powerboost	450	2	9	9
Mango-A-Go-Go	460	2	2	3
Banana Berry	470	2	5	5
Peach Pleasure	470	2	3	4
Raspberry Refresher	440	3	3	8
Razzmatazz power (32 oz.)	590	3	4	5
Peenya Kowlada power (32 oz.)	770	7	11	4

MALL FOOD (Smoothie King)

Menu Item	Calories	Total Fat (g)	Protein (g)	Fiber (g)
Smoothies (small—20 oz.—unless otherwise noted)				
Youth Fountain	270	0	3	5
Celestial Cherry High	290	0	1	4
Hawaiian Cafe Au Lei	290	0	10	0
GoGuava	300	0	1	2
Pineapple Pleasure	310	0	2	4
MangoFest	320	0	1	2
Peach Slice	340	0	5	3
Blackberry Dream	340	0	2	3
Lemon Twist, Banana	340	0	3	2
Caribbean Way	390	0	2	5
Light & Fluffy	390	0	2	4
Grape Expectations	400	0	3	2
Lemon Twist, Strawberry	400	0	3	2
Super Punch	430	0	2	6
Peach Slice Plus	470	0	4	5
Super Punch Plus	520	0	2	6
Grape Expectations II	530	0	4	4
Cranberry Cooler	540	0	1	3

MALL FOOD *(Smoothie King continued)* Menu Item	Calories	Total Fat (g)	Protein (g)	Fiber (g)
Cranberry Supreme	580	0	3	3
✔ Slim & Trim, Orange-Vanilla	200	1	5	1
✔ Slim & Trim, Vanilla	230	1	6	2
Pep Upper	330	1	3	5
Island Treat	330	1	2	5
Angel Food	330	1	6	4
Immune Builder	330	1	5	4
Muscle Punch Plus	340	1	6	5
Muscle Punch	340	1	6	4
Raspberry Sunrise	340	1	3	4
Slim & Trim Strawberry	360	1	7	3
Instant Vigor	360	1	2	2
Power Punch	430	1	6	4
Angel Food medium (32 oz.)	530	1	9	6
Angel Food king (40 oz.)	660	1	11	7
Slim & Trim Chocolate	270	2	12	3
Power Punch Plus	500	2	10	4
Yogurt D-Lite	340	4	13	2

MALL FOOD (Smoothie King continued) Menu Item	Calories	Total Fat (g)	Protein (g)	Fiber (g)
Coconut Surprise	460	6	8	5
Mo'cuccino	420	12	9	1
High Protein, Banana	410	14	34	6
Peanut Power	500	21	15	4
Peanut Power Plus Strawberry	630	21	15	5
The Hulk, Chocolate	850	29	23	6
The Hulk, Vanilla	850	29	23	5
Malt	890	41	17	0
Peanut Power Plus Grape, king (40 oz.)	1,400	42	32	7
The Hulk, Strawberry, king (40 oz.)	1,910	58	47	12

ICE CREAM, FROZEN YOGURT, ETC.

We've ranked ice cream and frozen yogurt from best to worst—that is, from least to most saturated fat, and toppings from least to most total fat.

MALL FOOD (Häagen-Dazs)

Menu Item

ICE CREAM, FROZEN YOGURT, ETC.

Ice Cream and Sorbet (1 scoop—½ cup—unless otherwise noted)	Calories	Total Fat (g)	Saturated Fat (g)
✔Sorbet	120	0	0
✔Lowfat Ice Cream, Coffee Fudge	170	3	2
✔Lowfat Ice Cream, Cookies & Fudge	180	3	2
✔Frozen Yogurt, Vanilla	200	5	3
Ice Cream, Pralines & Cream	290	18	9
Ice Cream, Dulce De Leche	290	17	10
Ice Cream, Cookies & Cream	270	17	11
Ice Cream, Vanilla	270	18	11
Ice Cream, Chocolate Swiss Almond	300	20	11
Ice Cream, Butter Pecan	310	23	11
Ice Cream, Cookie Dough Chip	310	20	12
Ice Cream, Vanilla (2 scoops—1 cup)	540	36	22
Ice Cream, Vanilla (3 scoops—1½ cups)	810	54	33

*Average of all flavors.

MALL FOOD *(TCBY)*

Menu Item	Calories	Total Fat (g)	Saturated Fat (g)
Frozen Yogurt (size of each item)			
✔ Kiddie Cup (3 fl. oz.)	110	3	2*
✔ Small Cup (6 fl. oz.)	200	5	3*
✔ Regular Cake Cone (6 fl. oz.)	210	5	3*
Regular Cup (8 fl. oz.)	270	6	4*
Regular Waffle Cone (8 fl. oz.)	380	6	4*
Large Cup (11 fl. oz.)	350	8	5*
Large Waffle Cone (11 fl. oz.)	460	8	5*
Toppings (1 scoop)			
Fruit Toppings	10	0	0
Waffle Cone Chips	10	1	N/A
Crumbled Fudge Brownies	50	1	N/A
Chocolate Chip Cookie Dough	60	3	N/A

MALL FOOD *(TCBY continued)*

Menu Item	Calories	Total Fat (g)	Saturated Fat (g)
Coconut	60	5	4*
M&M's	100	5	3*
Butterfinger Pieces	120	5	3*
Chocolate Sprinkles	140	6	N/A
Hot Fudge	140	7	N/A
Pecan Pieces	80	8	1*
Chocolate Topper	120	10	N/A
Walnuts in Syrup	160	10	1*

*CSPI estimate.
N/A = number not available

ITALIAN

MALL FOOD (Sbarro)

Menu Item	Calories	Total Fat (g)	Saturated Fat (g)	Sugars (g)
Pizza and Entrées (weight of each item)				
✔ Spaghetti with Sauce (18 oz.)*	630	18	*3*	1,260
Cheese Pizza (6 oz.)*	450	14	*7*	990
Pepperoni Pizza (6 oz.)*	510	21	*10*	1,240
Spinach & Broccoli Stuffed Pizza (11 oz.)*	710	26	*10*	1,490
Supreme Pizza (10 oz.)	600	25	12	1,580
Sausage Pizza (10 oz.)	640	29	14	1,560
Meat Lasagna (17 oz.)*	730	38	*17*	1,660
Sausage & Pepperoni Stuffed Pizza (11 oz.)*	880	44	*19*	2,230
Baked Ziti (14 oz.)	830	42	21	950

*Numbers from independent lab analyses.
Note: All pizza numbers are for one slice. Saturated fat numbers in *italics* include artery-clogging *trans* fat.

PRETZELS

We've ranked the pretzels and dipping sauces from best to worst—that is, from least to most total fat, then calories. The "Sugars" numbers include both refined sugars and (generally) much smaller amounts of naturally occurring sugars from fruit and milk. The U.S. Department of Agriculture's recommended limit for refined sugars is 40 grams, or 10 teaspoons, per day. (That's the amount in a typical 12-ounce soft drink.)

MALL FOOD (Auntie Anne's) Menu Item	Calories	Total Fat (g)	Sodium (mg)	Sugars (g)
Pretzels (4 oz.)				
✔ Jalapeño, no butter	270	0	780	8
✔ Sour Cream & Onion, no butter	310	0	920	9
✔ Garlic, no butter	320	0	830	9
✔ Cinnamon Sugar, no butter	350	0	410	16
✔ Original, no butter	340	1	900	10
✔ Almond, no butter	350	1	390	15
✔ Sesame, no butter	350	1	840	9
Glazin' Raisin, no butter	470	1	460	37
✔ Whole Wheat, no butter	350	2	1,100	10
✔ Parmesan Herb, no butter	390	3	780	10
Original, with butter	370	4	930	10
Glazin' Raisin, with butter	510	4	480	38
Jalapeno, with butter*	310	5	940	9

MALL FOOD *(Auntie Anne's continued)*

Menu Item	Calories	Total Fat (g)	Sodium (mg)	Sugars (g)
Sour Cream & Onion, with butter*	340	5	930	10
Garlic, with butter*	350	5	850	9
Whole Wheat, with butter	370	5	1,120	2
Almond, with butter*	400	8	400	15
Cinnamon Sugar, with butter*	450	9	430	26
Sesame, with butter*	410	12	860	9
Parmesan Herb, with butter*	440	13	660	10
Dipping Sauces (2 Tb.)				
Marinara Sauce	10	0	180	2
Sweet Mustard	60	2	120	8
Caramel Dip	140	3	110	21
Chocolate Flavored Dip	130	4	65	12
Light Cream Cheese*	70	6	140	1
Cheese Sauce*	100	8	510	3
Hot Salsa Cheese*	100	8	550	4
Strawberry Cream Cheese*	110	10	105	3

*Contains at least three grams of saturated fat.

STEAK AND POTATO

MALL FOOD *(The Great Steak and Potato Company)* Menu Item	Calories	Total Fat (g)	Saturated Fat (g)	Sodium (mg)
Sandwiches etc. (weight of each item)				
✔ Baked Potato with Broccoli and Cheese (12 oz.)	340	5	2	340
The Great Salad Experience with Chicken, without dressing (15 oz.)	260	9	5	490
✔ Chicken Teriyaki Sandwich (11 oz.)	580	17	5	1,470
Fresh Cut Fries, small (6 oz.)*	460	24	6	380
The Great Potato with Turkey (14 oz.)	610	28	6	620
Chicken Philadelphia Sandwich (10 oz.)	640	28	7	620
Turkey Philadelphia Sandwich (10 oz.)	690	28	7	290
Fresh Cut Fries, regular (7 oz.)*	540	29	7	440
The Veggie Delight Sandwich (9 oz.)	570	29	7	440
The Great Potato with Steak (14 oz.)	600	32	7	600
The Ham Delight Sandwich (11 oz.)	710	33	9	1,590
The Ham Explosion Sandwich (11 oz.)	710	33	9	1,590
The Great Steak Sandwich (11 oz.)	660	34	10	400
The Super Steak Sandwich (11 oz.)	660	34	10	400
Fresh Cut Fries, large (12 oz.)*	920	48	12	760
The Great Steak Sandwich, large, 12-inch (18 oz.)	1,070	55	16	610

* Our estimate.

Note: All sandwich numbers are for (7-inch) regular size, unless noted.
Except for Chicken Teriyaki, all sandwiches include mayo and cheese.

Chapter 18

Horror Show:
Movie Theater Snacks

t was not so long ago that a snack at the movies meant a modest box of popcorn or a small brown bag of M&Ms. At some point, number crunchers at the big theater chains realized that the snack concession was a cash cow that should be milked harder. They dramatically increased servings and prices. Cups for soft drinks turned into buckets, and patrons paid more and more for tubs of popcorn large enough to hold a small load of laundry. Candy bars, once a few bites' worth of junk, grew into hunks worthy of Paul Bunyan. And their captive audiences continued to buy. In fact, seven out of every ten moviegoers buy refreshments.

Movie Theater Popcorn

Everyone knows that candy carries a heavy load of sugar and calories. But popcorn—that movie classic—can be deceiving. Air-popped popcorn is a healthy snack. It's got lots of fiber, and it's low in fat and calories. But oil-popped popcorn is about as fatty as potato chips, and the popcorn served in the large theater chains is one of the worst foods you can buy. Why? Because so many theaters still pop their corn in highly saturated coconut oil. It's more than twice as saturated as lard, so buried in even a small serving (about 7 cups) of popcorn is not only 400 calories but a day's worth of saturated fat. That's equal to the saturated fat in two McDonald's Quarter Pounders. A large order (about 20 cups) has nearly three days' worth of saturated fat—and 1,160 calories. And that's without "butter." (Even though the topping is probably butterless, its partially hydrogenated soybean oil adds both artery-clogging saturated and *trans* fat.) By the time the server pumps a few squirts into your bucket, the calories climb to more than 1,600, and your arteries are stuck with three and a half days' worth of saturated fat.

These days some theaters pop their corn in partially hydro-genated vegetable oil (shortening). Most are not as low in satu-rated fat as the vegetable oils you use at home, and they're still high in calories, but they're not nearly as bad for the old ticker as coconut oil.

If you ask the kid behind the counter what type of oil your theater uses in the popper, you might get lucky. If the answer is coconut oil, or if he doesn't know, skip it.

Movie Theater Candy

We didn't have to analyze candy sold at movie theaters. The numbers are listed on the Nutrition Facts panel on the packages. Just keep in mind that a whole box or bar of some of these candies is brimming with sugar. How does 32 teaspoons in a 5½-ounce box of Junior Mints grab you? That's enough to supply roughly 500 calories—about par for the course in a box of movie-theater candy. A bag of Reese's Pieces has more than 1,000 calo-ries because it's got a hefty dose of fat mixed in with the sugar. That's why an entire theater-size box or bar of Buncha Crunch or KitKats supplies three-quarters of a day's saturated fat, while M&M's and Reese's Pieces have more than a day's worth. We've listed numbers for an entire box or bar. If you eat less (as we can only hope), divide accordingly.

Movie Theater Strategy

• **Bring your own air-popped popcorn.** Some theaters told us that they won't make a fuss if you don't show it to anybody.

• **Ask the manager to switch to nonhydrogenated liquid vegetable oil.** The popcorn won't be any lower in calories, but it also won't be as bad for your heart as popcorn popped in coconut oil or partially hydrogenated oils.

• **If you eat candy, choose the low-fat varieties and remember that less is better.** Low-fat Twizzlers may be loaded with sugar and calories, but at least they're kinder to your heart than chocolate candies.

Although the serving size for "small" (7 cups) and "large" (20 cups) is fairly consistent from chain to chain, the "medium" tends to fall around 11 or 16 cups. Popcorn is ranked from best to worst—that is, from least to most saturated fat. There are no Best Bites.

Reminder

Recommended limits for a 2,000-calorie diet:

Total fat: 65 grams
Saturated fat: 20 grams
Cholesterol: 300 milligrams
Sodium: 2,400 milligrams

POPCORN

POPPED IN COCONUT OIL	Calories	Total Fat (g)	Saturated Fat (g)
Kid's (5 cups)	300	20	*14*
Small (7 cups)	400	27	*19*
Medium (11 cups)	650	43	*31*
Medium (16 cups)	900	60	*43*
Large (20 cups)	1,160	77	*55*
POPPED IN COCONUT OIL WITH "BUTTER" TOPPING			
Kid's (5 cups)	470	37	*22*
Small (7 cups)	630	50	*29*
Medium (11 cups)	910	71	*41*
Medium (16 cups)	1,220	97	*56*
Large (20 cups)	1,640	126	*73*
POPPED IN VEGETABLE SHORTENING			
Small (7 cups)	360	22	*7*
Medium (11 cups)	630	38	*12*
Large (16 cups)	850	52	*16*

Note: Saturated-fat numbers in *italics* include artery-clogging *trans* fat.

The numbers in the chart are from the manufacturers. Saturated-fat numbers do not include *trans* fat; if they did, the saturated-fat numbers would be higher than those indicated. The "Sugars" numbers include both refined sugars and (generally) much smaller amounts of naturally occurring sugars from fruit and milk. The U.S. Department of Agriculture's recommended limit for refined sugars is 40 grams per day, or 10 teaspoons. (That's the amount in a typical 12-ounce soft drink.) Candy is ranked from best to worst—that is, from least to most saturated fat, then total fat, then sugar. There are no Best Bites.

CANDY Menu Item	Calories	Total Fat (g)	Saturated Fat (g)	Sugars (g)
Twizzlers Strawberry Twists (6 oz.)	560	2	0	64
Original Fruit Skittles (7 oz.)	770	9	0	140
Starburst Original Fruit Chews (7 oz.)	800	15	3	115
Milk Duds (4 oz.)	490	17	6	55
Reese's Peanut Butter Cups (2½ oz.)	370	21	7	32
Junior Mints (5½ oz.)	620	10	8	129
Whoppers (3 oz.)	360	14	11	46
Sno-Caps (3 oz.)	400	18	11	53
Raisinets (3½ oz.)	420	18	11	59
Butterfinger Mini Bars (4 oz.)	510	20	11	57
Goobers (3½ oz.)	530	34	12	43
Buncha Crunch (3 oz.)	480	25	15	48
KitKat (3½ oz.)	500	26	16	48
M&M's, Plain (5½ oz.)	770	39	16	77
M&M's, Milk Chocolate (5½ oz.)	800	34	23	103
Reese's Pieces (8 oz.)	1,140	54	36	120

Appendix

These are the major restaurant chains whose products are included in this book.

Applebee's
4551 West 107th St., Suite 100
Overland Park, KS 66207
888-59-APPLE (888-592-7753)
www.applebees.com

Au Bon Pain
Guest Services
19 Fid Kennedy Ave.
Boston, MA 02210
800-TALK-ABP (800-825-5227)
www.aubonpain.com

Auntie Anne's
Customer Service
160-A Route 41
P.O. Box 529
Gap, PA 17527
717-442-4766
www.auntieannes.com

Bakers Square
VICORP Restaurants, Inc.
400 West 48th Ave.
Denver, CO 80216
303-296-2121
www.vicorpinc.com/bsmainframe.html

Bennigan's
6500 International Pkwy.
Suite 1000
Plano, TX 75093
972-588-5000
www.bennigans.com

Big Boy
4199 Marcy St.
Warren, MI 48001
800-837-3003
www.bigboy.com

Blimpie
1775 The Exchange, Suite 600
Atlanta, GA 30339
800-447-6256
www.blimpie.com

Bob Evans
3776 South High St.
Columbus, OH 43207
800-939-2338
www.bobevans.com

Bugaboo Creek SteakHouse
RARE Hospitality International, Inc.
8215 Roswell Rd., Building 600
Atlanta, GA 30350
770-399-9595
www.bugaboocreeksteakhouse.com

Burger King
Consumer Relations
17777 Old Cutler Rd.
Miami, FL 33157
305-378-3535
www.burgerking.com

California Pizza Kitchen
Restaurant Support Center
6053 West Century Blvd., #1100
Los Angeles, CA 90045-6430
310-342-5000
www.cpk.com

Carrows
Carrows Restaurants
3355 Michelson Dr., Suite 350
Irvine, CA 92612
877-225-4161
www.carrows.com

Chart House
640 N LaSalle St., Suite 295
Chicago, IL 60710
312-266-1100
www.chart-house.com

The Cheesecake Factory
26950 Agoura Rd.
Calabasas Hills, CA 91301
818-871-3000
www.thecheesecakefactory.com

Chevys
CHEVYS Restaurant Support Center
2000 Powell St., Suite 200
Emeryville, CA 94608
800-4-CHEVYS (800-424-3897)
www.chevys.com

Chi-Chi's
10200 Linn Station Rd.
Louisville, KY 40223
800-436-6006
www.chi-chis.com

Chili's
Brinker International
6820 LBJ Freeway
Dallas, TX 75240
800-983-4637
www.chilis.com

Cinnabon
AFC Enterprises
Six Concourse Pkwy., Suite 1700
Atlanta, GA 30328
866-551-AFCE (866-551-2323)
www.cinnabon.com

Coco's
Coco's Bakery Restaurant
3355 Michelson Dr., Suite 350
Irvine, CA 92612
877-225-4161
www.cocosbakery.com

Country Kitchen
Country Kitchen International
801 Deming Way (53717)
P.O. Box 44434
Madison, WI 53744-4434
608-833-9633
www.visitcountrykitchen.com

Cracker Barrel
CBRL Group, Inc.
P.O. Box 787
Lebanon, TN 37088-0787
615-444-5533
www.crackerbarrel.com

Dairy Queen
American Dairy Queen Corporation
7505 Metro Blvd.
Minneapolis, MN 55439
952-830-0200
www.dairyqueen.com

Damon's
Damon's International, Inc.
4645 Executive Dr.
Columbus, OH 43220
614-442-7900
www.damons.com

Denny's
Denny's Guest Assurance
203 East Main St.
Box P-5-11
Spartanburg, SC 29319
800-733-6697
www.dennys.com

Domino's Pizza
Domino's Pizza LLC
Customer Care Center
30 Frank Lloyd Wright Dr.
P.O. Box 997
Ann Arbor, MI 48106
888-DOMINOS (888-366-4667)
www.dominos.com

Donatos Pizza
1 Easton Oval, Suite 200
Columbus, OH 43219
800-DONATOS (800-366-2867)
www.donatos.com

Don Pablo's
P.O. Box 725489
Atlanta, GA 31139
800-DPABLOS (800-372-2567)
www.donpablos.com

Dunkin' Donuts
Customer Service
125 Constitution Blvd.
Franklin, MA 02038-0249
1-877-8DD-COFFEE
(1-877-833-2633)
www.dunkindonuts.com

El Chico
Consolidated Restaurant Operations
12-200 Stemmons Freeway, Suite 100
Dallas, TX 75234
800-275-1337
www.elchico.com

El Torito
4001 Via Oro Ave., Suite 200
Long Beach, CA 90810
310-513-7500
www.eltorito.com

Friendly's
Friendly Ice Cream Corporation
1855 Boston Rd.
Wilbraham, MA 01095
413-543-2400
www.friendlys.com

Grady's American Grill
Quality Dining
4220 Edison Lakes Pkwy.
Mishawaka, IN 46545
800-589-3820

The Great Steak and Potato Company
Nicar Franchising, Inc.
188 North Brookwood Ave., Suite 100
Hamilton, OH 45013
513-896-9695
www.thegreatsteak.com

Häagen-Dazs
Consumer Relations
P.O. Box 1328
Minneapolis, MN 55440-1328
800-767-0120
www.haagendazs.com

Hard Rock Café
6100 Old Park Lane
Orlando, FL 32835
800-235-7625
www.hardrock.com

Houlihan's
Houlihan's Restaurant Group
P.O. Box 16000
Kansas City, MO 64112
816-756-2200
www.houlihans.com

Houston's
2425 East Camelback, Suite 200
Phoenix, AZ 85016
602-553-2111
www.houstons.com

Hungry Hunter
10200 Willow Creek Rd.
San Diego, CA 92131
800-570-9159
www.paragonsteakhouse.com

IHOP
IHOP Corp.
450 N. Brand Blvd.
Glendale, CA 91203
818-240-6055
www.ihop.com

Jamba Juice
Support Center
1700 17th St.
San Francisco, CA 94103
800-545-9972
www.jambajuice.com

Kentucky Fried Chicken
KFC Customer Service
P.O. Box 725489
Atlanta, GA 31139
800-225-5532
www.kfc.com

Landry's Seafood House
1510 West Loop South
Houston, TX 77027
713-850-1010
www.landrysseafoodhouse.com

Legal Sea Foods
33 Everett St.
Allston, MA 02134
800-EAT-FISH (800-328-3474)
www.legalseafoods.com

Little Caesars
Little Caesar Enterprises, Inc.
Fox Office Centre
2211 Woodward Ave.
Detroit, MI 48201
800-7-CAESAR (800-722-3727)
www.littlecaesars.com

Lone Star Steakhouse & Saloon
224 East Douglas St., Suite 700
Wichita, KS 67202
800-234-0888
www.lonestarsteakhouse.com

LongHorn Steakhouse
RARE Hospitality International, Inc.
8215 Roswell Rd., Building 600
Atlanta, GA 30350
770-399-9595
www.longhornsteakhouse.com

Marie Callender's
Marie Callender Pie Shops, Inc.
1100 Town & Country, Suite 1300
Orange, CA 92868
800-776-PIES (800-776-7437)
www.mcpies.com

McDonald's
Customer Service
McDonald's Plaza
Oakbrook, IL 60523
630-623-6198
www.mcdonalds.com

Mrs. Fields
Mrs. Fields Famous Brands
440 West Lawndale Dr.
Salt Lake City, UT 84115
800-COOKIES (800-266-5437)
www.mrsfields.com

The Olive Garden
P.O. Box 592037
Orlando, FL 32859-2037
800-331-2729
www.theolivegarden.com

Outback Steakhouse
2202 North West Shore Blvd., 5th Fl.
Tampa, FL 33607
813-282-1225
www.outbacksteakhouse.com

Panda Express
899 El Centro St.
South Pasadena, CA 91030
800-877-8988
www.pandaexpress.com

Papa John's
Papa John's International, Inc.
P.O. Box 99900
Louisville, KY 40269-9990
502-261-7272
www.papajohns.com

Perkins
6075 Poplar Ave., Suite 800
Memphis, TN 38119
800-GUEST-02 (800-483-7802)
www.perkinsrestaurants.com

Pizza Hut
Customer Service
14841 Dallas Pkwy.
Dallas, TX 75254
800-948-8488
www.pizzahut.com

Pizzeria Uno
Uno Restaurants, Inc.
100 Charles Park Rd.
Boston, MA 02132
617-323-9200
www.pizzeriauno.com

Planet Hollywood
Planet Hollywood Corporate
Headquarters
8669 Commodity Circle
Orlando, FL 32819
407-363-7827
www.planethollywood.com

Red Lobster
P.O. Box 593330
Orlando, FL 32859
800-LOBSTER (800-562-7837)
www.redlobster.com

Red Robin
Red Robin Gourmet Burgers
5575 DTC Pkwy., Suite 110
Greenwood Village, CO 80111
303-846-6000
www.redrobin.com

Ruby Tuesday
150 W. Church Ave.
Maryville, TN 37801
888-553-4352
www.ruby-tuesday.com

Rusty Pelican (TX)
1510 West Loop South
Houston, TX 77027
713-850-1010
www.landrysseafoodhouse.com

Rusty Pelican (CA)
Bubba Gump Shrimp Co.
940 Calle Negocio, Suite 250
San Clemente, CA 92673
949-366-6260
www.rustypelican.com

Sbarro
Customer Service
763 Larkfield Rd.
Commack, N.Y. 11725
631-715-4100
www.sbarro.com

Schlotzsky's Deli
Customer Service
203 Colorado St.
Austin, TX 78701-3922
800-846-BUNS (800-846-2867)
www.schlotzskys.com

Shoney's
Shoney's Guest Information Services
1717 Elm Hill Pike, Suite A10
Nashville, TN 37210
877-TELL-SHO (877-835-5746)
www.shoneysrestaurants.com

Smoothie King
Customer Service
2400 Veterans Blvd., #110
Kenner, LA 70062
800-577-4200
www.smoothieking.com

Starbucks
Starbucks Customer Relations
P.O. Box 3717
Seattle, WA 98124-3717
206-447-1575
www.starbucks.com

Steak and Ale Restaurant
6500 International Pkwy.
Suite 1000
Plano, TX 75093
800-727-TELL (800-727-8355)
www.steakandale.com

Stuart Anderson's
4410 El Camino Real, Suite 201
Los Altos, CA 94022
650-949-6400
www.stuartanderson.com

Subway
Subway World Headquarters
Customer Service
325 Bic Dr.
Milford, CT 06460
800-888-4848
www.subway.com

Taco Bell Corporation
Consumer Affairs
17901 Von Karman
Irvine, CA 92614
800-TACOBELL (800-822-6235)
www.tacobell.com

TCBY
Consumer Affairs
2855 East Cottonwood Pkwy., Suite 400
Salt Lake City, UT 84121-7050
800-343-5377
www.tcby.com

T.G.I. Friday's
Carlson Restaurants Worldwide Inc.
7540 LBJ Freeway
Dallas, TX 75251
800-FRIDAYS (800-374-3297)
www.tgifridays.com

Tony Roma's
RomaCorp Inc.
9304 Forest Lane, Suite 200
Dallas, TX 75243
800-286-7662
www.tonyromas.com

Vie de France
Vie de France Yamazaki, Inc.
2070 Chain Bridge Rd., Suite 500
Vienna, VA 22182-2536
703-442-9205
www.viedefrance.com

Village Inn
VICORP Restaurants, Inc
400 West 48th Ave.
Denver, CO 80216
303-296-2121
www.yourvillageinn.com

Waffle House
5986 Financial Dr.
Norcross, GA 30071
877-992-3353
www.wafflehouse.com

Wall Street Deli
Customer Service
One Independence Plaza, Suite 100
Birmingham, AL 35209
800-847-DELI (800-847-3354)
www.wallstreetdeli.com

Weathervane
31 Badger's Island West
Kittery, ME 03904
207-439-0335
www.weathervaneseafoods.com

Wendy's
Wendy's Customer Service
4288 W. Dublin-Granville Rd.
Dublin, OH 43017
614-764-3100
www.wendys.com

Index

NOW THAT YOU HAVE READ THE BOOK

Bring It with You!

CSPI's *Eating Smart Restaurant Guide* lists the calorie, fat, and saturated/trans fat content of almost 300 popular restaurant foods. It fits in purse or pocket, and its useful slide format lets you locate at a glance the information you need to decide what's best for your taste buds and your arteries.

Read the Newsletter

It's not always easy to know what's healthy to eat and what isn't. You can obtain the latest lifesaving information about the foods you eat in CSPI's Nutrition Action Healthletter. Our nutritionists help you discover exactly what's right (and wrong) with hundreds of brand-name foods. The lively writing in Nutrition Action is accompanied by full-color illustrations that help explain the vital information. Published ten times a year, each 16-page issue contains easy-to-use sections.

As *The New York Times* says, "Nutrition Action is the best known of the newsletters, probably because it is the most provocative...the information is accurate, well written and up to the minute." Subscribe today to the largest-circulation health newsletter in America. Nutrition Action comes with our no-questions-asked, money-back guarantee.

Visit www.restaurantconfidential.org

Please send me:

Eating Smart Restaurant Guide   _____@$4=_____

Subscription to *Nutrition Action Healthletter*   1 year_____@$24=_____
   2 years_____@$42=_____

More copies of *Restaurant Confidential*   _____@$12.95=_____

Postage & Handling
(except for *Nutrition Action Healthletter*)   _____@$2=_____

                   Total Enclosed=_____

Name _____

Street _____ **Apt.** _____

City _____ **State** _____ **ZIP** _____

Mail the coupon and a check for the total amount to:
Center for Science in the Public Interest orders
1875 Connecticut Avenue NW, Suite 300-A
Washington, DC 20009